A Textbook of
Paediatrics
in the Tropics and Sub-tropics

P.M.Barnes

MB(Edin.), FRCPEd, DCH, D.Obst.
Consultant Paediatrician, Bedford General
Hospital, Bedford, UK; Visiting Professor of
Paediatrics, Al-Arab Medical University,
Benghazi, Libya.
Formerly: Paediatric Registrar, University College
Hospital, Ibadan, Nigeria; Senior Registrar,
Mulago Hospital, Kampala, Uganda (seconded
from Hospital for Sick Children, Great Ormond
Street, London, UK); Paediatrician, Mofid
Children's Hospital, Teheran, Iran

Harjit Singh

MD, MNAMS, FIAMS, FIAP
Professor and Chairman, Department of
Paediatrics, Medical College and Hospital,
Rohtak, India.
Formerly: Professor of Paediatrics, El Fateh
Children's Hospital, Benghazi, Libya

A.J.H. Stephens

MRCGP, DCH, D.Obst.RCOG
Honorary Senior Lecturer in Child Health,
Liverpool School of Tropical Medicine, UK;
Visiting Professor of Paediatrics, Al-Arab Medical
University, Benghazi, Libya.
Formerly: Honorary Consultant Paediatrician,
Alder Hey Children's Hospital, Liverpool, UK;
Consultant Paediatrician and Medical
Superintendent, Arthur Davidson Children's
Hospital, Ndola, Zambia

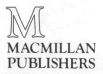

**MACMILLAN
PUBLISHERS**

First published 1990

Published by *Macmillan Publishers Ltd*
London and Basingstoke
Associated companies and representatives in Accra,
Auckland, Delhi, Dublin, Gaborone, Hamburg, Harare,
Hong Kong, Kuala Lumpur, Lagos, Manzini, Melbourne,
Mexico City, Nairobi, New York, Singapore, Tokyo

ISBN 0–333–53605–3 (hardcover)
ISBN 0–333–51590–0 (paperback)

Printed in Hong Kong

A CIP catalogue record for this book is available from the
British Library.

Pericarditis — Diphtheritic myocarditis —
Infective endocarditis — Endomyocardial
fibrosis — Hypertension — Cardiac
emergencies

12 Abdominal Disorders 145
The acute abdomen — The swollen
abdomen — Blood in the stool — Liver
disease — Cystic fibrosis — Chronic
diarrhoea — The vomiting child

13 Musculo-skeletal Disorders 155
Juvenile rheumatoid arthritis — Osteitis and
septic arthritis — Myositis and pyomyositis

14 Blood Disorders and Childhood 159
   Malignancies
Anaemia — Haemolytic anaemias —
Haemoglobinopathies — Sickling disorders —
Thalassaemia — Bleeding disorders in
children — Childhood malignancies —
The leukaemias — Lymphomas — Solid
tumours — Central nervous system tumours

15 Central Nervous System Disorders 187
Seizure disorders in children — Febrile
seizures — Management of the child with
convulsions — The unconscious child —
Cerebral palsy — Hydrocephalus —
Mental retardation — The child with a
handicap

16 Endocrine Disorders 207
Diabetes mellitus — Disorders of the thyroid
gland — Congenital adrenal hyperplasia
(adrenogenital syndrome) — The small child

17 Parasites 226
Worms — Parasites causing skin irrita-
tion — Lice and fleas — Amoebiasis
— Giardiasis — Schistosomiasis
(Bilharzia) — Leishmaniasis — Malaria

18 Skin Disorders 246
Pigmentary conditions — Naevi — Bacterial
skin infections — Napkin dermatitis —
Seborrhoeic dermatitis — Fungal infections —
Viral infections of the skin — Eczema

19 Eye Disorders 257
Diseases of the eyelid — Diseases of the
conjunctiva — Diseases of the cornea —
Diseases of the lens — Iridocyclitis —
Diseases of the retina — Onchocerciasis: river
blindness — Tumours of the eye

20 Accidents, Injuries and Child Abuse 263
Accidents and injuries — Child abuse

21 Notes on Prescribing for Children 272

   Recommended Further Reading 278
   Index 279

iv

Preface

The Declaration of Alma Ata by the World Health Organization in 1978 and the proclamation of 1979 as the International Year of the Child bear testimony to the serious concern and priority given to child health by the world community. Health problems vary not only with the socio-economic situation but have a geographical distribution as well. Child health care priorities will therefore vary from one part of the world to another. The Middle East shares with the Asian countries some of the problems of the developing world. Infections, diarrhoeal disease and malnutrition are common, even though the per capita income is high. Added to these are the genetic problems resulting from consanguinity.

These problems have to be tackled at the grass roots level and emphasis on basic child health care must be given in undergraduate training programmes in these regions. The larger textbooks are too complex and extensive for the needs of the undergraduate or general practitioner, and smaller texts with regional emphasis will continue to have an important role in medical education. It is an awareness of this regional approach that prompted the authors, all of whom have nearly three decades of clinical and academic experience in the Middle East, Asia and Africa, to compile the present volume. Much of the material is based on lectures given to undergraduates. Key words in the inclusion of topics have been the 'primary care approach' on a 'regional basis'. Day-to-day child health problems have been given priority over the more esoteric diseases, which have been left to the larger textbooks. Our aim has been to focus on the requirements of the undergraduate medical student and the generalist. The authors hope that they have succeeded in their endeavour.

After considerable thought, it was decided not to include neonatalogy in this book. It was felt that this had become a discipline in itself and warranted a separate textbook.

'In a room where a child is sleeping the lamp should be placed so that the light may be reflected from the mother's face on to the child's. Even as the Earth lends the Moon light borrowed from the Sun'.

(From an ancient Indian verse)

Acknowledgements

The authors would like to thank Dr Robin Broadland of the Liverpool School of Tropical Medicine for his help with the section on parasites causing skin irritation. We would also like to thank Miss Hazel Collard and Mrs Margaret Brown for their efficiency, speed and good humour in typing and retyping so much of the manuscript, Mrs Sheila Jones for editorial assistance, and Mrs Alice Barnes for her patience and tolerance.

The authors and publishers wish to acknowledge, with thanks, the following sources:
Bedford General Hospital for Figure 15.2;
Gower Medical Publishing Ltd for Figures 18.1, 18.3, 18.6 and 18.10;
Dr A.W. Ferguson for Figure 16.3;
Lepra, Farringdon House, 105/107 Farringdon Road, London EC1 3BT for Figures 6.5, 6.6 and 6.7;
Professor David Morley for Figure 5.3;
C. James Webb for Figures 3.4 and 16.2 and
The International Children's Centre, Paris for the extract on page 115.

The publishers have made every effort to trace the copyright holders, but if they have inadvertently overlooked any, they will be pleased to make the necessary arrangements at the first opportunity.

List of Abbreviations

ALL	acute lymphoblastic leukaemia
AML	acute myeloid leukaemia
ARF	acute renal failure
ASO titre	anti-streptolysin 'O' titre
ATP	adenosine triphosphate
BMT	bone marrow transplant
CRF	chronic renal failure
CT scan	computerized tomography scan
CVP	central venous pressure
DIC	disseminated intravascular coagulation
DNA	deoxyribonucleic acid
ECF	extracellular fluid
ELISA	enzyme-linked immunosorbent assay
ESR	erythrocyte sedimentation rate
GFR	glomerular filtration rate
HAV	hepatitis virus A
HBV	hepatitis virus B
IgA etc	immunoglobulins
i.m.	intramuscular
inj	injection
IT	intrathecal
ITP	idiopathic thrombocytopoenic purpura
i.v.	intravenous
i.v.p.	intravenous pyelogram
i.v.u.	intravenous urogram
MCNS	minimal change nephrotic syndrome
MCU	micturating cystourethrogram
m.i.c.	minimum inhibitory concentration
6MP	6 mercaptopurine
MTX	methotrexate
NS	nephrotic syndrome
PEM	protein−energy malnutrition
r.b.c.	red blood corpuscle
RBC	red blood cell count
RNA	ribonucleic acid
s.c.	subcutaneous
SLE	systemic lupus erythematosus
UTI	urinary tract infection
VCR	vincristine
VUR	vesico-ureteric reflux

Primary Health Care

WHO–UNICEF 1978

Primary Health Care is essential health care based on practical scientifically sound and socially acceptable methods. These should be made accessible to families in the community through their full participation and at a cost that they can afford. This should develop a spirit of self-reliance and self-determination.

From the beginning of their education, medical students are introduced to illness and care of the sick as it is encountered in hospital. In this way they see the middle and terminal stages of disease. They have little concept of the origin of disease which starts in the community. Even in advanced industrialized countries curative medicine takes precedence over preventative medicine, and as treatments become more sophisticated and expensive, more and more of national financial resources are diverted towards these treatments and treatment centres and less and less towards the preventative services. For example, in some relatively poor countries facilities and finances are directed towards the production of units for carrying out open and closed heart surgery for the replacement of heart valves damaged by rheumatic fever, instead of devoting that money and energy towards eradicating rheumatic fever from the community.

Primary health care is aimed at the early detection and prevention of disease, and in this way many diseases will be eradicated.

In the United Kingdom, primary health care is based on the general medical practitioner (GP) who is based in, and serves, the community and the good practitioner is involved in detection and prevention of disease. This system is developing towards the concept of a primary health care team in which the GP is an important member and a new form of primary health care is evolving. Other European countries are developing similar systems. In many of the socialist countries of Eastern Europe,

Cuba and China, primary health care is based on the polyclinic and the results produced by this system are beginning to bear fruit. These countries cannot afford sophisticated medical care and even the training of doctors is expensive but the cost of training primary health care workers is not.

The problem in developing countries

After independence, most governments made commitments to improve health care for their people. In many developing countries only about 25 per cent of the population obtained any sort of medical care. This percentage existed around the large towns, but most of the population lived in the rural areas. In many central African countries, particularly Zambia, Zimbabwe and Malawi, the British Colonial Medical Service had started a network of Health Care Clinics based on the District Hospitals. The various mission hospitals which tended to work in the rural areas were outside this system. In Zambia, (then Northern Rhodesia) the main towns were supplied by a general hospital and this was the apex of the health care pyramid (Figure 1.1).

The general hospitals covered all specialities and were served by as many as 30 or 40 doctors of all grades. District hospitals tended to have one or two surgeons and one or two physicians with anaesthetists. The rural hospitals often only had one doctor, who also supervised the rural health clinics. The rural health clinics were manned by one or two medical assistants. Medical assistants were generally male indigenous medical workers, who had two to three years' training in schools situated near the general hospital. Their main task was in diagnosis and treatment of minor ailments. The French and Belgians had similar systems in Africa, although medical assistants tended to be given more responsibility.

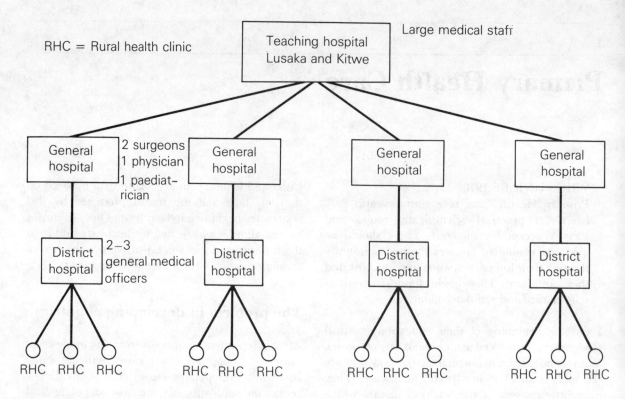

RHC = Rural health clinic

Teaching hospital
Lusaka and Kitwe

Large medical staff

General hospital

2 surgeons
1 physician
1 paediat-
rician

General hospital

General hospital

General hospital

District hospital

2–3 general medical officers

District hospital

District hospital

District hospital

RHC RHC RHC

RHC RHC RHC

RHC RHC RHC

RHC RHC RHC

Figure 1.1 The health care pyramid

During the colonial period, few, if any, indigenous personnel were trained as doctors and almost all of the hospital staffing came from the colonial power. There was not a shortage of doctors, particularly after the two World Wars. However, the best well-trained medical staff tended to stay in the general hospitals. Doctors with less training and experience gravitated to the rural hospitals. Financing the health services was concentrated in the central areas and little went to the periphery. Similar systems were present in other parts of the world under colonial rule.

After independence, most countries carried on with the system, building medical schools and employing expatriate doctors to fill in the gaps left by the colonial powers. Seventy per cent of the health budget continued to be spent on the centre and large prestige hospitals were being built. These could not be staffed. The money began to run out and many of the new governments had to rethink their health policies.

Some of the newly oil-rich Arab countries have not yet had to do this, as they have been able to afford to build expensive hospitals completely staffed by expatriate groups (Americans, Yugoslavs, Poles and Irish) to bridge the period until their own people can man the hospitals at a satisfactory level of competence. Some of these countries, because of the size of the population, will probably never be able to do this. These countries are a minority and probably not typical of the problems in developing countries.

Rethinking on health care

Cuba and China have shown that a health service based on primary health care (PHC) which stresses prevention and community-based care can produce excellent results. To achieve this, the countries had to have a socialist government based on the one-party system. Doctors were to be part of a health team with no special status. In the Cameroons, at a fairly early stage after independence, the Government decided to train nurses, medical assistants and medical students in the same school. The idea was that they should get to know and respect each other at an early stage in their careers. All the hospitals in the area of the medical school had one storey, similar to those in the rural areas.

In Tanzania, where finances were very tight, it was decided to base the health service on primary health care at a village level. Malnutrition and infection were the main problems for the children, particularly those under the age of five. Each village health team incorporated an agricultural unit to ensure greatest use was made of the local soil and crops. These primary health care units were run by committees made up of senior local citizens who were Party members, because it was very important that the policies of the Government were carried out at a basic level.

The three most important aspects of health at this level were nutrition, maternal and child health, infection and health education. Most infectious diseases can be controlled provided immunization is total and effective. Many developing countries now realize that central hospital care creates dependence and care for only a few. The main focus must be on the common health problems of the community.

This requires a revolution in health care thought, producing complete involvement of the individual in his own care and this may take one or two generations to bring about. It is very important (although perhaps sad to say) that the doctor is no longer considered as Deity but as an important but *equal* member of a primary health care team. More money should be allocated to the training of health workers as this would be cheaper and more cost-effective than spending vast sums of money training more doctors.

In Libya, for example, effective primary health care is being developed and based on the polyclinic. These polyclinics are staffed at the moment by general practitioners and community physicians. Immunization programmes are based on the polyclinics.

Primary health care in the South and Central American countries, as well as those in the Pacific, is beginning to produce results with regard to the increase in health and happiness of the countries.

Unfortunately, wars, civil wars and natural disasters can instantly destroy a decade a progress.

Further reading

Ebrahim, G.J. and Rankin, J.P. (1988). *Primary Health Care*. Macmillan, London and Basingstoke.

King, M., King, F. and Martdipoero, S. (1978). *Primary Child Care Book I* and *Book II*. Oxford Medical Publications, Oxford.

WHO (1985). *Review of Primary Health Care*. WHO, Geneva.

Growth and Development

Definition

Growth is referred to as an increase in cell number and size and *development* as an increase in functional capacity.

Growth and development occur simultaneously. *Maturation* and *learning* are intimately associated.

Maturation is a sophistication of growth and development that ultimately permits the function of the organism.

Learning is an alteration of behaviour resulting from experience.

Principles of normal growth and development

1. The process of growth and development is continuous from conception to maturity.
2. The sequence is the same for all children but the rate may vary from child to child.
3. Development is directly related to the maturation of the nervous system and generalized mass activity is replaced by specific individual responses.
4. Development is in the 'head to tail' direction.
5. Certain primitive reflexes have to be lost before the corresponding voluntary movement is acquired.

Heredity and genetics

Potential growth and development are governed by an interplay of inherited genes. This genetic expression can be modified by a number of environmental factors.

Prenatal environment

These factors are:
1. maternal infections − rubella, cytomegalic inclusion disease, syphilis, toxoplasmosis
2. maternal endocrine disorders − diabetes mellitus, hypothyroidism
3. maternal nutritional disorders
4. genetic disorders − isoimmunization disorders,

metabolic disorders e.g. Down's syndrome

Postnatal environment

Poor nutrition, increased incidence of acute and chronic illness, inadequate medical supervision and care, crowded and inefficient housing and sanitation, non-supportive psychological inputs.

Sex

Till adolescence girls are shorter than boys. During 11−14 years girls shoot up, and are taller. After that boys shoot up and are then taller. Boys are heavier than girls. Girls mature sexually 2 to 2½ years earlier than boys. Boys have more advanced muscular development.

Endocrine system

A number of hormones are linked directly or indirectly with growth and development, mainly the pituitary gland, thyroid gland, gonads and adrenals.

Nutrition

Causes of inadequate nutrition may extend from uterine life to adulthood, e.g. placental dysfunction, chronic illness and disease, inadequate intake, maternal neglect.

Disease

Chronic disease states regardless of etiology can cause growth failure, e.g. cystic fibrosis, renal disorders, intestinal malabsorption, infectious diseases. When the condition improves the rate of growth may be accelerated, i.e. 'catch up growth', but in certain severe and prolonged illnesses the child may never regain normal growth.

Periods of growth and development

Intrauterine

Embryonic − organogenesis first 12 weeks

Fetal 28 weeks − previable
28−38 weeks − viable (premature)
38 weeks − full term.

Extrauterine
Neonatal − 1 month
Infancy − 1 year
Preschool − 5 years
Early school years − 10−12 years
Adolescent

Growth curves of different tissues

General
1. relative rapid growth during infancy with a gradual deceleration until about the fourth year
2. a slow but uniform period of growth till puberty
3. a prominent adolescent growth spurt
4. a relatively gradual decrease in the rate of growth until completion of maturity

General includes respiratory and digestive, kidney, aortic and pulmonary trunks, musculative, blood volume.

Neural
Brain and head − 70−89 per cent of brain growth occurs in the first 2 years of life. By 5 years 90 per cent of adult weight. By 10 years 95 per cent of adult weight.

Genital
Reproductive system − growth spurt during adolescence and 100 per cent growth achieved by 20 years.

Lymphoid
Thymus, lymph nodes − hypertrophy till 12 years up to 180−200 per cent and then regresses to 100 per cent by 20 years.

Growth patterns
When normal growth values are plotted on a graph a bell-shaped curve results, denoting that most values cluster about the mean value.

Percentile
The value of growth of each child can be read in terms of percentile, e.g. if we say a child is at the 25th percentile for weight, that means that 25 per cent of children have less weight than this child.

Standard deviation
Describes the degree of dispersion of the observed value as they deviate from the mean value.

Values lying between
+1SD to −1SD   68 per cent of all values
+2SD to −2SD   95 per cent of all values
+3SD to −3SD   99.7 per cent of all values

Such measures of growth as percentile will indicate the status of the child in relation to other children of the same age. Sequential measurement of the same child will indicate the normal or abnormal dynamics of the process through which each child is achieving his or her growth potential.

Types of growth data

1. Longitudinal studies: same child is used at each age for data collection, better but time-consuming and tedious.
2. Cross sectional: all children of one age group are studied at one time.

Areas of growth and development

Physical growth and development is measured in terms of:

1. weight
2. height
3. head circumference
4. body proportions
5. osseus maturation
6. dental development
7. anthropometry

Weight

- a full term newborn weighs 2.5 kg or more
- weight is lost − about 10 per cent in the first 10 days of life
- after this, weight gain is 20 g/day for five months
- then 15 g/day until one year of age
- birth weight is doubled by five to six months
- tripled by one year of age
- 2.5 kg gain in the second year of life
- 2 kg gain each year in the third, fourth and fifth years of life
- up to 10 years in girls ⎫ weight gain is
- up to 12 years in boys ⎬ 3−3½ kg per year

- after this adolescent growth begins

Weech's Formula	Weight in kg
Weight at birth	3.25 kg
3−12 months	$\dfrac{\text{age (months)} + 9}{2}$
1−6 years	age (years) $\times$ 2 + 8
6−12 years	$\dfrac{\text{age (years)} \times 7 - 5}{2}$
Height at birth	50 cm
1 year	75 cm
2−12 years	age (years) $\times$ 6 + 77 = height in cm

Height

- average length at birth — 50 cm
- in 1st year increases by — 25−30 cm, so becomes 75 cm
- in 2nd year increases by — 12 cm
- in 3rd, 4th and 5th years — 8 to 6 cm per year
- up to 10 years in girls — 6 cm per year
- up to 13 years in boys — 6 cm per year

Head circumference

- birth — 34−35 cm — head is larger than chest at birth
- 6 months — 44 cm — equal at one year
- 1 year — 47 cm — chest exceeds head circumference after one year
- 2nd year — 49 cm
- in the first year — head circumference increases by 12−13 cm
- in the second year — head circumference increases by only 2−2.5 cm
- by the end of 1st year brain is 2/3rd of adult size
- by the end of 2nd year brain is 4/5th of adult size
- by the end of 12 years brain is equal to adult size
- by the end of 5th year — 51 cm
- between 5 and 12 years — 53−54 cm
- anterior fontanelle is open at birth, goes on increasing until 6 months and then decreases progressively and closes anytime from 9−18 months — usually at 18 months.
- posterior fontanelle closes from birth to 4 months.

Body proportions

- head forms ½ of total height at 2nd fetal month

¼ of total height at birth
⅛ of total height in adults
- upper segment to lower segment ratios: − US:LS
  US − head to symphysis pubis
  LS − symphysis pubis to heel
- US:LS at birth − 1.7 to 1
- US decreases by 0.1 every year for first three years
- US decreases by 0.1 every third year after that
- ratio becomes 1:1 at 12 years of age
- infantile ratios are retained in hypothyroidism − relative preponderance of growth at the cephalad part of the body in fetal life and infancy and later; followed by caudal growth of trunk and extremeties is termed as cephalocaudal progression
- sitting height − 70 per cent of body length at birth
  − 57 per cent at three years
  − 52 per cent at menarche in girls at 15 years in boys

Osseous maturation

- fetal ossification begins at five months
- sequence is first in clavicles, membraneous bone of skull, long bones and spine
- five ossification centres are present in 90 per cent of cases at birth − these are:
  − distal femoral epiphyses
  − proximal tibial epiphyses
  − talus
  − calcaneus
  − cuboid

Bone age is a good index of general growth and can be judged by X-rays. Hand and wrist are useful till 10 years of age for judging bone age, in infancy X-ray of leg is useful.

Girls are more advanced than boys in skeletal maturation.

X-ray wrist:
At birth −	no ossification centres
1 year −	hamate (4 months)
	capitate (6 months)
	epiphysis radius
2 years −	same
3 years −	triquetium appears
	− all epiphysis metacarpals
	− all epiphysis phalanges
4 years −	lunate appears

5 years – trapezium appears
6 years – trapezoid
        – epiphysis ulna
10 years – pisiform
11 years – styloid of ulna

Dental development

Decidous teeth – 20	*Average time of eruption*
Central incisors – lower	6–7 months
– upper	
Lateral incisors – lower	9 months
– upper	
First molar	12 months
Canines	18 months
Second molar	24 months
At end of 1st year	6–8 teeth on average
At end of 2nd year	14–16 teeth
By 2½ years	20 teeth usually erupt

Permanent dentition – 32	*Average time of eruption*
1st molar – lower	6th year
– upper	
Central incisors – lower	6th year
– upper	6th–7th year
Lateral incisors – lower	7th year
– upper	8th year
Canines – lower	10th year
– upper	10th–11th year
1st premolar – upper	10th year
– lower	10th–12th year
2nd premolar – upper	11th year
– lower	11th–12th year
2nd molar – lower	11th–12th year
– upper	12th year
3rd molar	20 years

Anthropometry

This is measurement of skin fold thickness. Fifty per cent of body fat is present in the subcutaneous tissue and there is a correlation between fat content and skin thickness. These measurements can be carried out with skin fold calipers commonly at the triceps and subscapular region. Such measurements are complex, time-consuming and subject to errors, hence not preferred over height and weight, though they give a good idea of the general nutritional status.

Growth charts

These are valuable charts to measure height, weight

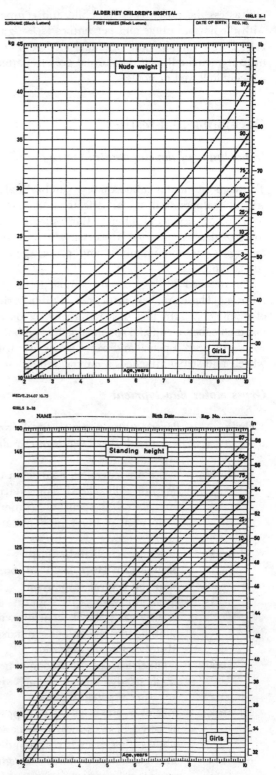

Figure 2.1 Percentile graph developed from the bell shaped curve. These graphs are used to compare heights and weights of children

and assess the progress of the child and compare with the normal range and percentiles (see Figure 2.1). It is a valuable and practical method. Serial measurements tell us if the normal growth pattern is being followed or not.

Developmental testing

Importance of developmental testing

To diagnose mental subnormality, cerebral palsy, severe deafness and visual defects, and certain neurological defects of infancy. Early diagnosis in some of these conditions is necessary to give better treatment and prognosis and proper genetic counselling.

For detailed testing, certain simple items are required. These are: bell, rattle, pencil torch, a ring of diameter 6.5 cm tied to a red string, colourful one inch cubes, a cup and spoon, a pellet and bottle with wide neck, a pencil and paper, a few toys with wheels and string attached, a mirror, a doll, etc.

Gross motor development

Birth	— flexed attitude, turns head from side to side, head lag, Moro's reflex present
4 weeks	— legs more extended, holds chin up on prone, lifts head momentarily on ventral suspension (prone), tonic neck posture, predominates till 12 weeks.
8 weeks	— raises head slightly further on prone, can keep head in body plane on ventral suspension
12 weeks	— chest up with arm support on prone, early head control with bobbing movement, back rounded. Moro's reflex disappearing.
16 weeks	— symmetrical posture predominates, head steady, enjoys sitting with full truncal support
28 weeks	— rolls over, sits briefly with support of pelvis, leans forward on hands while sitting, back is still rounded
40 weeks	— sits alone well, back straight, crawls, pulls to standing position
52 weeks	— cruises—walks holding one hand on furniture

15 months	— walks alone, crawls upstairs
18 months	— runs, stiffly, walks upstairs with one hand held
24 months	— runs well, walks up and down stairs one step at a time, opens doors, climbs on furniture
30 months	— jumps
36 months	— goes upstairs alternating feet, rides tricycle, stands momentarily on one foot
48 months	— hops on one foot, climbs well, throws ball overhead
60 months	— skips

Fine motor and adaptive

These are fine motor movements which need a lot of co-ordinated movements and adaptive function, e.g. eye movements. NB dolls eye movements.

4 weeks	— follows moving object but less than 180°
12 weeks	— follows moving object up to 180°

Dangling red ring

4 weeks	— regards
15 weeks	— reaches for dangling ring
18 weeks	— carries ring to mouth, closes on dangling ring

Pellet behaviour

16 weeks	— sees pellet but makes no move at it
28 weeks	— rakes at pellet
40 weeks	— picks up pellet with crude pincer grasp
52 weeks	— picks up pellet with fine pincer grasp
15 months	— inserts pellet in bottle
18 months	— dumps pellet from bottle

Grasp behaviour

ulnar palmar prehension	— 22 weeks
radial palmar prehension	— 26 weeks
pincer grasp inferior	— 34 weeks
pincer grasp superior	— 38—40 weeks

Cube behaviour

16 weeks	— regards cube
28 weeks	— reaches out and grasps it, transfers it from one hand to the other
40 weeks	— releases object (cube) grasped by other person

52 weeks — releases object (cube) to other person on request
15 months — tower of two cubes
18 months — tower of three cubes
24 months — tower of six cubes
30 months — tower of eight cubes
36 months — tower of nine cubes
48 months — imitates construction of gate of five cubes

Mirror image approach
mirror image approach (regards it) — 22 weeks
smiles at mirror image — 26 weeks
playful response to mirror — 30 weeks

Writing
15 months — makes a line with crayon
18 months — imitates scribbling and vertical stroke
24 months — imitates circular scribbling and horizontal stroke
30 months — makes horizontal and vertical stroke, but generally will not join them to make a cross
36 months — copies a circle and cross

Language
12 weeks — cooing sounds, aah ngah
28 weeks — polysyllable vowel sounds formed, ah, ooh, eeh
40 weeks — repetitive consonant sounds (ma-ma, da-da) without meaning
52 weeks — a few words besides ma-ma, da-da
15 months — jargon, follows simple commands, names a few familiar objects, e.g. ball, bottle
18 months — 10 words (average), names pictures
24 months — puts three words together (subject, verb, object), small sentences
30 months — refers to self by pronoun 'I', knows full name
36 months — knows age and sex, counts three objects correctly
48 months — counts up to four correctly, tells a story

Social behaviour
4 weeks — visual preference for human face
6 weeks — social smile
8 weeks — listens to voice and coos
12 weeks — sustained social contact, listens to music
16 weeks — laughs aloud, shows displeasure if social contact is broken, excited at sight of food
28 weeks — prefers mother, responds to changes in emotional content on social contact
40 weeks — responds to sound of name, waves bye—bye, plays peek-a-boo
52 weeks — plays simple ball games, adjusts posture on dressing
15 months — indicates desire and needs by pointing
18 months — feeds self, seeks help when in trouble, may complain when wet or soiled
24 months — eats with spoon well, helps to undress, tells immediate experiences, listens to stories with pictures, verbalizes toilet needs
30 months — helps put things away.
36 months — helps in dressing, plays simple games with other children.
48 months — role-playing, goes to toilet alone.
60 months — dresses and undresses, asks lots of questions, domestic role-playing.

Special senses
A newborn baby can hear, smell, taste and see at birth.

Further reading

Illingworth, R.S. (1987). *The Development of the Infant and Young Child Normal and Abnormal*. Churchill Livingstone, New York.
Brook, Charles (1982). *Growth Assessment in Childhood and Adolescence*. Blackwell, Oxford.

3

Nutrition

The period of life where nutrition is most important is in infancy and childhood. Feeding patterns achieved in this period affect the health and growth of the child's whole life.

Children require more nutrition per unit weight than adults and are more likely to suffer from inadequate nutrition than adults.

An adult to some extent can control his nutritional requirements himself but children are entirely dependent on adults and so can be abused and neglected in this field as in others.

Fetal nutrition

Maternal nutrition affecting the fetus

Infant feeding begins at conception, and so the nutrition of the mother can affect the nutrition of the baby. It has been said that the fetus is a parasite of the mother, living off the nutrition of the mother. Severely malnourished mothers can produce normal-sized babies but this is not as common as was once thought. Mothers do loose protein during pregnancy, and in the lactating period, and cases of kwashiorkor have been reported in India in adult women who have had repeated pregnancies.

It is not possible to control the diet of women in most developing countries, but it must be remembered that a high-protein, low-calorie increase in the maternal diet can lead to early premature births and often severe birth weight depression. A well balanced, normal diet is all that is required for the mother during pregnancy and this is probably the most difficult to obtain.

Other factors affecting fetal nutrition

The fetus may become malnourished in the uterus, resulting in 'small for dates' babies. The condition is known under the general term of 'placental insufficiency' and the causes of this are numerous.

Maternal ill-health is probably the commonest cause of fetal malnutrition in developing countries, starting with maternal malnutrition, chronic renal disease, pre-eclamptic toxaemia and multiple pregnancies. Smoking, alcoholism and severe physical exercise are less common causes, as they are all socially unacceptable in many areas, certainly in the Middle East.

Most of these conditions cause placental infarction, which directly affects placental function, which in turn controls fetal nutrition and oxygenation.

Infant feeding

The joint WHO/UNICEF meeting on infant feeding held at Geneva in October, 1979 stated,

> poor infant feeding practices and their consequences are one of the world's major problems and a serious obstacle to social and economic development. Breast feeding is an integral part of the normal reproductive process and should, therefore, be encouraged. For this reason it is the responsibility of society to promote breast feeding and to protect pregnant and lactating mothers from any influences that could disrupt it.

It has been established that the decline in breast feeding in a community, with a rise in artificial infant feeding, results in an increase in gastroenteritis and marasmus in that community.

These are the main consequences of poor infant feeding practices and they can be overcome by a return to breast feeding in urban areas where it has declined in the past few years. What happens in urban areas today may spread to rural areas tomorrow.

Reflexes associated with breast feeding baby

The following reflexes are all present at birth in a full-term baby: rooting reflex, sucking reflex, and swallowing reflex.

The rooting reflex

This is a 'searching' reflex. When the baby's cheek is stimulated by touch, the lips will turn to the stimulated side. When a baby is 'put to the breast' he should be allowed to find the nipple himself by this method. The baby should not be forced onto the nipple by the mother or the nurse. He will resist this.

The sucking reflex

This is self-explanatory. The baby's lips surround the areola tissue of the mother's nipple. Within the alveoli are the saccules full of milk. The act of emptying the saccules starts the first of the maternal reflexes (see below).

At the same time the nipple (which contains erectile tissue – see Figure 3.1) extends upwards in the baby's mouth to come in contact with the hard palate.

The swallowing reflex

This is self-explanatory and is present in all normal full-term babies. It may be absent in pre-term babies, and these would have to be tube-fed. It is started by the contact of milk from the erectile nipple onto the hard palate. In bottle fed babies the bottle teat comes into contact with the soft palate, and may result in rejection of the milk (regurgitation).

Maternal reflexes

The mother's reflexes are the prolactin reflex and the let down reflex (see Figure 3.2).

Breast/bottle feeding

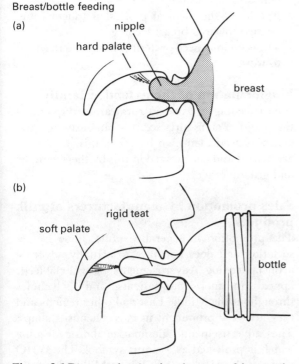

Figure 3.1 Diagram showing the advantage of the erectile tissue in the nipple compared with the rigid teat of the artificially fed baby in infant feeding; (a) erectile tissue of human nipple squirts milk onto the hard palate, (b) bottle teat squirts milk onto soft palate resulting in choking, air swallowing and regurgitation.

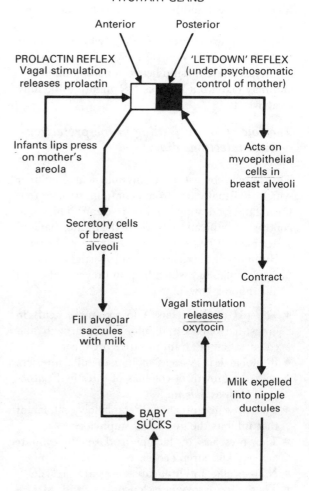

Figure 3.2 Diagrams showing the pathways of the prolactin and 'let-down' reflexes

11

Prolactin reflex

The act of the infant's lips pressing on the areola of the mother's nipple produces vagal stimulation of the anterior pituitary gland with the release of the hormone prolactin. Prolactin acts on the secretory cells of the breast alveoli and the alveolar saccules are filled with milk.

'Let down' reflex

The act of sucking produces vagal stimulation of the posterior pituitary gland with the release of the hormone oxytocin. This stimulates the myoepithelial cells lining the alveoli of the breast tissue to contract and expel the milk into the nipple ductules. This 'let down' reflex is also under psychosomatic control of the mother's central nervous system. If the mother is tense and nervous, the reflex may be inhibited and breast feeding will not be established. If she is relaxed and happy it is easily established.

The natural art of breast feeding, which has been neglected in many countries, depends upon a good and relaxed relationship between mother and baby and may take from 2 weeks to 1 month to be fully established.

The role of breast feeding in the protection against infectious diarrhoea

The human breast is a physiological container which is virtually free from contamination, so that the infant food supply remains clean. This is in contrast to artificial feeds where the bottle, teat and water may all be heavily infected with pathogens.

Human milk also has unique properties not found in cow's milk, and which help to prevent infection in the infant's bowel.

- The pH of the colon is lower (more acid) in breast-fed babies and inhibits the growth and colonization of Gram-negative organisms.
- Bifidobacteria present in human milk interfere with the growth of colonies of intestinal pathogens such as *Shigella*.
- The presence of an anti-staphylococcal factor that inhibits the growth of staphylococci.
- The presence of lactoperoxidase thiocyanate actively kills streptococci.
- Non-specific antiviral substances are present.
- There are lysozymes, leucocytes and macrophages present that produce active phagocytosis of bacteria.

- Lactoferrin. This has a greater affinity for free serum iron than bacteria thus depriving the bacteria of iron vitally needed for growth and reproduction. This results in effective bacteriostasis.
- The presence of large amounts of secretory IgA and smaller amounts of IgG and IgM as antibodies to Gram-negative pathogens in the small bowel also contributes to host defence.

Cow's milk has none of these properties. On the contrary, there is reason to believe that there are factors in cow's milk which promote the growth of Gram-negative organisms. In the weaning of calves these bacteria help break down cellulose during the process of rumination.

The reasons for the decline in breast feeding

The following causes can be said to have influenced the decline in breast feeding:

1. The fragmentation of the extended village family as a result of urbanization.
2. Sales promotion by manufacturers of milk products and soft drinks.
3. Apathy of the medical profession (doctors and nurses) towards breast feeding.
4. The economic need or desire of mothers to go out to work.

Fragmentation of the extended family

Breast feeding is usual in rural areas throughout the world. Young girls see it at an early age and expect to feed their own babies in this way. They are helped and encouraged in this by their mothers and grandmothers.

Sales promotion by manufacturers of milk products

The promotion is generally subtle, done by association and does not have to actually advocate artificial feeding. Advertisements for artificial feeds appear in most out-patients and polyclinics throughout the Middle East and other regions and they are very prominent in most chemist's shops. The advertisements glamourize bottle feeding which is projected as a status symbol. The WHO Code on the Marketing of Breast Milk Substitutes sets out guidelines to prevent such unscrupulous use of advertising.

In the developed countries breast feeding is now being encouraged.

Apathy of the medical profession (doctors and nurses) towards breast feeding

Most paediatricians are aware of this attitude among some of their colleagues and consider it a disgrace to the profession. It may not be easy to help a young mother to continue breast feeding in a busy urban clinic, but there is no doubt that the extra effort will help reduce the incidence of gastroenteritis and marasmus.

The economic need or desire of mothers to go out to work

In this more emancipated age, more and more young mothers in urban areas desire or need to undertake employment immediately after the birth of their child. Few work places have facilities for the mother to feed her baby, and in consequence the child is left at home with a neighbour who feeds it artificially.

It is possible that the problem of working mothers in relation to the decline in breast feeding has been overemphasized, but it is a factor that has to be considered, particularly in connection with the fragmentation of the family unit by urbanization.

How to encourage breast feeding

It is only in the last 100 years or so that cow's milk has been used regularly as a substitute for human milk in the feeding of human infants, although ass's milk and goat's milk were mentioned in biblical times.

There is no contra-indication to breast feeding. Mothers with active pulmonary tuberculosis should continue feeding their babies having been given treatment themselves.

In the case of maternal death, the practice of wet nursing, usually by a young nursing mother who has a good milk supply, is used extensively in most rural areas in India, Africa, South America and the Far East and was common practice in Europe up to the turn of the century. However, it has never been employed in one or two countries where it is culturally unacceptable.

Encouragement of mothers to return to breast feeding can be given at both government level and at a personal level.

At government level

Advertisements by food firms could be forbidden in clinics and public places (WHO Code on the Marketing of Breast Milk Substitutes). This has been carried out successfully in Zambia for many years.

Active educational programmes should be carried out by means of the media, particularly the radio. Transistor radios are owned by almost everyone in urban areas. The use of television is also important, and can be used in clinics for educational purposes.

At a personal level

Mothers separated from their home and tribal background come to the nurse or doctor at the clinic or outpatients for help. To help a mother establish breast feeding, a knowledge of its physiology is essential and many general physicians have forgotten it. It is helpful to explain the principles in simple terms to mothers who are struggling with feeding.

Artificial feeding

There are occasions where it may not be possible to breast feed a baby. In these cases artificial feeding should be employed under supervision of the medical staff in much the same way as antibiotics are used. The dosage must be correct. In Papua New Guinea, artificial milk can only be obtained on a doctor's prescription. In Iraq a feeding bottle cannot be obtained without a doctor's prescription.

Although bottle feeding may appear easy, the bottle and teat are easily infected and cup and spoon feeding is recommended. In most developing countries powdered milk, in the form of full cream, is used and reconstituted with water. Table 3.1 compares the food and energy contents of 100 ml of

Table 3.1 *Analysis of milk per 100 ml reconstituted feed*

	Protein g	Fat g	CHO g	Kilojoules
Breast milk	1.5	3.5	7.0	273
Cow's milk	3.5	4.4	4.5	273
Full cream powdered milk	3.3	3.4	4.8	265
Full cream evaporated milk	3.0	3.0	4.8	260

Table 3.2 *Nutrition, fluid and electrolytes aproximate daily needs*

Age (years)	Fluids (ml/kg)	Kilojoules (per kg)	Protein (g/kg)
0–1	150	420	3.0
1–3	100	378	2.5
3–6	90	336	2.0
7–12	70	294	2.0

reconstituted full cream powdered milk. Table 3.2 shows the daily fluid electrolyte and energy requirements of an infant from birth to the age of 12 years.

When reconstituting powdered milk the powder should be heaped slightly in the spoon and levelled off with a knife, but not packed, as this latter method could easily double the dose of powder.

Many formula milks have a high solute load (high in sodium). Low solute loads are preferable but they are expensive. High solute feeds, because of the high sodium, make the baby thirsty and he cries. The mother thinks he is hungry and gives him more feed. This will raise the serum osmality considerably, producing the state of hypernatraemia.

In some countries local water may have a high salt content and if used to reconstitute powdered milk will increase its sodium content. If the mother boils this water, the sodium content will be increased even more.

Weaning

This is the process of introducing any non-milk food into the infant diet irrespective of whether or not breast or bottle feeding continues.

It is generally accepted that milk is insufficient for sustained growth and development after the sixth month of life, but this is disputed by some. However, it is certain that milk alone is quite adequate up to the age of 4 months and it is fairly certain that the gut immunological system cannot cope with other forms of protein up to this age. In many rural areas in developing countries, babies seem to thrive on breast milk alone up to the age of a year. This was the norm in rural England over 100 years ago. However, most infants find it difficult to tolerate the extra quantity of fluid required to sustain growth after the age of 6 months on milk alone.

Principles of weaning

The whole weaning process may last for 3 months. By the age of 1 year the child should be coping with an adult-type diet.

1. It is important that breast feeding or formula feeding should continue as long as possible during the weaning process.
2. After the age of 6 months, tissue deposition requires a more varied diet than previously and the idea of weaning is to introduce these extra amino-acids, minerals, vitamins and iron early into the infant's diet.
3. An infant does not take easily to a new taste or form of diet and refusal and rejection are common. Patience is needed and although the baby may not need the extra food before the age of 6 months, it is preferable to start the weaning process at 4 months.
4. After the age of 6 months teeth are due to appear and the baby will feel the desire to bite on things. By this time his weaning food may contain more solids to encourage this. Biscuits and rusks may be taken at 9 to 12 months.
5. The introduction of Vitamins C and D is important at the start of the weaning process.
6. Cereals should be the first food. They should be given in liquid form, mixed with milk or water. Rice is a preferable cereal because wheat-based cereal may induce a gluten enteropathy in a sensitive individual.
7. By the age of 6 to 7 months, the introduced cereals should be given four times per day.
8. Other weaning foods may include:
   - eggs or cheese mashed in potato
   - banana mashed in milk
   - minced meat
   and towards the end of the weaning process:
   - hard rusks
   - bread portions
9. Initially the weaning food should be given by spoon by the mother. Later the child will try to feed himself. Note that this can be a wasteful process with food.
10. Protein requirements of a 12-month-old child is contained in 750 ml of cow's milk, and en-

ergy requirements in about twice that amount. (Breast-milk has only half the protein content of cow's milk but contains the same amount of energy.) A weaning child at this age can tolerate 750 ml milk per day and can therefore obtain the large proportion of food for growth and energy from his milk. Weaning foods provide the extra energy, vitamins and minerals not present in cow's milk.

When supervising the diet of a child in developing countries, the importance of milk in the diet of an infant and toddler is paramount. Strict attention should be paid to the cleanliness of milk supplies.

Hazards of weaning

1. *Weaning diarrhoea.* This is generally caused by bacteria introduced from infected water or utensils, but may be as a result of food allergy.
2. *Food allergy.* This is caused by the introduction of certain proteins, generally in the weaning diet, into an infant digestive system that is not immunologically prepared for it. The commonest disorder of this type is the gluten-sensitive enteropathy.
3. *Malnutrition* due to failure to introduce sufficient quantity of essential nutrients such as Vitamin C (scurvy), Vitamin D (rickets), protein (protein−energy malnutrition) and total deficiency of all nutrients causing marasmus.
4. *Hypernatraemia* resulting from too much sodium in the weaning food.

It is important that babies should not be fed between the four meals a day routine, and all weaning babies should be personally fed.

Constructing a diet for children

Feeding the under fives

The highest incidence in malnutrition in most developing countries is in this period and fortunately most of the aid and advice to these countries is directed along lines to prevent this.

Ideally three to four meals per day should be offered to the child. Energy and protein requirements are shown in Table 3.2. Unfortunately, a child will eat chiefly to satisfy his calorie requirements. Whether his protein requirements (the most important element of his diet) are satisfied depends on the overall protein/energy ratio of his food. This should be approximately 2 g protein/420 kJ.

There are four main constituents to the construction of a diet for a growing child.

1. *The staple.* This is the main source of carbohydrate e.g. rice, wheat, maize, cassava (this contains hardly any protein). All these cereals lack the essential amino acid lysine.
2. *Vegetable proteins.* These are legumes and include peas, beans, lentils, chicken peas, groundnuts, soyabeans. They all lack the essential amino acid methionine.
3. *Animal proteins.* These include meat, fish, eggs, chicken, liver, milk, cheese, yoghurt. They are all well balanced and have a high content of essential amino acids. Some should be included in all meals.
4. *Dark green vegetables.* These include french beans, spinach, aubergine (egg plant), cabbage. These are an excellent source of vitamin A precursors, vitamin B, vitamin C, iron and some protein.

Various combinations of these constituents will make for a good mixed and varied diet. Actual ingredients will depend on seasonable variations.

1. staple + vegetable protein + milk
2. staple + animal protein + dark green vegetables
3. staple + animal protein + vegetable protein
4. staple + vegetable protein + animal protein + dark green vegetable

It can be seen that each meal must contain a staple and some source of animal protein.

The following staple foods have a high level protein/energy ratio:

Wheat	3.6 g/420 kJ
Maize	3.1 g/420 kJ
Rice	2.0 g/420 kJ
Potato	2.5 g/420 kJ
Yam	2.0 g/420 kJ
Cassava	0.5 g/420 kJ
Couscous	2.5 g/420 kJ

The following vegetables have a good supply of protein:

Legumes	7.5 g/420 kJ
Soyabeans	9.0 g/420 kJ
Broad beans	5.7 g/420 kJ

The protein content of some animal products is:

Fish   18 g/420 kJ
Lamb   12 g/420 kJ
Chicken   14 g/420 kJ

Dark green vegetables have a similar protein content to European potatoes.

When constructing a diet for advice to a government involved in health education, it is very important to assess the local foods available. It is seldom necessary to import or grow new types of food.

Feeding school children and teenagers

The same principles may be used as for the under fives provided it is realized that a young teenager may require the same calorie intake as a manual worker engaged in heavy labour.

Malnutrition

Protein—energy malnutrition is the most prevalent form of malnutrition in the world. It is estimated that 2.5 per cent of the under fives are severely malnourished and 20 per cent moderately malnourished. This means that there are approximately 100 000 000 moderate to severely malnourished children in the world.

A child will grow and develop normally if his diet consists of the right quality and quantity of protein, carbohydrate, fat and vitamins.

Malnutrition in childhood will result if the child receives improper quantity and quality of food. In an affluent society this takes the form of obesity due to excessive food intake and on unbalanced diet.

Malnutrition in developing countries is classed under the heading of protein—energy malnutrition (PEM). Protein—energy malnutrition covers a wide spectrum of deficiency in nutrition ranging from marasmus and the underweight child to kwashiorkor. The first sign of PEM is poor weight gain.

There have been many classifications of PEM, none entirely satisfactory. The most widely used is the Wellcome Classification. However, in South America the Gomez Classification is preferred. In order to understand these classifications it is necessary to have a knowledge of the centile chart system on which they are based.

The centile charts

The Boston and Tanner Charts are the most widely used. The Boston Charts are the basis of the Wellcome, Gomez and Waterlow Classifications.

In Boston in the 1950s and 1960s a large number of normal children were measured by weight and height from birth to 18 years, and their growth curves plotted on centile charts. It was found that the largest number of children followed the 50th centile. Smaller children followed centiles below this and larger children followed centiles above. The lowest acceptable centile for normal growth was the 3rd, and the highest the 97th. The Wellcome, Waterlow and Gomez Classifications are based on the Boston 50th centile. There have not, as yet, been centile charts devised for most developing countries. Although there are differences in the charts of boys and girls, it is reasonable to use a single chart for both sexes in demonstrating the principles of malnutrition.

Other growth measurements have also been charted in the same way, including 'mid-arm circumference', 'skin fold thickness', 'head circumference' and 'crown to rump length'.

The first three of these form the basis of other nutritional measurements (see below).

Use of height and weight centile charts

Weight and height are probably the best measurements in assessing the growth of an infant or toddler.

In developing countries the centile charts are of limited value, as it is not easy to measure heights accurately (as opposed to the accurate measurement of weight, which is feasible) and accurate age is difficult to assess over the age of one year. The measurement of weight is the basis of the Wellcome and Gomez Classifications.

Used correctly these charts are very helpful, provided it is remembered:

1. that a single weight is valueless
2. a stationary weight over a period of one to two months in a child under five years indicates a serious problem

Regular measurement of weight still remains the simplest and most satisfactory method of assessing the growth of a child in developing countries. Other methods have been devised and are mentioned below.

Protein—energy malnutrition classifications

The Wellcome Classification

Table 3.3 *The Wellcome Classification*

Weight % of 50th centile	Oedema	
	Present	*Absent*
80—60	Kwashiorkor	Underweight child
60	Marasmic kwashiorkor	Marasmus

The Gomez Classification

This is based on weight for age using the Boston 50th centile standards as a reference.

Between 75 and 90 per cent of the 50th centile is classed as first degree malnutrition, 60 to 75 per cent second degree malnutrition and 60 per cent or less as third degree.

This definition does not differentiate between the different forms of PEM and is best used as a classification of the nutritional status of a community.

The Waterlow Classification

There is a reasonably constant relationship between weight and height in early childhood. Using both weight and height helps to free us from some constraints of not noting the age.

The child whose weight is proportionate to height is unlikely to have an acute nutritional problem.

Other classifications have been based on clinical features alone and have not been found to be very helpful.

Clinical syndromes

Marasmus

Marasmus is probably the commonest form of PEM in most parts of the world. Its highest incidence is in infancy, particularly in areas where there is a failure of breast feeding, and the syndrome results in total lack of calorie intake. In many cases marasmus is a result of feeding mismanagement and not necessarily of poverty. Marasmus will always be present at any age group in famine areas where total food supply is deficient or absent. This is the result of a balanced response to starvation.

Signs of marasmus

A marasmic child literally 'eats himself' (Figure 3.3). Because of inadequate calorie intake he uses up his 'pool' of carbohydrate, fat and first-class protein. As a result of this there is marked muscle and tissue wasting with growth retardation (due to lack of calories) but no oedema or fatty liver, as the protein he uses (from his own muscle) is the right type to protect liver function and the serum proteins remain within normal limits. The serum biochemistry is generally within normal limits but there is a reduced excretion of hydroxyproline in the urine due to a low turnover of collagen.

There are also mental changes and the infant with marasmus is alert but irritable. The appetite is generally good. Hair is sparse and brittle.

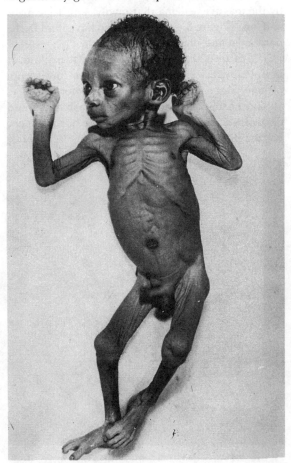

Figure 3.3 The gross wasting in a child with marasmus

Recovery under treatment is slow and management tedious.

Kwashiorkor

Kwashiorkor occurs in an older age group compared with marasmus, generally in the weaning period. In some Middle Eastern countries the age of onset may be as late as three years. It results from an inbalanced response to starvation. The exact aetiology is not known and food toxins may be implicated.

The incidence is lower than marasmus, and epidemics may occur at the start of the rainy season in some countries. The condition is rarer than marasmus.

Signs of kwashiorkor

A child with kwashiorkor has been given a diet very low in protein but often with normal calorie intake. Despite this he suffers from height loss with muscle and tissue wasting. This wasting is masked by the massive oedema that involves his legs, arms and face (Figure 3.4). He may also have fluid in the peritoneal and pleural cavities.

The cause of the oedema is not easy to explain. It is not always directly related to the low serum protein, and sodium retention is a factor.

Skin changes are common in kwashiorkor and dermatoses resembling second degree burns appear on the limbs and abdomen (Figure 3.5). Hair

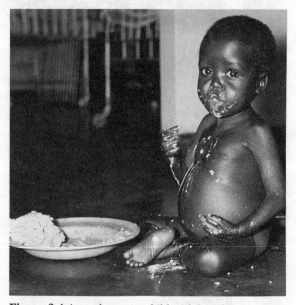

Figure 3.4 An oedematous child with kwashiorkor feeding on high protein diet

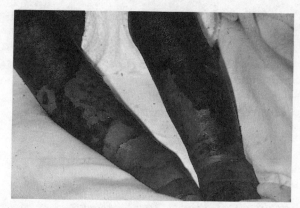

Figure 3.5 Severe dermatosis, resembling third degree burns, in a child with kwashiorkor

changes are more severe than in marasmus and may involve loss of pigment resulting in fair or red hair in black children. The hair itself is crinkly and brittle.

Mental changes

Children with kwashiorkor have no appetite and are drowsy and depressed with little interest in their surroundings. The first signs of recovery, even before the oedema has gone, is a smile.

The liver is always enlarged due to fatty infiltration. In severe or malignant kwashiorkor diarrhoea, hypoglycaemia, hypothermia and low serum potassium and magnesium occur and are likely to kill the child. Almost all children with kwashiorkor have diarrhoea and, despite the oedema, may be dehydrated. Unlike marasmic children, kwashiorkor children are drowsy, apathetic and have no appetite. Growth retardation occurs but is not so severe as in marasmus. The serum biochemistry is grossly abnormal with very low levels of serum protein (serum albumin may be as low as 0.5 g/100 ml; serum transferrin less than 0.45 mmol/l; serum lipoproteins less than 4 g/l; serum cholesterol less than 2.5 mmol/l; serum pseudocholesterase less than 1.5 iu/ml; serum potassium less than 3.0 mmol/l; and serum magnesium less than 0.5 mmol/l).

However, the serum cortisol levels are high. Serum iron and red cell folate are also low due to malabsorption. Whereas it is important to give folic acid in the early days of treatment, it is dangerous to give iron because of the low level of serum transferrin.

Recovery under correct treatment is relatively rapid but mortality rate is high.

Marasmic kwaskiorkor

This is an intermediate stage. The features of both marasmus and kwashiorkor are present to a lesser degree (Figure 3.6). The duration of the illness is longer than in kwashiorkor. Oedema generally remains in the legs only and dermatoses are not so common. Hepatomegaly due to fatty infiltration is however a common sign and growth retardation is more marked than in kwashiorkor, probably because the condition is of much longer duration. The child tends to be reasonably happy and eats well. In many areas this condition is more common than kwashiorkor.

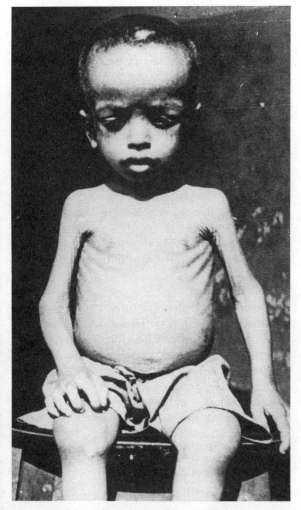

Figure 3.6 A child with marasmic kwashiorkor, he has pedal oedema and some oedema of the eyelids — the rest of his body resembles a child with marasmus

Severe or malignant kwashiorkor

Some children develop kwashiorkor rapidly and die within 24 to 48 hours or admission to hospital. These children are generally drowsy or even unconscious on admission. They frequently have septicaemia and hypoglycaemia which does not respond to treatment. They also become hypothermic and are difficult to resuscitate. Infection which may start in the skin ulcers, rapidly enters the bloodstream to cause septicaemia.

The organisms involved are Gram-negative bacteria such as *Escherichia coli*, *Pseudomonas* and *Proteus*. These organisms are similar to those affecting newborn babies and cause disease because of a similar deficiency in defence mechanisms. As in kwashiorkor the liver can be very large due to fatty infiltration.

Other measures for assessment of nutritional state

Weight for height

Various formulae have been devised but Rao and Singh in India in 1970 found the following formula to be useful:

$$\frac{\text{Weight}}{\text{Height}^2} \times 100$$

This formula is useful because it does not depend on a knowledge of the age of the child. Its main disadvantage is that malnutrition is not the only cause of growth retardation. Recurrent infection without significant malnutrition may also cause this.

The mean value found in normal children is 0.16 and for those with evidence of PEM the value is between 0.12 and 0.14. This formula only holds good for children between the ages of 1 to 5 years.

Height

Measurement of height alone is of little value in the assessment of acute malnutrition as it is not possible to lose height. Stationary height or a height that does not follow the normal growth course can be a useful indicator of prolonged malnutrition.

Skin fold measurements

These measurements involve the assessment of depletion of subcutaneous fat over the triceps of subscapular areas. Calipers are used in measuring skinfold thickness in these areas by the 'pinching' method. The calipers are extremely expensive and the measurements are only of value in skilled hands. However, normal standards are required for comparison.

Mid upper arm circumference
This is a measurement of muscle wasting and loss of subcutaneous fat. It is useful in children between the ages of 1 and 4 years and only requires a non-stretchable tape measure. It has been used in nutritional surveys but is only really of value when used in conjunction with skinfold thickness. To some extent the measurement is age dependent. There is little increase in arm circumference between 1 and 4 years and therefore this measurement is relatively free from age constraints.

Normal range

Age	Arm circumference
12 months	15.8 cm
24 months	16.2 cm
36 months	16.5 cm
48 months	16.7 cm

Thus arm circumference

12.5 cm	=	severe malnutrition
12.5−14 cm	=	moderate
14−16.5 cm	=	normal

Disadvantages

1. accurate measurement essential
2. because of narrow limits this is a rather insensitive index
3. the standards given above are not universally accepted

Mid arm/head circumference ratio
The normal ratio for a child under the age of 5 years is 0.331. Levels between 0.280 and 0.31 show mild PEM, 0.250 and 0.279 show moderate PEM and less than 0.250 severe PEM.

Summary of measures of assessment of nutritional states

Under one year of age
Weight and length used in conjunction with a centile chart.

One year to five years
1. Mid-arm circumference
2. Weight for height (Rao and Singh, 1970)

The management of malnutrition

Marasmus

Problems
1. infection
2. dehydration
3. anaemia
4. anorexia

Treatment
1. resuscitation
2. rehabilitation
3. convalescence

Resuscitation

Infection

- pneumonia (chiefly pneumococcal)
- tuberculosis, NB Mantoux test will probably be negative
- intestinal parasites

The cause of the infection should be diagnosed and the appropriate therapy given.

Dehydration
As for acute gastro-enteritis (see page 31). Rate and quantity depending on the degree of dehydration. The nasogastric route is suitable except when shock is present.

However, a small blood transfusion (10 ml/kg/actual weight) often helps to initiate recovery.

Rehabilitation
This diet will be high in calorie and protein content. Under the age of 1 year this should be mixture of milk and cereal with a high protein high calorie powder (e.g. Casilan™ (Farley)) added. Later the diet should contain protein in the form of minced chicken, pulses and eggs.

Carbohydrates in the form of rice or wheat cereal will be added to this. The proportion of these ingredients should be:

cereals	6 parts
protein	4 parts
sugar	2 parts

As in kwashiorkor the calories should be given in the quantity of 420 kJ/kg/day and the protein content in the quantity of 3 g/kg/day.

In very sick infants, and all marasmic babies under the age of 1 year, feeds should be given 2-hourly and by the nasogastric route. This should control anorexia, and after 2 to 3 weeks the route should be changed from the nasogastric to bottle, spoon and cup.

The diet should be calculated as per expected weight rather than actual weight, e.g. a 6-month-old baby (birth weight 3 kg) weighing only 3 kg should have his diet calculated as if he weighed 6 kg. When calculating fluid requirement (e.g. assessing dehydration or blood transfusion) actual weight is used.

Convalescence

Progress should be measured by weekly weighing. Failure to respond to treatment:

- incorrectly calculated calorie intake
- insufficient food given by ancillary staff
- unsuspected congenital abnormality
- cross-infection in the ward (particularly salmonellosis)

Acute kwashiorkor

Problems

1. infection
2. dehydration
3. anorexia
4. derangement of metabolic processes

Treatment

1. resuscitation
2. rehabilitation
3. convalescence

Resuscitation

Infection

- septicaemia and meningitis
- urinary tract infection
- malaria
- intestinal parasites and small bowel, bacterial overgrowth

N.B. Treat all severe cases as septicaemia, if laboratory facilities are not available.

Infection should be controlled by the appropriate therapy.

Dehydration

Fluid should be given by the nasogastric route. Rate 180 ml/kg/day. However, blood transfusion should be given if the following conditions exist:

- severe infection
- severe anaemia
- as a source of nutrients if appetite is very poor.

Quantity of blood should be small — 10 ml/kg actual weight.

Rehabilitation

The aim is to control anorexia and derangement of metabolic processes by diet. In severe cases it is important to start with a low calorie/low protein diet — 336 kJ/kg/day including 3 g/protein/kg/day. Added to this should be magnesium 3 mg/kg/day, potassium 0.5 g/day and folic acid 5 mg/day. Oral iron should not be included in the diet until the convalescent period when the serum transferrin levels should be approaching normal levels. Feeds should be given hourly at first via the nasogastric route. After 5 days the calories should be increased to 420 kJ/kg/day and the protein content increased gradually until the level of at least 7 g/kg/day is reached. This level should be continued throughout the convalescent period. Feeds should be given every 2–3 hours after the first week and for some time at this rate.

Extra protein is given in the form of a high-protein powdered milk (e.g. Casilan) and boiled eggs.

Convalescence

The target should be a total weight gain of 2–4 kg in 10 weeks for a child weighing 10 kg at the commencement of treatment. Parents must be involved in all dietary treatment from the start.

Failure to respond:

- insufficient food intake
- undetected or untreated infection or infestation NB particularly tuberculosis
- unsuspected congenital or acquired heart disease.

The underweight child

This form of PEM is the commonest in any country. Typically there is a general loss of subcutaneous fat with some muscle wasting although not as severe as that found in marasmus. There is also growth retardation. Any age group from 1 year onwards may be involved, but it is commoner in the neglected group of children over the age of 5 years. Many treated cases of marasmus and kwashiorkor may proceed to this condition.

The obese child

An obese child is one whose weight is several centiles above his height and generally results from excessive energy intake over energy output. It is a form of malnutrition associated with an increase in affluence in the family and the country.

Artificially fed babies tend to obesity generally as a result of improperly prepared feeds. Some babies tend to slim spontaneously in late infancy. In many others obesity in infancy may persist to adulthood.

Some male adolescents slim spontaneously during the puberty spurt, despite excessive food intake. This is not so with female adolescents, who do not have the same growth spurt. Moderately obese children may lose weight with moderate food intake reduction. Gross obesity in childhood is very difficult to treat.

When confronted with an obese child, all pathological causes of obesity should be excluded. These generally comprise only one to two per cent of cases.

A very good dietary and family history should be taken. Time taken on the first interview and examination is very important. Most fat children are on the defensive and respond well if they feel a genuine interest is being taken in them. An optimistic outlook is important but no promises should be made. Rapport between child and physician is more important than in most illnesses.

Management of nutritional obesity
It is important to realize that complete reduction may not be possible, so aim at a loss of 500 g per week. Treatment of obesity is not possible unless the child is seen and weighed at regular intervals, by the same physician, of not more than two months.

There is no advantage in using 'special' diets. A well balanced diet is essential but quantity must be reduced to 4200—6300 kJ after the age of 5 years. Appetite must never be satisfied. Diet must never contain sweets, sugars or pastries. Brown bread is preferable to white bread, as it contains more fibre per equivalent weight.

Increase in energy output is important. This includes walking to school, cycling and swimming.

Follow-up at monthly intervals. At follow-ups take a 24-hour dietary recall before informing the child and parents of present weight. An obese child is not usually a happy child.

Vitamins

Vitamin A (retinol)

- Fat soluble
- Occurs in these foods in its activated form:
  - butter
  - eggs
  - fish (cod liver oil)
- A pigment, carotene, occurs in many fruit and vegetables, particularly paw paw and carrots. Carotene is converted into vitamin A in the lining of the small bowel.

Deficiency of vitamin A in children
Deficiency results in a change in shape of the epithelial surfaces of all parts of the body. The cells flatten and 'pile up'. This is noticeable in the throat and larynx, but much more seriously in the sclera of the eye. This condition is known as xerophthalmia.

Vitamin A deficiency is one of the accompaniments of cystic fibrosis and of PEM in areas where vitamin A sources are deficient.

Treatment
- Prevention — 700 μg daily
- Mild deficiency — 2000 μg daily for 10 days
- Severe deficiency with eye involvement — 35 000 μg i.v. stat followed by 1000 μg daily for 10 days

Toxicity
- Acute — vomiting and raised intracranial pressure
- Chronic — anorexia, failure to thrive, hepatomegaly and cirrhosis of the liver. Tender bony swelling with midshaft hyperostosis

Vitamin B complex

This is the name given to a number of water soluble vitamins. Only three are important to those dealing with children in developing countries:
- thiamine
- nicotinic acid, and
- riboflavine.

Thiamine

- The human body does not require large amounts of this vitamin.
- All animal and plant tissues have traces of the vitamin.
- The largest sources come from the seeds of plants. The greatest amounts occur in:
  - wheat
  - pulses
  - millet
- In animal tissues, pork has the highest quantity.
- In rice thiamine occurs in the husks, and weight for weight, contains only a quarter of the amount in wheat or pork.
- As the vitamin is water soluble, excessive boiling will remove it entirely from the food.

Deficiency of thiamine in children

The children at greatest risk are those whose sole diet is rice that has been polished and boiled for a long time. This vitamin is involved in the breakdown of carbohydrate. Deficiency causes the accumulation of a toxic substance (lactic acid) which damages the heart in young babies and the nervous system in older children and adults. This disease is known as beriberi and although now very rare in older children and adults, it is still quite common in infants in some parts of Asia. Acute heart failure develops with fluid in the lungs and this is called 'wet' beriberi.

Nicotinic acid

- Nicotinic acid occurs abundantly in the following:
  - beef, mutton, pork and fish
  - wheat, maize, millet, rice and sorghum
  - liver and kidney
- Less abundantly in the following foods:
  - pulses, oatmeal, nuts and fruit
- In very small amounts in the following foods:
  - eggs, milk, cheese, vegetables and fruit

Deficiency of nicotinic acid in children

Nicotinic acid is known as the 'pellagra-preventing' vitamin. Pellagra is a disease of obscure origin known as the disease of the three Ds, 'dermatitis, diarrhoea and dementia'. The dermatitis only occurs when the skin is exposed to sunlight. The disease is not common in children. Deficiency of nicotinic acid alone does not cause pellagra as other foods are also 'pellagra-preventing'.

Riboflavin

This vitamin occurs in reasonable quantities in the 'expensive foods': milk, eggs, cheese, liver and green vegetables.

Deficiency occurs in most types of PEM and causes only minor conditions such as angular stomatitis and cheilosis.

Vitamin C (ascorbic acid)

- This is a water soluble vitamin.
- Only a small quantity is required in the diet.
- It occurs abundantly in the following:
  - citrus fruits
  - green vegetables and
  - skin of potatoes.

Deficiency of vitamin C in children

Deficiency is now rare in children. Vitamin C is involved in maintaining the health of the connective tissue and also in uptake of iron in the red cells.

Deficiency causes scurvy, a bleeding disease due to increased fragility of capillaries. This results in widespread bleeding, particularly the gums, in the skin and beneath the periosteum of long bones, resulting in painful bones. The disease is now rare in children. In babies the painful limbs may appear to be paralysed.

Vitamin D (cholecalciferol)

- Vitamin D is fat soluble.
- Occurs in the following foods:
  - fish oils
  - margarine
  - cheese
  - eggs,
  - butter
  - milk

These sources are 'expensive foods' and very many children receive little or none from their diet. However, the precursors of the vitamin occur in the stratum granulosum of the skin. Through the action of ultraviolet light from the sun the precursors are converted into cholecalciferol (vitamin D).

Deficiency of vitamin D in children

Rickets is a disease of calcium and phosphorus metabolism resulting from a deficiency of one of the regulatory hormones 1,25-dihydroxycholecalciferol, the active component of vitamin D.

Most of the body's calcium and phosphate are in the bone and in children this is retained for skeletal growth. The child has to adapt calcium and phosphate absorption and reabsorption to the needs of skeletal growth despite alterations in diet. The level of ionized plasma calcium must also be maintained at a constant level for normal neuromuscular function. To control this Ca^+ and P^+ metabolism several regulatory hormones are required. The chief of these are:

1. parathyroid hormone
2. 1,25-dihydroxycholecalciferol

Parathyroid hormone (PTH)

This acts on specific cell membrane receptors linked to adenyl cyclose in kidney, bone and gut. This action sets up a reaction which transmits the stimulus within the cell

Action in the kidney

1. Calcium. PTH increases the reabsorption of calcium and raises the renal calcium threshold.
2. Phosphate. PTH decreases the reabsorption of phosphate and lowers the renal threshold of phosphate. This allows the same excretion of phosphate at a lower plasma concentration.
3. 1,25-dihydroxycholecalciferol (1,25-DHCC). PTH stimulates renal production of 1,25-DHCC from the plasma precursor 25-HCC (25-hydroxycholecalciferol).

Action on the bone

PTH increases bone resorption of calcium and both Ca^+ and P^+ may be released into the circulation. Increased mineralization is coupled to resorption resulting in excessive osteoid calcification and raised serum alkaline phosphatose.

Action on the gut

PTH acts on 1,25-DHCC to increase absorption of Ca and P from the gut.

PTH is produced in the four parathyroid glands and its secretion is controlled by the level of ionized calcium in the plasma. The constant level of plasma is controlled by a negative feedback.

1,25-Dihydroxycholecalciferol (1,25-DHCC)

This is the endocrine form of vitamin D and is transported to specific nucleus receptors in the cells of the gut and bones.

Action on the gut

The active transport of Ca and P is increased in the presence of the hormones.

Action on bone

Remineralization of uncalcified bone is carried out by 1,25-DHCC. It involves increased bone resorption and mineralization involving extracellular Ca and phosphate.

Control of 1,25-DHCC production

Vitamin D precursors in the skin are converted to cholecalciferol which then undergoes hydroxylation in the liver to 25-hydroxycholecalciferol. This then undergoes further hydroxylation in the kidney where the enzyme 1-α-hydroxylase converts this to 1,25-dihydroxycholecalciferol. (See Figure 3.7.) Homeostasis of this process is controlled in the short term by levels of calcium, phosphate, PTH, and 1,25-DHCC (negative feed-back), and in the long term by growth hormone, prolactin, and sex hormones.

Rickets

The main source of vitamin D is in the skin and has to be activated by the action of ultraviolet light (UVL). Melanin in the skin protects the child from over-production of cholecalciferol when the sources of UVL are strong. Should a heavily pigmented child be removed from the source of UVL during the growing period of life, he will develop rickets. Many black children and children of Moslem parents are kept away from sunlight often for the first year of life. Children in industrial areas in temperate climates often do not get sufficient sunlight to produce sufficient cholecalciferol despite the lack of protective pigment. These children will also get rickets. Sufficient vitamin D can be added to the diet but foods rich in vitamin D, such as cow's milk, butter, eggs, cheese and fish are expensive.

Rickets may be present at birth, but this is not nutritional in the accepted sense.

Skeletal rickets

1. Early signs (from birth to one year)
   • Skull — the skull is thinned due to large unossified areas and feels like a ping-pong ball, indenting to finger pressure and then springing back to normal shape. This is called craniotabes. However, it may even be present in normal infants.
   • Long bones — widening occurs at the epiphyses (where growing cartilage joins preformed bones — the area of osteoid tissue) in the wrist and knees, widening is due to excessive pro-

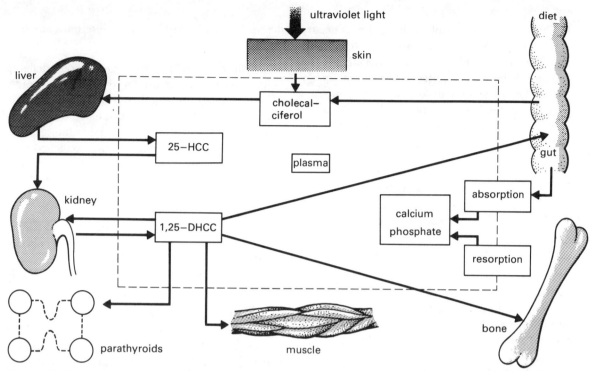

Figure 3.7 The metabolism of Vitamin D as described in the text

duction of osteoid tissue. In the ankle it is felt as doubling of the medial maleolus. This also occurs at the costochondrial junction of the ribs. This latter forms 'beading' of the ribs and is called a 'Rickety Rosary'. (See Figures 3.8 and 3.9)

2. Later signs (one year onwards)
   - Skull — there is delay in closure of the sutures (after 18 months this is abnormal). 'Bossing' of the skull due to calcification of excessive osteoid tissue. This condition, together with widening of the sutures, may be mistaken for the skull of a child with sickle cell disease or thalassaemia. It may even be mistaken for hydrocephalus.
   - Dentition is delayed, but many normal children have no teeth at one year.
   - Rib cage — the bones are soft and the commonest defect in most developing countries results in a transverse depression across the lower rib cage (at the level of the attachment of the diaphragm). It is caused by the pull of the diaphragmatic muscle on the soft rib cage. This is known as 'Harrison's sulcus'.

   The child may also have a 'pigeon' chest or a funnel chest, but rickets is not the only cause of these conditions.

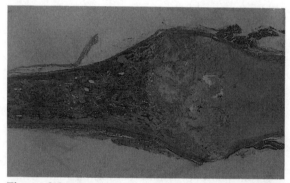

Figure 3.8 A histological section of the costochondrial junction of the rib of a small baby with rickets, the swelling of the junction is caused by proliferation of the osteoid tissue

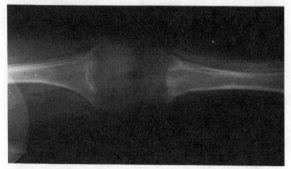

Figure 3.9 An X-ray of the wrist of a child with florid active rickets

- Limbs — deformities of the lower limbs occur when the child starts to walk and are due to weight or muscle acting on softened bones. The soft bones of the femur and tibia 'bow' and the ankles may disappear altogether, resulting in the child walking on the lower ends of his tibia. Bowing may also be seen occasionally in the forearms if the infant bears weight on upper limbs during crawling.

  Due to pressure on the ball and socket joint of the femur and pelvis, the pelvis is also deformed and becomes contracted.

- Later, the spinal vertebra may collapse due to softness and muscle pull, resulting in curvature of the spine, scoliosis, as well as kyphosis and lordosis.

In many Muslim countries these deformities do not occur because the child is generally exposed to sunlight after the age of 6 months and the rickets heal before the infants stand and bear weight.

Extra-skeletal signs of rickets
1. loss of muscle tone resulting in swollen abdomen and umbilical hernia
2. diarrhoea
3. pneumonia
4. tetany ('fits') due to low levels of calcium in the blood. (muscle spasm resembling fits)

Biochemistry of rickets
- serum calcium may be normal (Range 8.8–11 ml) or low (< 8 mg/100 ml). If low tetany will occur
- serum phosphorus may be normal (3.5–6 mg/100 ml)
- serum alkaline phosphotase is raised (> 25 KA units) — However raised values do occur in normal growing children
- serum 25-DHCC is low (< 10 ng/ml).

Treatment
Either:
1. 300 000 international units of vitamin D intramuscularly in one single dose, repeated in 2 weeks, or
2. 2000 international units orally daily for 1 month followed by 1000 international units orally daily for 3 months.

(The maintenance dose, which is also the normal dose for normal nutrition, is 400 international units daily.)

3. A synthetic product, 1α-hydroxycholecalciferol, has recently been produced which is rapidly hydroxylated in the liver to 1,25-dihydroxycholecalciferol thus overcoming the impaired action of 1-α-hydroxylase in the kidney. It also has the advantage of being rapidly removed from the system when therapy is discontinued. The dose for children under 20 kg is 0.05 g/kg/day.

Signs of response to treatment:

1. loss of pain in affected limbs in 2 to 3 weeks
2. swollen wrists, knees and ankles return to normal within 4 to 6 weeks (see Figure 3.10)
3. ossification lines of osteoid tissue visible in X-ray pictures present after 4 weeks

A child who is responding to treatment becomes more cheerful and lively within 2 to 3 weeks.

Some children with rickets do not appear to have restricted exposure to sunlight and it would seem that there is a rachitic factor in the diet which prevents the absorption of calcium and vitamin D. Flour prepared from high extract wheat may be a factor, and it is also possible that genetic factors may be involved resulting in low levels of serum 25-hydroxycholecalciferol.

Toxicity of vitamin D
Signs of this are anorexia, constipation, polydipsia, polyuria, failure to thrive, metastatic calcification and renal calcinosis.

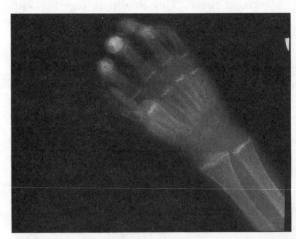

Figure 3.10 An X-ray of the wrist of a child with healing rickets, note the white dense area of calcification

Nutritional rehabilitation and re-education

Most cases of protein energy malnutrition occur in areas where food is in short supply, water is contaminated and there is gross overcrowding. The result of a famine situation following war, floods or other disasters is the production of refugees. Many of these cannot be helped and will die. Others will slowly improve with the help of feeding centres, medical aid, clean water and improvement in the health of the mothers, which will occur when famine relief arrives.

The problem

In many developing countries, there is a steady flow of severely malnourished children into out-patients and hospitals. Many of these result from ignorance of correct feeding practices and foods for their children. Knowledge of personal hygiene is poor and many do not connect dirty water with gastro-enteritis, the infection most likely to restart the vicious cycle of malnutrition. It is therefore useless to correct the nutrition of the child in hospital, improve his health and weight, and then send him back home to the same environment from which he will shortly return as malnourished as before.

The solution

This problem, which is largely one of education, has been tackled in many ways with varying results.

Education at hospital

Many hospitals in Africa and India have hostels for the mothers of sick children. These mothers help with the care of their children and see them get better under correct feeding and treatment in a relatively hygienic environment. They have faith in the nurses and doctors, relate the improvement of their child to the medical staff and, of course, blame them if the child dies.

Many hospitals run health and nutritional courses in the hospital for mothers who have time on their hands. These courses are run by senior nurses who may or may not have much enthusiasm for teaching. The mothers are often bored and cannot relate the teaching to their own problem. Sometimes the teaching is even carried out through an interpreter. I personally feel that this approach is of very little value.

Nutritional rehabilitation units

These units are based away from hospital and not connected with them. (See Figure 3.11.) Most of the mothers and children who attend come from the Polyclinic or Rural Health Clinic that is situated near the Rehabilitation Unit. Few are referred from the hospital. However, in Central Africa some hospitals set up their own units, situated outside the hospital compound and not staffed by the hospital's nurses, being a separate unit. These units are generally used as recovery shelters for children who have been treated in hospital. This is not really the function of a Nutritional Rehabilitation Unit.

The function of a Nutritional Rehabilitation Unit

The idea is to take a group of mothers, with moderately malnourished children, into a residential unit (Figure 3.12). The unit ideally is like a small village compound which is self-contained, with its own vegetable plot, possibly one or two cows and quarters for staff and mothers. The staff are trained in nutrition and general nursing but there is no doctor or white-coated worker in the area. In Uganda, in one such unit, a doctor visited once per week for minor complaints. The mothers are

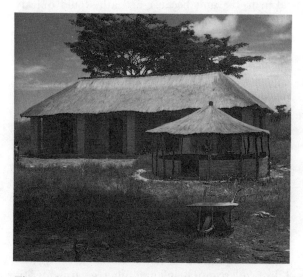

Figure 3.11 A small Nutritional Rehabilitation Unit in the Zambian Flying Doctors Service showing the cooking nsaka in the foreground and the residential hut incorporating a small lecture room in the background

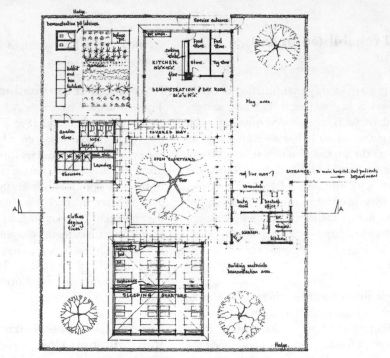

Figure 3.12 Plan of a custom-built residential unit which is self-contained with resident staff, this unit was to be situated near a village and away from hospital

instructed in housekeeping, hygiene and shopping in the nearby village. In this way their children gradually improved but the mothers realize that they, and not the hospital, are achieving this.

There have been many variations of this principle and it is one of the main stays of primary health care. It is very important that no very sick child is taken to the unit because a death would quickly bring the scheme to an end. It is hoped that the mothers, on returning home to their village, would set an example to others. However, this is a little idealistic due to the influence of grandmothers and village headmen. An attempt to overcome this in Uganda was made by choosing senior ladies from neighbouring villages to help in the care of the children.

Education through the television
Television is now almost universal in the urban areas of most developing countries (the Rehabilitation Units are difficult to organize in the urban areas) and many governments run health programmes daily on their main TV channels. This can be very effective and has been of great help in Libya with regard to infant feeding, gastro-enteritis and obesity. Often the doctors and nurses who appear on these programmes are well-known to many of the viewers because of the close community.

Conclusion

Many of the nutritional and infectious diseases problems in the Third World can be solved at very little cost but a great deal of energy and enthusiasm on the part of the protagonists of the various schemes. Government backing is essential. It has at last been recognized in many countries that health education is an essential part of the secondary school curriculum and this is a step forward for the future.

Further reading

Golden, M.H.N. (1988). The pathogenesis of the kwashiorkor syndrome. In: (eds R. Pounder and P. Chiodini) *Advances in Medicine*, **23**, Journal of the Royal College of Physicians of London.

Poskitt, E.M.E. (1988). *Practical Paediatric Nutrition*. Butterworths, Guildford.

Rao, K.V. and Singh, D. (1970). Metabolism in kwashiorkor. *American Journal of Clinical Nutrition*, **23**, 83.

WHO (1981). *The Treatment and Management of Severe Kwashiorkor*. WHO, Geneva.

WHO (1981). *WHO Code on the Marketing of Breast Milk Substitutes*. WHO, Geneva.

4

Fluids, Electrolytes and Dehydration

Water is for life, milk is for food and tea is for pleasure.

(Tuareg proverb, Sahel)

At birth, water constitutes about 80 per cent of body weight, and this decreases to 60 per cent during the first 2 years of life. Fluid balance during this time is always precarious partly because of the considerably increased fluid requirements of the infant in proportion to body weight and partly because of the relative immaturity of the kidney which cannot handle excessive solute (sodium) loads (Table 4.1).

Table 4.1 *Maintenance basal requirements at different ages*

Body weight		Daily fluid Requirement (ml/kg)
Newborn	3.5 kg	150
1 year	10 kg	100−120
	20 kg	80
	40 kg	60
Adult	65 kg	45

To maintain a steady state, water intake must balance physiological output in the form of:

- urinary loss = 50−100 ml/kg/day.
- faecal loss = 10 ml/kg/day.
- insensible losses (expired air, sweating, etc.) 400 ml/m^2/day.

Fluid and electrolyte losses are considerably increased during fever, gastro-enteritis and hypermetabolic states.

Maintenance of the body's fluid balance involves basically two mechanisms, namely water intake, regulated by the thirst centre of the hypothalamus and water reabsorption in the distal and collecting tubules of the kidney, regulated by the antidiuretic hormone (ADH). This in turn is dependent on adequate renal function which itself depends on an adequate renal blood flow.

Disturbances of fluid balance

Any significant change in body fluids is reflected as changes in circulating plasma volume. A decrease or increase of up to 5 per cent causes few symptoms or physical signs although there may be subtle changes in urinary output, but changes approaching 15 per cent in body fluid balance become life threatening. In practice overhydration is seldom a clinical problem, it is most likely to happen as a result of excessive, too rapid and uncontrolled or overzealous administration of intravenous fluids, or less often in situations associated with the inappropriate secretion of ADH, such as meningitis, encephalitis or traumatic head injury. The result is a decrease in osmolarity and electrolyte concentration, especially sodium. Clinically 'water overload' and generalized oedema may develop and there are profound effects on the central nervous system, causing cerebral oedema and convulsions, and the cardiovascular system leading to heart failure. Management of water overload primarily requires fluid restriction.

Dehydration is a state of negative fluid balance resulting from either decreased intake or, more commonly, from excessive losses. In infants and young children, by far the commonest causes are losses from the gastrointestinal tract through vomiting and diarrhoea, insensible losses due to fever or an increased respiratory rate, or in the urine. Anorexia accompanying many illnesses further reduces fluid intake and increases dehydration. Dehydration always causes significant electrolyte disturbances, most readily reflected in serum sodium status.

Assessment of dehydration

This is essential to plan treatment and fluid replacement and is based on the clinical assessment of the severity or degree of dehydration and accompanying electrolyte disturbance as reflected in serum sodium levels.

Severity of dehydration

Conventionally, dehydration is graded into mild, moderate or severe. These are based on weight loss and estimated as follows:

mild — less than 5 per cent body weight loss
— few or no physical signs

moderate — 5–10 per cent body weight loss
— signs of dehydration

severe — 10–15 per cent body weight loss
— signs of dehydration, peripheral circulatory failure and shock

The clinical signs of dehydration are given in Table 4.2.

This reflects a balanced loss of sodium and water and is the commonest form of dehydration seen in well nourished infants.

Hypotonic (Hyponatraemic)

Serum sodium is less than 130 mmol/l. This may follow correction of dehydration with fluids of low electrolyte content or if a young child is given only water to drink. Malnourished children with chronic salt depletion tend to get hypotonic dehydration and it is the commonest form of dehydration in countries where diarrhoeal disease is associated with malnutrition. Patients with bacilliary dysentery or cholera may have faecal sodium losses in excess of fluid losses.

Hypertonic (Hypernatraemic)

Serum sodium is more than 150 mmol/l. This is the least common but most serious form and occurs when fluid losses exceed sodium loss. Such situations may arise with high fevers or high environmental temperatures or hyperventilation. An

Table 4.2   *Clinical assessment of dehydration*

Sign	Mild	Moderate	Severe
Loss of skin turgor or elasticity	None or +	+ to ++	+++
Sunken eyes	None	+ to ++	+++
Depressed anterior fontanelle	None or +	++	+++
Thirst	+	++	+ or none
Dry mouth and teeth	None or slight	Dry	Very dry and parched
Mental changes	None	Restlessness	Restlessness
		Apathy	Total apathy, stupor or coma
Signs of peripheral circulatory failure and shock:			
• weak pulse and tachycardia	None	+	+++
• hypotension	None	None or +	++
• peripheral cyanosis and cold extremities	None	None	+++

Type of dehydration

Three types are recognized depending on the sodium status. The normal serum sodium level is between 130 and 145 mmol/l.

Isotonic (isonatraemic)

Serum sodium is between 130 and 145 mmol/l.

increased sodium intake from the use of high solute unmodified infant milk formulae, combined with fluid losses from fever or diarrhoea, is probably the commonest cause and is aggravated by the inability of the infant's kidney to handle a high sodium load. Other contributory causes include a high sodium content in the drinking water (in certain areas) or the use of replacement fluids containing electrolytes in excess of requirements.

Table 4.3 *Clinical assessment of type of dehydration*

Sign	Isotonic	Hypotonic	Hypertonic
Skin:			
Colour	Grey	Grey	Grey
Temperature	Cold	Cold	Cold or hot
Turgor	Decreased	Decreased/clammy	Thickened 'doughy'
Mucous membranes (mouth)	Dry	Clammy	Very dry and parched
Eyeballs	Soft and sunken	Sunken	Sunken
Anterior fontanelle	Sunken	Sunken	Sunken
Pulse	Rapid	Rapid	Moderate increase

Note: The signs are similar in isotonic and hypotonic dehydration but tend to be more severe in the hypotonic form.

Some of the physical signs associated with the different types of dehydration are summarized in Table 4.3.

Treatment of dehydration in acute diarrhoea

There are many ways of doing this, some are quite unnecessarily complicated. The following regime which is practical, easy and simple to follow, is recommended:

- estimate the degree and type of dehydration as above
- calculate the fluid deficit
- weigh the child — if a recent normal weight is known, this will help in giving a more accurate estimate of the fluid deficit.
- measure serum electrolytes.
- calculate the fluid requirements for the first 24 hours, based on:
  - replacing the estimated deficit
  - plus normal maintenance requirements
  - plus an allowance for ongoing abnormal losses

Example

An infant showing signs of severe dehydration weighs 9 kg on admission.

- estimated weight loss = 10 per cent
- true weight is therefore 10 kg
- deficit = 1 kg = 1000 ml
- maintenance fluids for next 24 hours = 10(kg) × 100(ml/kg) = 1000 ml
- total fluid requirements = deficit 1000 ml

plus maintenance = 1000 ml
= 2000 ml

- an extra allowance may have to be made if severe ongoing losses as diarrhoea or vomiting persist

Route of administration

All patients with mild dehydration and many with moderate degrees do well with oral rehydration therapy, even if there is a mild degree of vomiting. Give small amounts frequently by cup and spoon, or from a bottle. In some cases of moderate dehydration with anorexia and refusal to drink, it may be necessary to pass a nasogastric tube but care must be taken not to give too large a volume of fluid too quickly by this route.

All patients with severe dehydration, peripheral circulatory failure, severe matabolic electrolyte disturbance, paralytic ileus and persistent vomiting require intravenous therapy. Patients with moderate dehydration whose condition fails to improve with oral rehydration or is deteriorating should be changed to intravenous fluids.

Choice and type of fluid

Oral rehydration

Intravenous therapy is expensive, can only be given in a hospital setting, carries a risk of serious complications and needs constant medical and nursing attention. Considering the magnitude of diarrhoeal disease in many countries and limited resources available, liberal intravenous therapy is a luxury which the countries where such disorders abound, can ill afford. Oral rehydration, on the other hand, is cheap, effective in most situations and can be used in a field as well as hospital setting. Every effort, therefore, must be made to manage patients on oral fluids.

The WHO oral rehydration salts (ORS) when reconstituted from the sachets supplied by UNICEF provide a satisfactory rehydration fluid. The composition of each sachet is:

NaCl	3.5 g
KCl	1.5 g
NaHCO$_3$	2.5 g
glucose	20.0 g

When dissolved in one litre of boiled, cooled water, it provides Na$^+$ 90 mmol/l, K$^+$ 20 mmol/l and bicarbonate 30 mmol/l, i.e., approximately equivalent to slightly more than half normal saline. The sodium content of ORS needs to be reduced therefore, in areas where the drinking water has a high sodium content.

A home-made preparation can be made by adding a level teaspoonful of salt and a level tablespoonful of sugar to 500 ml of cooled boiled water. This, of course, contains no potassium or bicarbonate.

Intravenous fluids

A bewildering variety of intravenous fluids exists, but therapy can be kept simple using normal (0.9 per cent) saline and 5 per cent dextrose in various combinations, and adding potassium chloride and sodium bicarbonate 8.4 per cent or one-sixth molar lactate as required.

All patients in shock and with peripheral circulatory failure need to be given plasma initially (or a plasma expander such as dextran or gelatin e.g Haemaccel^{TM} at a rate of 20 ml/kg over the first 2 hours, or until the circulation improves. (If plasma, or a substitute is unavailable, then normal saline has to be used.)

In severe dehydration normal saline or Darrow's solution, both of which contain 150 mmol/l of sodium, should be given only for the first 2 hours, otherwise excessive sodium retention and oedema may develop. After the first 2 hours further rehydration and maintenance should be continued with either 0.18 per cent saline in 4.3 per cent of dextrose or one-third normal saline in 5 per cent dextrose. Dextrose has a double function, firstly in providing calories, and secondly in facilitating the sodium pump in the assimilation and utilization of sodium.

Rate of fluid administration

Mild dehydration
Give half the calculated amount over the first 8 hours and the remainder spread evenly over the next 16 hours.

Moderate dehydration
If the child is not vomiting, give oral fluids at a rate of 20 ml/kg for the first hour or two and then continue as for mild dehydration. If the child is vomiting, proceed as for mild dehydration giving small amounts of fluid at frequent intervals.

Severe dehydration
Give one-third requirements (deficit plus maintenance) in first 6 hours. Give one-third over next 6 hours (7–12 hours). Give one-third over remaining 12 hours (13–24 hours).

An alternative regime is to give half over first 8 hours, and half over remaining 16 hours.

An exception to these rules is hypenatraemic dehydration where the deficit must be corrected more slowly to avoid the risk of cerebral oedema (see below for details of management).

Babies
An approximate guide to the fluid requirements for babies less than 10 kg in weight is as follows:

- average requirements for normal child = 120 ml/kg/day orally
- mild dehydration (less than 5 per cent weight loss) = 150 ml/kg/day orally
- moderate dehydration (5–10 per cent weight loss) = 200 ml/kg/day orally
- severe dehydration (10–15 per cent weight loss) = 250 ml/kg/day intravenously

Follow-up

Continual assessment of the state of hydration and further losses, together with a review of fluid requirements, is necessary every few hours for successful management. It is important not only to treat dehydration effectively, but equally important not to overhydrate the patient.

If diarrhoea continues after 24 hours, the child must be reassessed, serum electrolytes repeated and fluid requirements calculated for the next 24 hours.

Breast feeding should be continued immediately the child stops vomiting. It is important that some of the fluid in the second day, if possible, should be milk as the child now needs the extra calories and protein especially if there is already evidence of malnutrition.

Correction of electrolyte disturbances

This must be done concurrently with rehydration. The major disturbances are due to an excessive loss of base and potassium in diarrhoeal fluid resulting in a metabolic acidosis and hypokalaemia. Details of management are given below under the appropriate electrolyte disturbance.

Hypernatraemic dehydration

Clinically there may be relatively few signs of dehydration, and the skin feels firm or like dough, or even hard and scleremic due to intracellular dehydration. Rehydration must be carried out slowly to avoid the complications of cerebral oedema and convulsions, giving between two-thirds and three-quarters of the calculated fluid requirements in the first 24 hours. Serum sodium should not be allowed to fall by more than 10 mmol/l in the first 24 hours and it is advisable to correct the deficit over 48 hours.

If the child is in shock, this should be corrected in the usual way using plasma 20 ml/kg over the first 2 hours, then returning to the slower rate. In hypertonic dehydration, correction of the potassium deficit and acidosis is more urgent than in other types of dehydration and early administration of both potassium and bicarbonate may be necessary. Some patients may also be hyperglycaemic and if so 2.5 per cent dextrose solutions should be used. Convulsions may be controlled with phenobarbitone or diazepam. In very severe cases (sodium > 165 mmol/l) peritoneal dialysis with glucose solution may be tried.

Electrolyte disturbances

Sodium

Sodium is the main cation of the extracellular fluid and is the principal solute that maintains extracellular fluid volume. The kidney plays a major role in maintaining sodium balance although in early infancy the limited concentrating capacity of the kidney restricts its ability to excrete a large sodium load and readily results in the development of hypernatraemia.

Hyponatraemia (serum sodium less than 130 mmol/l)

The main causes are:
1. *Low intake* (uncommon).
2. Increased *urinary losses* (urinary sodium greater than 20 mmol/l) due to diuretic excess, mineralocorticoid deficiency and adrenal insufficiency, osmotic diuresis (glycerol, urea, mannitol) or salt losing nephritis.
3. *Non-renal losses* (urinary sodium less than 20 mmol/l) such as in diarrhoea or vomiting.
4. Dilutional *hyponatraemia*, occurring in any condition leading to abnormal fluid retention, such as congestive heart failure, nephrotic syndrome, and syndrome of inappropriate antidiuretic hormone secretion, seen in disorders of the CNS such as meningitis, encephalitis and following trauma. Serum sodium is also artifactually lowered in hyperglycaemia by producing an osmotic gradient and drawing water from within the cells into the extracellular fluid. Mild degrees of hyponatraemia cause few symptoms until the serum sodium falls below 120 mmol/l when convulsions may occur. Other symptoms include weakness, hypotension and peripheral circulatory failure. It is essential to distinguish between dilutional hyponatramia and that due to excessive loss of salt. Dilutional hyponatraemia must be treated by rigorous restriction of water intake to about 50 per cent to 60 per cent of normal intake until normal serum sodium levels are restored. Symptomatic hyponatraemia is treated by giving normal saline and in extreme cases 3 per cent sodium chloride may be given. A dose of 12 ml/kg of 3 per cent sodium chloride will raise serum sodium by about 10 mmol/l; it should be raised slowly at a rate not exceeding 5 – 10 mmol/l over about 4 hours.

Hypernatraemia

Serum sodium levels of over 150 mmol/l occur as part of hypertonic dehydration (see hypernatraemic dehydration) or from salt poisoning. The infant kidney is unable to handle excessive sodium loads, partly because of the relatively low GFR in the infant kidney, and partly because of immature tubular function; as a result the maximum osmolality achieved after fluid deprivation is lower in infancy as compared with older children. High serum sodium levels cause a shift of water from intracellular fluid into the extracellular compartment, causing cellular dehydration. Brain cells are especially sensitive to these changes, and with serum sodium levels over 160 mmol/l not only is mortality very high, with coma, convulsions and cerebral thrombosis, but permanent brain damage is a common sequel in survivors. Hyperglycaemia occurs in some patients. For details of treatment, see hypernatraemic dehydration. Sodium retention also occurs in renal failure, or due to the effects on renal function of disorders such as congestive heart failure, and is secondary to increased aldosterone production. This results in sodium retention and potassium depletion. Sodium retention leads to extracellular fluid retention and oedema, reflected in a rapid increase in body weight. Serum sodium levels are, however, usually normal because of the concomitant fluid retention. Central venous pressure monitoring is a sensitive index of cardiac response to sodium overload.

Potassium

Potassium is the main intracellular cation, and only a small fraction of total body potassium is present in the extracellular compartment. The intracellular concentration of potassium is 150 mmol/l; in extracellular fluids it is between 4 and 5 mmol/l. Disturbances of potassium therefore have profound effects on body function at cellular level.

The main source of potassium is the diet and the principal loss is through the urine. Requirements during the growing years of early life are relatively large, 2 to 3 mmol/kg/day in infancy. Potassium balance is regulated by the kidney, and unlike sodium, it can handle potassium without difficulty. Glomerular function, unless severely compromised, does not affect potassium and regulation is mainly at tubular level. In the proximal tubule potassium absorption is virtually complete, and in the distal and collecting tubules it is actively secreted under control by aldosterone. At intestinal level, potassium is exchanged for sodium in the colon.

Hypokalaemia

Hypokalaemia occurs when serum levels are less

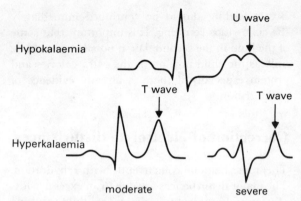

Figure 4.1 ECG changes in hypokalaemia and hyperkalaemia

than 3.5 mmol/l. In general a fall of 1 mmol/l reflects a loss of between 5 per cent and 10 per cent of body potassium. A urinary potassium of less than 10 mmol/l indicates severe potassium depletion. Causes of hypokalaemia include chronic starvation; diarrhoea; vomiting; prolonged diuretic therapy; diabetic ketoacidosis; endocrine disturbances such as Cushing's disease and hyperaldosteronism, and renal tubular acidosis.

Hypokalaemia produces a marked effect on muscle function, reflected clinically in muscle weakness, cramps, flaccid paralysis and paralytic ileus. The effects on cardiac muscle are seen in the ECG changes which show a decrease in T wave voltage, appearance of U waves, ST segment changes and prolonged QT interval, followed by arrhythmias (see Figure 4.1). Chronic potassium depletion also impairs the concentrating ability of the kidneys.

Management
Potassium supplements should be given when the serum potassium falls below 3.5 mmol/l; orally as either potassium chloride solution 0.25−0.5 g (3.5−7.0 mmol) 6-hourly or fresh fruit juice, and continued for several days. If serum potassium is very low, less than 2.5 mmol/l, potassium should be given intravenously, adding not more than 20 mmol to a 500 ml bottle of intravenous fluid (maximum 40 mmol/l). Potassium chloride 1 g is approximately equivalent to 13 mmol. Potassium should not normally be added to rehydrating fluids until the child has begun to pass urine, and should never be given as a bolus injection.

Hyperkalaemia

Hyperkalaemia occurs when serum potassium exceeds 5.5 mmol/l, and is generally the result of impaired renal function; less often it is due to decreased aldosterone production as in congenital adrenal hyperplasia and adrenal insufficiency. It is rarely caused by an increased intake.

Clinically, it leads to confusion, muscular weakness, paraesthesias and ascending paralysis; in profound hyperkalaemia ventricular fibrillation may cause death. ECG changes include tall tented T waves, widening of the QRS complex, an increased PR interval and depressed ST segment (see Figure 4.1).

Management
Conservative management in the form of restricted intake is sufficient when serum levels are below 6.5 mmol/l. With levels of 7.5 mmol/l or above, active management is necessary. Measures include:

- Administration of 10 per cent *calcium gluconate* 0.2 to 0.5 ml/kg intravenously, slowly under ECG monitoring.
- *Sodium bicarbonate* 1 to 2 ml/kg of 8.4 per cent solution intravenously, given slowly over 5– 10 minutes and dextrose with insulin – 10 or 20 per cent dextrose to provide 0.5 g/kg with 0.3 units soluble insulin per gram of glucose. The solution is infused over 2 hours. Care is needed in small infants, who may become hypoglycaemic.
- *Cation exchange resin.* This can be given as a 10 per cent oral suspension or a 15 per cent retention enema, retained for 30 to 60 minutes and then evacuated with normal saline. Treatment with 1.0 g/kg of resin should lower serum potassium by about 1 mEq/l, and can be repeated every 1 to 3 hours.
- If the above measures fail to reduce or control hyperkalaemia, then *peritoneal dialysis* should be carried out.

Magnesium

This metabolically important cation is a constituent of body enzymes including ATPase. Normal serum levels are between 1.5 and 1.8 mmol/l. Magnesium is absorbed mainly in the upper gastrointestinal tract. Vitamin D, parathormone and sodium absorption increase magnesium absorption, while increased intestinal motility, calcium and phosphate decrease absorption.

Hypomagnesaemia occurs when serum levels fall below 1 mmol/l. The most common causes are disturbances of nutrition including protein-energy malnutrition, long-term parenteral nutrition, malabsorption states and diabetic ketoacidosis. It is also seen occasionally in newborn infants. Clinical features resemble those of hypocalcaemia, with tetany and convulsions. Treatment is by giving magnesium sulphate 50 per cent solution, 0.1– 0.2 ml/kg slowly intravenously every 12 hours, for up to 48 hours. In neonatal transient hypomagnesaemia, one injection is usually sufficient.

Acid-base balance

Several mechanisms interact to maintain a constant body pH, namely the body buffers, the gaseous exchanges, in the lungs and the release of CO_2 from bicarbonate, and the kidneys. Haemoglobin is the major buffer of blood, plasma proteins are involved to a lesser extent and proteins also act as intracellular buffers. Bicarbonate and phosphate have an important role in plasma, interstitial fluid and intracellular fluids.

Lactic acid, pyruvic acid, inorganic and other non-volatile acids are to a large extent buffered by cations, mainly sodium (Na^+) which is retained in the proximal tubule by exchange for hydrogen ion (H^+). Some exchange also occurs in the distal tubule. Acidification of the urine thus helps to conserve cations.

Metabolic acidosis
The commonest cause is excessive loss of base in diarrhoeal fluid. Other important causes are an excessive production of hydrogen ions as in diabetic ketoacidosis or decreased excretion as in renal failure and renal tubular acidosis and in salicylate poisoning. Severe acidosis is characterized clinically by deep rapid respiration (Kussmaul breathing), though this is not always seen in infants under 3 months of age even when severely acidotic. Peripheral circulatory failure and pulmonary oedema may also occur.

Management
Mild to moderate degrees of acidosis require no specific treatment other than rehydration and correction of other electrolyte imbalances, leaving the kidney to make the necessary adjustments.

Severe acidosis (bicarbonate $\leqslant 10 \, \text{mol/l}$) or with Kussmaul respiration requires correction with sodium bicarbonate, calculated as:

dose of $NaHCO_3$ (mmol) = base deficit $\times$ 0.4 $\times$ body weight (kg)
1 ml 8.4% $NaHCO_3$ = 1 mmol

Half of the dose can be given slowly as an infusion with normal saline or 5 per cent dextrose over the first hour, and the remainder infused slowly over the next few hours. Sodium bicarbonate should never be given as a rapid bolus injection. In clinically severe acidosis, when facilities for monitoring electrolytes are not available a dose of 1 mmol/kg body weight should be given.

Metabolic alkalosis

Results from excessive loss of chloride due to vomiting (hypochloraemic alkalosis), excessive bicarbonate administration or from excessive renal absorption of bicarbonate in potassium depletion and primary hyperaldosteronism. Urinary chloride is low (less than 10 mmol/l) in hypochloraemic alkalosis, and is high (over 20 mmol/l) in potassium depletion due to hyperaldosteronism. Paradoxical aciduria with systemic alkalosis is associated with potassium depletion. Patients present with slow and shallow breathing and may develop tetany.

Management

Management consists of correcting the underlying cause. If alkalosis is severe enough to interfere with vital functions it may be corrected by giving ammonium chloride as a 2 per cent solution in the following dose:

NH_4Cl (mmol) = bicarbonate excess $\times$ 0.2 $\times$ wt (kg)
1 ml 20% NH_4Cl solution = 4 mmol

Potassium losses should also be corrected.

5

Infectious Diseases

Infectious diseases are the commonest causes of death and debility in childhood. There is a vicious circle in relation to infectious diseases and malnutrition. The two conditions work together to the detriment of the child's health, particularly those under the age of 5 years.

The commonest acute diseases are described in this chapter, but the two, slowly developing diseases, tuberculosis and leprosy, are discussed in a separate chapter as they have features not present in most acute infectious diseases. Their development is slow but their convalescence after treatment is slower.

Measles

Measles is a highly infectious disease caused by an RNS virus similar to the para-influenzal group. The virus may invade every system in the body, but the respiratory tract and the skin are the most commonly affected.

Mode of spread

This is by droplet infection and the respiratory tract is the system most commonly invaded but infection may be introduced via the conjunctiva. After initial involvement a viraemia develops and every system, including the central nervous system, will become infected.

Incubation period

This is from 12 to 24 days.

Prodromal signs and symptoms

For 4 to 6 days after infection the child will have a persistent fever, nasal catarrh, bronchitis and photophobia. (See Figure 5.1.) At the end of this period an extensive rash may be seen on the inside of the mouth and cheek. It consists of fine white spots, on an inflamed mucous membrane. The rash is the internal rash of measles and the spots are

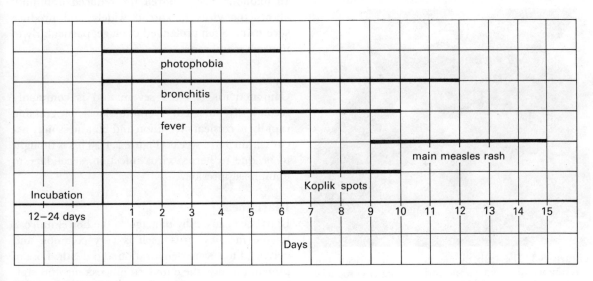

Figure 5.1 Development of measles

known as Koplik spots. It may be present through-out the whole gastrointestinal tract and last about 2 to 4 days.

Clinical course

After the prodromal period the main rash of measles appears. This is the external rash which starts behind the ears and consists of small, dull, raised (can be felt) red spots (Figure 5.2). This rash spreads all over the trunk and limbs often joining together to form large, velvety red areas. At the same time the eyes become inflamed and the child complains of the light. After about 5 days the external rash fades and the skin peels (Figure 5.3).

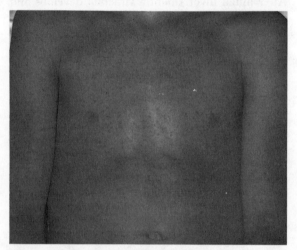

Figure 5.2 The rash of early measles in an English boy

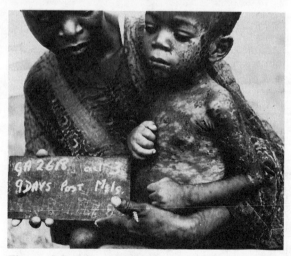

Figure 5.3 The rash of measles in an African boy showing its raised nature and early scaling (Reproduced courtesy of Prof. David Morley)

In light skinned children a brown stain remains where the rash was for 7 more days. The eyes clear up at the same time as the rash and the cough may last another 2 to 3 weeks.

Diagnosis

During the late prodromal period the virus may be isolated from the blood, nasal discharge, conjunctival secretions and urine. After the main rash has been present for 2 to 4 days the virus becomes very difficult to isolate. Neutralizing antibodies develop during the disease. Two samples of blood must be taken, one in the early stages and the second 2 weeks later. A rising titre is diagnostic. In subacute sclerosing panencephalitis a very high titre is present several years after the initial infection. Antibodies are also present in the central nervous system.

Differential diagnosis

Atypical measles may occur in children who have been immunized and this may resemble rubella. Infective mononucleosis rash resembles measles but there is an absence of catarrhal symptoms. This is also the case with other enteroviruses with the exception of respiratory syncitial virus with bronchiolitis.

Complications

In malnourished children the reduced immunity allows the virus to spread widely and produce severe and often prolonged damage, particularly to mucous membranes.

Eyes
Conjunctivitis is often severe and is commonly secondarily infected. Keratomalacia progressing rapidly to corneal ulceration and blindness may occur within 3 to 4 weeks (Figure 5.4). This is thought to be due to herpes virus infection, secondary to immunosuppresion.

Diarrhoea
Diarrhoea caused by damage to the bowel mucosa by the measles virus itself is very common and may lead to severe dehydration and death. Loss of protein through the damaged mucosa may precipitate kwashiorkor.

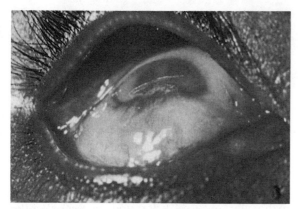

Figure 5.4 The eye of a malnourished three-year-old child with 'phthisis bulbae' resulting from keratomalacia. It resulted from an untreated conjunctivitis in measles, affecting a malnourished boy with Vitamin A deficiency and developed within three weeks of the onset of measles

Respiratory tract
A cough is a normal accompaniment of measles and in some cases may resemble whooping cough.

Upper respiratory tract
Inflammation of the larynx may be severe resulting in inspiratory stridor (croup) and is a very serious and difficult problem to manage. Without expert nursing, sudden respiratory obstruction and death may occur.

Lower respiratory tract
Pneumonia caused by the virus alone may be seen early on in the illness. A secondary bacterial pneumonia is more common and may occur any time from a week to 2 to 3 weeks after the onset of the illness. Rupture of alveoli, probably due to the severe cough and dehydration, may cause air to escape into the lung (causing cysts), the mediastinum (pneumomediastinum) or pleura (pneumothorax) and may track up the neck causing surgical emphysema.

Thrombocytopenic purpura
Thrombocytopenia may occur after the appearance of the measles rash producing 'haemorrhagic' measles.

Central nervous system
Convulsions in measles are relatively common, and these are pyrexial convulsions. Encephalomyelitis with high mortality and morbidity is rare and generally presents about 10–12 days after the rash appears. It may present with increasing drowsiness ending in coma, or with convulsions and neurological defects.

EEGs are not very helpful as the findings are abnormal in uncomplicated cases of measles.

A rare condition associated with the measles virus is known as subacute sclerosing panencephalitis. This is a progressive degenerative neurological disease which is invariably fatal. It may present in late childhood, many years after the initial attack of measles, which may be mild. It may be due to a reactivated virus that has lain dormant in the central nervous system but the exact aetiology is not known.

Prognosis

The prognosis is good in uncomplicated measles in a well-nourished child and mortality rate is under one per cent. In these cases the chief cause of death is measles encephalitis. In malnourished children the prognosis is not good and mortality rate can be as high as 50 per cent. The chief cause of death in these cases are from involvement of the respiratory tract.

Management

Conjunctivitis
1. keep clean, swabbing with clean water or saline
2. tetracycline or chloramphenicol eye ointment (tetracycline may be of value in areas endemic for trachoma)
3. vitamin A oral/i.m.

A close watch must be kept on the eyes for signs of ulceration. See vitamin A deficiency on page 22.

Diarrhoea
See section on rehydration page 31.

Respiratory tract
See section on respiratory tract page 105.

Nutrition
Many children will be malnourished, or marginally so, and with the devastating effect measles can have on nutrition close attention must be paid to maintaining an adequate diet (see section on convalescent kwashiorkor diet page 21).

Encephalitis

There is no specific therapy for this condition apart from general nursing care of the unconscious child. Steroid therapy has been tried without success.

Cancrum orus

Mouth hygiene in early measles is very important to prevent this condition developing. Once established, systemic penicillin may help but general toxaemia and death is common and rapid. Severe cases that survive need plastic surgery.

Prevention

Passive immunity

Children who are at risk from some debilitating disease such as diabetes or fibrocystic disease may be given hyperimmune gamma globulin during an epidemic. If given before measles has been contracted it will give protection for from 3 to 6 months. If given while the child is incubating the disease the child will develop a mild form of measles.

Active immunity

A child with measles ceases to be infectious about 7 days after the main rash appears.

Special notes

In severe malnutrition the measles virus may remain active for a much longer period than in a well-nourished child and an overwhelming viraemia will result in death. In borderline malnutrition measles may precipitate kwashiorkor. Measles is an immunosuppressant disease and may possibly reactivate a healed primary tuberculous complex, but for the same reason the Mantoux test will remain negative for 6 weeks after the attack of measles. A child with a nephrotic syndrome might go into remission after an attack of measles but they may also succumb to the disease.

Mumps

Mumps is an infection of the salivary glands — commonly the parotid glands — caused by a paramyxo virus. The virus gives transplacental immunity and so a mother who has had mumps protects her child from the disease for the first 6 months of life.

Incubation period

This is 8 to 37 days. Normal range 17—21 days.

Mode of spread

By droplet infection. Viraemia occurs and all organs may be infected but the parotid and other salivary glands are most commonly involved. Virus is shed in the saliva one week before and one week after the parotid swelling.

Clinical

1. Characterized by swollen and tender salivary glands. Swelling is caused by:
   - oedema
   - hyperaemia
   - acinar cell necrosis
   - swollen ductal glands
   - mononuclear cell necrosis

   The damage is probably the result of virus/antibody reaction.
2. Fever, vomiting and headache for one to two days.
3. The swollen glands may be bilateral or unilateral. Duration of swelling is variable but may peak by three to four days and then subside slowly by the end of the week.

Diagnosis

1. Look for swelling of Stenson or Wharton's duct.
2. Serum amylase may be raised (particularly if there is pancreatitis or epididimo-orchitis — see below).

Treatment

1. bed rest
2. fluids
3. oral hygiene

Complications

1. *Neurological*
   - meningitis
   - encephalitis

These may present without parotitis and may be associated with deafness, optic neuritis or diabetes insipidus. Prognosis is generally good. Virus may be isolated from the CSF.
2. *Epididimo-orchitis*. Generally occurs post-pubertal and often presents in an epidemic without parotitis. The condition is extremely painful and may require morphine. Does not generally cause sterility.
3. *Pancreatitis*. Generally occurs without parotitis, is mild and is often a biochemical diagnosis. (Serum amylase values very high.) Characterized by vague central abdominal pain during a mumps epidemic.
4. *Myocarditis*. Rare but prognosis is generally good.

Prevention

Immunization against mumps has not been generally considered necessary in the past but a measles/mumps/rubella (MMR) vaccine is now available. It is a live attenuated vaccine and given in one dose, 0.5 ml i.m. or s.c.

Rubella

Rubella is an infection caused by an arborvirus and infects children at any age after 6 months. If infected in early pregnancy, a mother may deliver a damaged baby (see intra-uterine infections).

Mode of spread

By droplet infection and occurs in epidemic and endemic spread.

Incubation period

This is from 14 to 21 days.

Clinical

1. *May be symptom and sign free*. Diagnosis made by serology.
2. *Adenopathy*. This will be generalized, starting in the sub-occipital area.
3. *Rash*. This may be in the form of a transient rash but generally is in the form of pink macules, starting on the face and spreading over the whole trunk. Duration is seldom more than three days.

4. *Conjunctivitis*. This is mild and lasts only one to two days.
5. *Fever* occasionally occurs but precedes the rash.
6. *Arthralgia*. This starts before the rash, simulates juvenile rheumatoid arthritis but is transient and seldom lasts more than a week, with no permanent damage.

Complications

1. *Thrombocytopenia purpura*. Prognosis is generally good.
2. *Encephalitis*. Probably an immunological response. Rare and generally not serious.

Prevention

Important in girls before the menarche, in order to prevent her developing the rubella syndrome in pregnancy.

It is a live attenuated vaccine and may be given singly or in combination with measles and mumps (MMR).

Infantum roseola

A fairly common infection between the age of 3 months and 2 years (highest incidence 3 to 6 months). The aetiology is unknown but is probably caused by a virus which has not been isolated.

Clinical

1. fever for 2 to 3 days
2. followed by rubella-type rash lasting 1 to 2 days
3. rash preceded by marked occipal and cervical adenitis
4. convulsions may occur but are rare

Treatment

Supportive — illness seldom lasts more than 3 to 4 days.

Pertussis (whooping cough)

Pertussis is a highly infectious disease, caused by the organism *Bordetella pertussis*, affecting the respiratory tract of infants and children.

There is no transplacental immunity, and infection may occur from birth. It is most serious with highest incidence of mortality under the age of 3 months. As with measles, the commonest age of infection is between 6 months and 2 years, the age when these children are most at risk from malnutrition.

Mode of spread

This is by droplet infection.

Incubation period

This is from 7 to 10 days.

Prodromal signs and symptoms

There are signs of upper respiratory tract infection with a runny discharge from the nose (coryzal phase). The discharge is clear, thick mucus. This stage lasts 7 days, during which period it is most infectious.

Clinical course

The infection spreads down the respiratory tract to the bronchioles and the exudate is thick and sticky. The child has a short, sharp cough to try to dislodge the mucus. Eventually he is forced to take a deep breath through a larynx which is closed in spasm. This results in the typical 'whoop' and is associated with vomiting which is serious in malnourished children. Even in fit children the whole episode is very exhausting. Spasms occur frequently and may be provoked by eating, emotion or may occur spontaneously. The cough may last from 4 to 6 weeks. The child is only slightly infectious during the first week of the whoop. Spasmodic coughing may go on for many months. This is largely due to habit. (See Figure 5.5.)

In infants under 3 months of age the clinical picture is different, and the main features are those of cough and spells of apnoea. Death is frequent during the apnoeic spells.

Diagnosis

This is generally made on clinical grounds. The organism collected by per nasal swabs can be isolated in experienced laboratories. Most children with whooping cough have a lymphocyte count over 20 000 per mm^3. The reason for this is not known, but it is helpful in diagnosis.

Differential diagnosis

In infants whooping cough can resemble the various enteroviral infections, particularly that caused by the respiratory syncitial virus. The chlamydial virus may also produce a syndrome in young infants resembling whooping cough. In older children the cough of fibrocystic disease is very similar and an inhaled foreign body in a small bronchiole may present a problem of diagnosis.

Complications

In malnourished children the persistent vomiting may lead to severe protein energy malnutrition.

Eyes
Rupture of small vessels in the sclera produce large

Weeks				
1 2	3 4 5 6 7 8	9 10 11 12	Up to three years	
Catarrh	Paroxysms	Convalescing	Recurrence of spasmodic cough after URT infection	

Nasal discharge

Cough +	++++		++++ +++ ++ ++ ++ ++	+ + + + +
		Paroxysms with vomiting		+ +

Cough plate +ve

High lymphocytosis

Figure 5.5 Development of whooping cough in children over six months of age

42

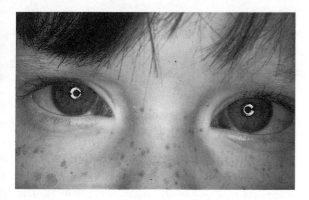

Figure 5.6 Ecchymoses in the sclera of a child with whooping cough

ecchymoses (Figure 5.6). These are not serious and require no treatment.

Brain and brain stem

Occasionally persistent coughing may cause small vessels to rupture, resulting in neurological damage including hemiplegia. Rarely, encephalitis occurs about 10 days after the onset of the illness as in measles.

Lungs

Rupture of alveoli may occur during bouts of coughing resulting in pneumothorax and pneumomediastinum (Figure 5.7). In the latter case, air may pass up into the tissues around the neck, causing surgical emphysema. A severe pneumonia may occur a week to 10 days after the onset of the coughing. This is due to secondary bacterial infection. Bronchiectasis may occur later but is a very rare complication.

Intestinal tract

Increased intra-abdominal pressure during coughing may cause herniae and prolapse of the rectum. Occasionally there may be a breakdown of a healed primary tuberculous complex with the development of active tuberculosis.

Prognosis

Pertussis is a serious disease and mortality rate is high under the age of 3 months. Morbidity and mortality are high in the older malnourished child.

Management

The cough

Any baby under 3 months must be admitted to hospital and the cot kept near to the ward sister's station. Oxygen and suction must be readily available. The upper respiratory tract must be sucked out regularly. Apneoic spells, which are particularly common in infants under the age of 6 months, are managed by Ambu bagging and giving oxygen.

In older children there is no treatment for the cough but malnourished children must be re-fed after vomiting with a high calorie feed in which corn oil gives the calories and dried skimmed milk the protein. No cough medicine is effective.

Respiratory tract complications

See under section on respiratory tract page 105.

Intestinal tract

Herniae and prolapsed rectal mucosa may have to be treated surgically.

Eyes

Sub-conjunctival haemorrhages need no treatment.

Antibiotics and whooping cough

Bordetella pertussis is sensitive to chloramphenicol, erythromycin and co-trimoxazole. However, this is only so during the coryzal phase, which is a phase rarely seen by the doctor in developing countries. During the first 2 weeks of the whooping phase antibiotics may reduce the excretion of the bacillus without affecting the course of the illness. Therefore it is reasonable to give a 10-day course of one of the antibiotics to the infected child if there are babies in the home.

Prevention

Specific active immunization is given in a vaccine combined with diphtheria and tetanus (the triple antigen). The vaccine contains whole killed organisms. The schedule varies with countries but the initial dose should not be given later than 3 months of age.

A 10-day course of erythromycin and co-trimoxazole should also be given to the uninfected babies in families where older children have the disease.

Special notes

Like measles, whooping cough can be a severe problem in malnourished children.

Varicella (chicken-pox)

Varicella is a highly infectious disease, common in children of all ages including the neonatal period. It is caused by the varicella-zoster virus. The same virus causes herpes zoster (shingles). In an epidemic of varicella some children may develop herpes zoster.

Mode of spread

This is by droplet infection.

Incubation period

This is approximately 14 days.

Prodromal signs and symptoms

There is seldom severe systemic upset and the child usually presents with a fever, lasting 1—2 days.

Clinical course

The rash appears in crops, usually on the trunk, thighs and upper arms as well as the face, hair and mucous membrane of the mouth and throat. The 'spots' appear on the first day and spread rapidly. They start as a macule (raised inflamed area of the skin) form a papule which vesiculates (forms a blister) which encrusts forming a scab. Vesiculation occurs within a few hours of macule formation.

Fresh crops occur daily for the next 4 to 5 days. All scabs have fallen off by the end of 3 weeks. (See Figure 5.7.)

Diagnosis

This is made from the clinical picture but can be confirmed by isolating the virus from the vesicle.

Differential diagnosis

Before the eradication of smallpox the differential diagnosis was one of the most difficult in clinical medicine. Papular urticaria produces a similar rash, but there is no systemic upset. Follicles seldom appear in the hair or mouth, as in varicella.

Complications

Secondary infection of the lesions

The rash is extremely itchy and secondary staphylococcal or streptococcal infection occurs. This can cause isolated boils which when healed will leave scar formation. The lesions in the mouth form small superficial ulcers which heal quickly without problems.

Encephalitis

This is a rare complication which occurs about 8 days after the onset of the rash. It generally involves the cerebellum resulting in ataxia. The condition is generally benign with complete recovery.

Pneumonia

This is an extremely rare complication in childhood, although it does occur in malnourished children. The condition is severe and often fatal. It is probably the cause of death in children who develop varicella while on steroid therapy (see below). It

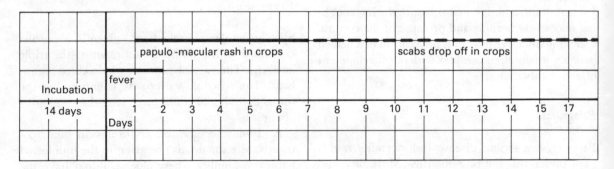

Figure 5.7 Development of varicella

takes the form of a bronchopneumonia and the chest X-ray resembles that of a case of miliary tuberculosis.

Prognosis

This is good in healthy children.

Management

There is no treatment for the disease, apart from symptomatic treatment of the rash. It is important to prevent the child from scratching the lesions. However, it must be stressed that varicella is a benign illness in most cases.

Prevention

There is no active immunization for varicella but children at risk may be given some passive immunity from hyperimmune gammaglobulin.

Special notes

Most children on long-term steroid therapy (e.g. the leukaemias) may succumb to a varicella infection. Some antiviral agents (not readily available in most developing countries) may help. Should a child be at risk during the outbreak of an epidemic, hyperimmune gammaglobulin can give some protection for a period of 6 weeks.

Streptococcal disease

The haemolytic *Streptococcus* is an organism which produces a great deal of debility in children in developing countries in areas where there is much overcrowding. The bacterium is associated with two serious diseases, rheumatic fever and acute glomerular nephritis. Infection seldom occurs before the age of 3 months, but after that age is common throughout childhood. There are many strains, some benign and others more serious, being associated with the two diseases mentioned above. Figure 5.8 summarizes the development of haemolytic streptococcus.

Mode of spread

Droplet through the throat, causing acute tonsilitis, or through abrasions in the skin, resulting in impetigo.

Incubation period

This is 2−3 days.

Prodromal signs and symptoms

There are few.

Clinical course

Acute sore throat
The bacteria at first infect the throat, and the onset of very high fever and debility is sudden, generally accompanied by enlarged and inflamed tonsils. The tonsillar glands in the neck may also be enlarged. There is often a white membrane, easily removed, on the tonsils and the tongue may be furred with red papillae showing through. With antibiotic treatment the fever and sore throat subsides within 48 hours and the child becomes well within 3 to 4 days. Without antibiotic treatment, abscesses may occur in the tonsils known as 'quinzy'

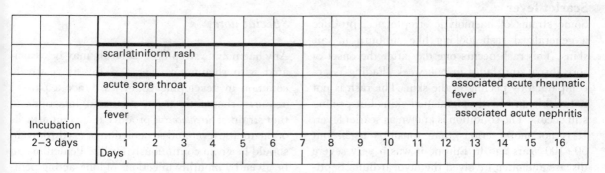

Figure 5.8 Development of haemolytic streptococcus

and these have to be opened to prevent upper respiratory obstruction. Quinzy may be due to a highly invasive *Streptococcus*.

Impetigo

Impetigo is a skin condition (see page 248) that is caused by *Streptococcus* or *Staphylococcus*. There is no constitutional upset as in the streptococcal sore throat, but it may be associated with acute nephritis. It is not associated with the scarlet fever rash.

Diagnosis

This can only be made by isolating the organisms from a throat swab or swab from the impetigo lesion. However the anti-streptolysin titre of antibodies is a help in diagnosis, provided blood samples are taken at the onset of the disease and 10 days later (in the convalescent period). A rising titre is diagnostic.

Differential diagnosis

Many virus infections produce severely inflamed tonsils and the tonsillar fauces but they do not generally produce a membrane. This is not so in infectious mononucleosis, however, where the clinical picture in the throat may be similar but there will be other signs of glandular fever, and the disease is not common in young children, as with haemolytic *Streptococcus*. Diptheria produces a membrane on the fauces but the throat does not look so red and the fever is low grade. However, the child is generally toxic.

Complications

Scarlet fever

Some strains of haemolytic streptococci produce a generalized rash looking like sunburn in fair skins. This rash occurs one day after the onset of sore throat and fades in one week. Fading is accompanied by peeling of the skin. The rash is not noticeable on heavily pigmented skins but peeling still occurs. The condition is known as scarlet fever. It is not more serious than tonsilitis itself, but 50–100 years ago in Europe it was a very severe disease and often involved the myocardium. Septicaemia was also common.

Rheumatic fever

Has a similar immunological association which affects the muscles, tendons, joints and heart of the host about 10 days to 3 weeks after the onset of the infection. This condition is known as rheumatic fever. There is no specific rheumatogenic strain so re-infection is common with further damage, particularly to the heart, from any strain of haemolytic *Streptococcus*. Rheumatic fever is dealt with in chapter on cardiology (see page 129).

Acute glomerulonephritis

These are specific strains of the haemolytic *Streptococcus* which produce immunological complexes that circulate in the blood stream and settle in the kidneys causing an acute glomerulonephritis, about 10 days after the initial infection. This strain is comparatively rare and re-infection with further damage to the kidney is very rare (see chapter on renal disease page 91).

Prognosis

This is good in the treated, uncomplicated case but the complications often have a poor prognosis.

Management

The haemolytic streptococcal infection responds satisfactorily to a full 10-day course of penicillin. Should the patient be sensitive to penicillin, then erythromycin is as effective. This treatment should be given to cases with impetigo as well as acute sore throat.

Prevention

In all cases that develop rheumatic fever prophylactic penicillin should be given for life (see below).

Special notes

Any haemolytic streptococcal strain may be associated with rheumatic fever and this is relatively common in developing countries. Once a patient acquires rheumatic fever, recurrent infections of that strain of *Streptococcus* produce recurrent attacks of rheumatic fever and so penicillin or erythromycin should be given continuously for life. Penicillin can be given by monthly injections of long-acting penicillin. Erythromycin would have to be taken by mouth. The strain of the bacteria associated with acute glomerular nephritis is relatively uncommon; long-term antibiotic treatment is not necessary and only the initial 10 day course of penicillin or erythromycin is required.

Diphtheria

Diphtheria is a disease caused by the bacteria called *Corynebacterium diphtheriae*. There are three strains:

1. gravis, producing serious disease;
2. intermedius, producing a less severe form of disease; and
3. mitis, which produces a mild form of disease.

The disease affects children of all ages, from 6 months to adulthood. The bacteria produces a tough membrane at the site of the infection. If this is in the throat and pharynx it may cause upper respiratory obstruction, which could result in death within the first week of the infection. During this period the tough membrane protects the bacterium which produces a toxin that enters the blood stream and causes damage to the heart muscle 10 to 14 days after the infection. The toxin takes a long time to invade the nervous system and this does not show itself until 5 to 7 weeks.

Involvement of the heart and nervous system is most likely to occur in gravis strain infections and least likely in mitis. All strains produce membrane. Figure 5.9 outlines the development of the disease.

Mode of spread

This may be either by droplet infection via the nasopharynx, or through an abrasion in the skin or through the conjunctiva.

Incubation period

This is from 2 to 7 days.

Prodromal signs and symptoms

The child may have a low grade fever for 2 to 3 days, but quite severe constitutional upset. Bradycardia may be present.

Clinical course

This depends on the site of infection:

1. *The nares* — presenting as a bloody nasal discharge.
2. *Tonsils* — slow mild onset over 2 to 3 days with slight fever, mild sore throat with very enlarged cervical glands. The child appears very much sicker than a child with streptococcal sore throat who will have, however, a much higher fever.
3. *Pharynx and larynx* — again presents with low grade fever but, as the membrane spreads, develops 'croup' with signs of upper respiratory obstruction.
4. *Skin* — presents as a chronic ulcer on the hand or leg which does not heal.
5. The *conjunctiva* may also be a site of membrane formation.

The infection from sites (1), (2) and (3) may produce upper respiratory tract obstruction, which can kill the child if it is not relieved.

All sites may produce toxin which may result in heart and nervous system damage.

Diagnosis

If diphtheria is suspected swabs should be taken from the lesion after removing some membrane.

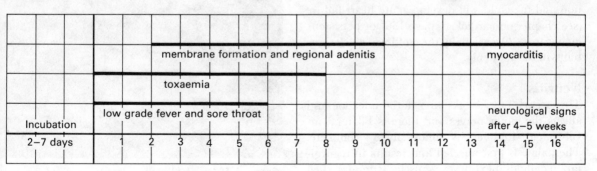

Figure 5.9 Development of diphtheria

This will confirm the diagnosis but treatment should be started before the result of the swab is known. In some areas children may present with neurological complications.

The Schick test
This test will show whether a person is susceptible to the diphtheria bacillus (i.e. one who has not previously been infected or immunized). It is an important test for those who have to nurse a child with diphtheria.

Susceptible persons should be immunized before caring for cases during an epidemic. In performing the test 0.1 ml of the toxin is given under the skin. A positive result is read 72 hours later and shows itself as a red area 10 mm across. A positive result means the person is susceptible to the germ.

Differential diagnosis
The discharging nostril may be mistaken for an infected foreign body. However, in diphtheria the discharge is bilateral and the child is very toxic. Infected impetigo around the nares may also present a problem. The throat lesion may resemble that of the haemolytic *Streptococcus*, infective mononucleosis and any viral sore throat, which could also present as croup. Swabs of the discharges should confirm the diagnosis.

The neurological complications (see below) may resemble acute poliomyelitis and bulbar palsy. The neurological lesion has bilateral involvement (unlike in poliomyelitis). The myocardial complication has to be differentiated from viral myocarditis and this is not always possible.

Complications (Toxin)

Myocarditis
This occurs approximately 2 weeks after the infection and the child will develop acute heart failure (see chapter on cardiology page 136) or persistent tachycardia. Occasionally the child will show signs but will die suddenly.

Neuritis
This occurs 3 to 7 weeks after initial infection and affects the motor nerves and there is bilateral involvement. Recovery is almost always complete. The palate is first affected and results in regurgitation of fluids, next the eye muscles (squints), then the diaphragm (with respiratory distress) and finally the upper and lower limbs. Often the initial infection is mild and unrecognized and the child presents with neurological complications. Bulbar palsy may occur.

Prognosis

Infants have a higher mortality rate than older children. The prognosis of those with gravis strain is worse than those with mitis. Prognosis is improved by early diagnosis and early recognition of the need for tracheostomy (Figure 5.10).

Management

Chemo- and immunotherapy

Chemotherapy
The bacillus is sensitive to penicillin and erythromycin and so the patient should have a 10-day course of either drug.

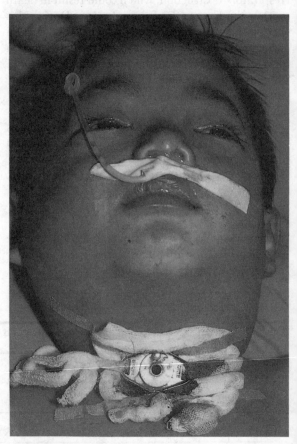

Figure 5.10 A child with a tracheostomy following laryngeal membranous diphtheria

Antitoxin

Dose of antitoxin depends on the site and extent of the membrane.

1. membrane not extending below the tonsil 20 000 units antitoxin i.m.
2. more extensive membrane spreading below the tonsil and causing respiratory obstruction 100 000 units i.v.

There is no need to give more than one dose.

Croup (laryngo-tracheo-bronchitis)

See section on upper respiratory obstruction page 113. Early tracheotomy may be life-saving.

Myocarditis

Diuretics if in heart failure (see section on heart failure page 127). N.B. The myocardium is extremely sensitive to digoxin and so half the recommended dose should be given.

Neuritis

This is self-limiting, although death can come from respiratory failure when respiratory muscles are involved and requires respiratory support until recovery is complete.

Prevention

Full immunization is needed to eliminate the disease. This has been successful in USA and Europe. The disease, for the same reason, is now becoming rare in those countries that have comprehensive immunization schedules (see section on immunization page 78). A patient with the carrier state is not affected by immuno-therapy but is generally cleared by a course of penicillin for 3 weeks.

Poliomyelitis

Poliomyelitis is one of the oldest recorded infectious diseases and case histories have been reported from the times of the Egyptian Pharoahs 3000 years ago.

It is a very common disease in developing countries, particularly in urban areas where hygiene is poor. The disease affects anterior horn cells of the spinal cord and brain stem nerves, resulting in irreversible paralysis and wasting of the muscles supplied by these. The cause is an RNA enterovirus. There are three main types of the virus but each types has many strains. Most epidemics are caused by type I.

The commonest age group to be affected is that under the age of 5 years, and most children at the age of 5 in any area where hygiene is poor may be infected asymptomatically. Five per cent of all cases occur from birth to 6 months. There may also be a genetic susceptibility to paralytic polio. More than 10 per cent of all cases under the age of 1 year are fatal as opposed to a mortality rate of 50 per cent over the age of 40.

Mode of spread

The virus may infect the child by droplet infection via the nasopharyngeal route but more commonly the spread is via the oral—faecal route emphasizing that the disease is one associated with poor hygiene. After entering the body the virus passes onto the regional lymph nodes. In the nasopharyngeal area the infectivity of the pharyngeal secretions disappears rapidly. However, in the regional lymph nodes of the intestinal wall there is continual excretion into the bowel for several months. The virus passes into the blood stream from the regional nodes and may pass into the central nervous system via the selective action of the blood—brain barrier but the exact passage to the anterior horn cells is not properly understood.

Passage of the virus along the neural pathways from the periphery to the central nervous system is not very likely.

Incubation period

This is between 7 and 21 days.

Prodromal signs and symptoms

After infection the child develops an illness with high fever, headache and sore throat. This lasts for about 2 to 4 days. This is followed by the development of stiff neck, photophobia and muscle pain in the limbs. This period lasts for a further 2 to 4 days. (See Figure 5.11)

Clinical course

The illness may present in one of the following ways:

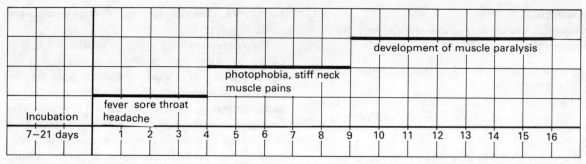

Figure 5.11 The development of poliomyelitis

1. sub-clinical
2. non-paralytic
3. paralytic

Sub-clinical

In sub-clinical attacks (by far the most common type of infection), the child does not even appear ill but develops antibodies to the infecting strain of virus, which protect him from that strain.

Non-paralytic

The prodromal signs and symptoms only are present and the patient is symptom-free about 10 days after this period, the illness resembling influenza.

Paralytic

This type of the illness, which is the most serious, commences as for the non-paralytic form, but after the second phase, instead of getting better the patient develops paralysis. The paralysis is generally unilateral, affects the large muscles more commonly than the small and the legs more commonly than the arms. There is no sensory loss, but paralysis affects large groups of muscles and the patient can retain reasonable function of the limbs after the convalescent phase but may be paralysed for life.

If the brain stem is affected, the muscles involved in swallowing and respiration (diaphragm and intercostal) are paralysed and the patient will die of respiratory failure if respiratory support is not available. Even if respiratory support apparatus is available the patient may have to spend the rest of his life in it. Bulbar palsy will require postural drainage and suction.

Infection from one strain of the virus gives lifelong immunity from that strain but no protection against other strains.

Diagnosis

The virus can be isolated and identified from throat swabs in the early stages of the illness and from the faeces several weeks after the onset. Isolation from the CSF is difficult. Tests for neutralizing antibodies and compliment fixation and serum should be taken at the onset of the illness and 2 weeks later to test for a significant rising titre.

Differential diagnosis

Non-paralytic polio cannot be differentiated from aseptic-meningitis on clinical grounds. Paralytic polio resembles paralytic episodes of other enteroviruses such as Coxsackie A and several ECHO viruses.

Other conditions causing unilateral paralysis such as acute polyneuritis, mumps and infective mononucleosis. It is very important therefore during an epidemic to confirm diagnosis by virus isolation or serological tests.

Prognosis

This depends on the muscle activity of the child before illness during an epidemic (the greater the activity the worse the prognosis). The use of provocation drugs, etc. (see below) during an epidemic will also worsen the prognosis.

Management

In the preparalytic stage bed rest is essential and analgesics should be given.

All cases of paralytic polio should be followed up. Improvement of use of the paralysed limb may continue until 2 years after the infection but complete recovery does not occur and the limb will be thinner than the normal one due to disuse atrophy.

Following up these cases prevents the development of contractural deformities by early splinting of the limb in the position of best use.

The use of crutches and surgical boots

Crutches (Figure 5.12) and boots can be made locally but the following guidelines should be observed:

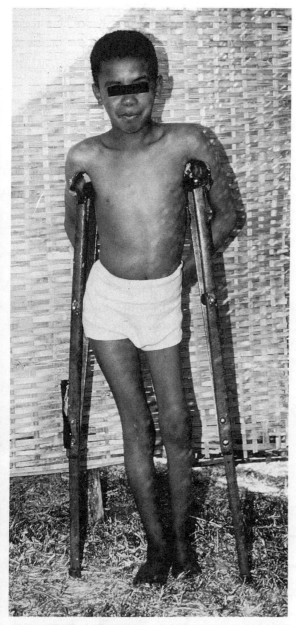

Figure 5.12 A child using crutches to aid walking, his left leg is the affected one

1. Children 4 years of age and under are too young for the fitting of boots and too weak for the use of crutches.
2. The child must be able to sit without support from his hands (back muscles).
3. Extensor muscles of one hip should be active so that the crutch can be swung forward.
4. The child can still walk with crutches if both hip extensors are paralysed but must have full power in both arms and trunk (see 2 above).
5. Crutches cannot be fitted if flexion deformities and contractures are present. Those have to be corrected first by surgery.

Prevention

Polio vaccination of an area must cover most of the people in the area and vaccination must be a continuous process (see section on immunization page 78). N.B. It is important to vaccinate polio victims as they will have protection from only one strain and successful immunization covers all or most strains of the virus.

Special notes

The following drugs and infections will increase by up to ten times the risk of a child developing poliomyelitis during an epidemic:

1. diphtheria/pertussis/tetanus vaccine
2. toxocara infections
3. penicillin injections
4. steroids
5. tonsillectomy
6. dapsone (for the treatment of leprosy)

Typhoid fever

Typhoid fever has a world-wide distribution but occurs most commonly in tropical and subtropical countries. The infecting organism is one of the species of bacteria known as *Salmonella*. Over 1000 strains of *Salmonella* have been discovered. Most of these are pathogenic to man and animals, with reservoirs in man and animals. *Salmonella typhi* (the organism causing typhoid fever) and paratyphoid A, B, and C are the only members of the species that are solely pathogenic to man although paratyphoid B may be pathogenic to cattle. The reservoir will therefore be only in man. Paratyphoid A,

B and C produce a mild form of typhoid fever and will not be discussed further.

Although the source of infection is a human carrier who is often symptom-free, the vehicle of the bacteria is food or water. Heavy doses are found in food and light doses in drink. The bacillus is excreted in the faeces or urine of the carrier.

Mode of spread

The bacillus passes into the stomach from the ingestion of food or water where small amounts are destroyed by the gastric acid. If the dose is large the bacteria pass into the small intestines where they invade the lining and enter the lymphatics via the Peyer's patches. Invasion may occur within minutes of infection. Here they multiply rapidly and pass into the blood stream and signs and symptoms of typhoid develop. Any organ of the body may be invaded.

Incubation period

This is between 7 and 14 days.

Prodromal signs and symptoms

The onset of the illness may be sudden with high fever, meningismus and even circulatory collapse. The condition resembles septicaemia. In small children diarrhoea and vomiting may be a feature in the prodromal phase. Bradycardia and constipation, a feature in the adult disease, is not common in children.

Clinical course

The fever may last for 2 to 3 weeks and a persistent dry cough occurs after the first week (Figure 5.13).

By the second week there is some abdominal tenderness and the spleen is always palpable and 'rose spots', a petechial-type rash resembling flea bites, occur in 20 per cent of all cases. They occur in crops on the trunk, do not itch and contain the typhoid bacillus.

Abdominal distension develops by the second week and the child looses weight, is listless and looks ill. The fever is present sometimes up to the fourth week, but in uncomplicated cases the fever falls by lysis and there is slow recovery. Relapses do occur, and most cases secrete the bacillus in the faeces for a further 3 months after recovery. These children are not carriers.

Diagnosis

Bacteriology
Blood culture may be positive in the early days of the infection. The organism remains in the blood for several days after the start of antibiotics. It is now recognized that the stool and urine cultures are positive within the first 10 days of infection.

Serology
The Widal reaction may be a help if taken early in the illness and the patient has not been immunized or does not live in an area where typhoid is common. The detection of rising titres of anti-O and anti-H agglutins are diagnostic. Elevation of titres fall to zero within 6 months of infection or TAB immunization.

Differential diagnosis
Typhoid fever must be distinguished from other *Salmonella* infections. Brucellosis, bacterial meningitis and even tuberculosis should also be suspected, but early blood culture and serial serology will confirm the diagnosis.

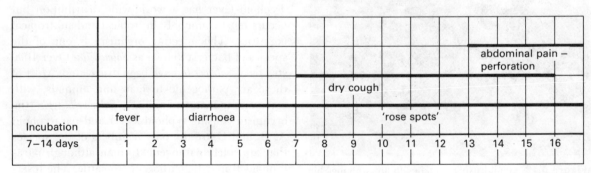

Figure 5.13 The development of typhoid fever

Complications

There are very many involving almost every system but they are rare if antibiotics are started early in the disease. In the early stages a toxic myocarditis is common but it clears up when the infection is controlled. Meningitis also occurs. Urinary tract infection is common.

The other common complications involve the gut and occur in the third and fourth weeks. They are intestinal haemorrhage and intestinal perforation, pneumonia, and erythema, which occur during the septicaemia stage, and osteitis late in the disease (Figure 5.14).

Prognosis

Before the introduction of chloramphenicol the mortality rate was quite high. Now it still remains around 1 per cent. Death generally occurs within

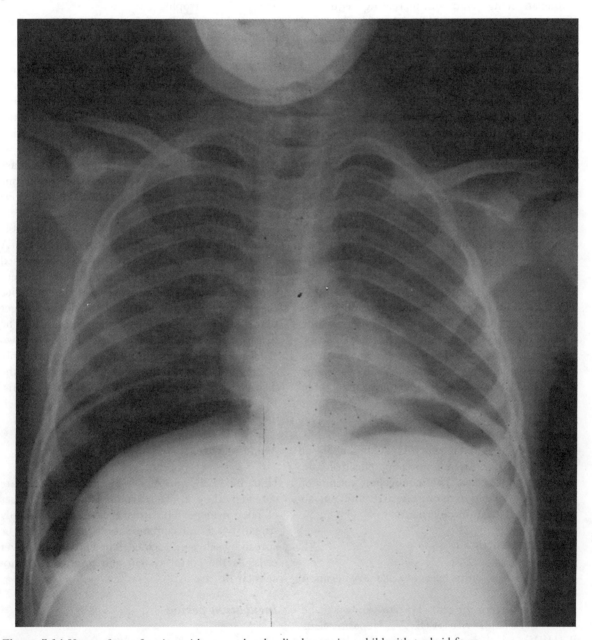

Figure 5.14 X-ray of a perforation with gas under the diaphragm in a child with typhoid fever

the first 48 hours often before a diagnosis has been made. Late deaths are generally due to perforation. Infants and young children are at greatest risk.

Management

Fluid replacement together with antibiotic therapy is the most effective treatment. Most patients are dehydrated due to high fever. The antibiotic of choice is chloramphenicol, although drug-resistant strains are being found with increasing frequency. Co-trimoxazole, amoxycillin and cefotaxime are alternatives. Antibiotics should be used in full doses for 14 days. Chloramphenicol should be tried first and the others used only if the patient fails to respond.

The typhoid bacillus lives in the gall-bladder of the carrier and is slowly excreted. Cholecystectomy may, but not always, produce elimination of the organism.

A four-week course of co-trimoxazole, two tablets twice a day, is sometimes successful in eradication. It is important to realize that all who have had typhoid fever may secrete the bacteria for up to 3 months after clinical cure. Carriers are only classed as such if they secrete for periods longer than this.

Prevention

This is a disease of poor hygiene and during an epidemic the source of the infection and possible carriers must be found before the outbreak can be controlled. Most cases have positive stools for at least 3 months after an attack. A carrier is one whose stools remain positive for more than three months.

Immunization

Vaccines such as TAB which has components of para A and para B are not very effective and extremely unpleasant. The monovalent vaccine of salmonella typhoid is more effective and not so unpleasant if given intradermally.

Viral hepatitis

The term viral hepatitis refers to a primary infection of the liver.

Five distinct viral agents are now known to be involved. Hepatitis virus A (HAV), Hepatitis virus B (HBV), which have been positively identified, and three non-identified agents which have characteristics distinct from virus A and virus B known as non-A, non-B and delta virus. When non-A and non-B have been positively identified, it is possible that they will be called virus C and virus D.

Hepatitis A has been recognized for at least a thousand years and has been known under many names such as infectious hepatitis, epidemic jaundice and acute catarrhal jaundice. Acute fulminating forms of the disease have been referred to as acute yellow atrophy.

Viral hepatitis B used to be known as serum hepatitis and was first recognized in 1883 as being related to the transfer by needle of an organism causing jaundice during a vaccination programme. Subsequently it was observed to occur during immunization programmes, VD clinics involving injections, and blood transfusion. Clinically the disease was seen to differ from infectious hepatitis by the length of its incubation period (90 days as opposed to from 30 to 40) and its frequent increase in severity. Like hepatitis A it has had numerous names including serum jaundice, homologous serum jaundice and post vaccinal jaundice.

In the middle of the 1970s, when it was possible to identify positively the viruses causing hepatitis A and B, it was found that hepatitis was also caused by unidentifiable agents immunologically different from those causing hepatitis A and B. The jaundice these agents caused had an incubation period longer than that of hepatitis A and shorter than B. The disease also was milder on average. There were two separate agents transmitting the disease, probably by the oral—faecal route as in hepatitis A and the diseases were known as non-A and non-B hepatitis. Recently another virus has been suspected, associated with HBV and known as delta virus.

Mode of spread

Hepatitis A, B, non-A, non-B and delta virus are spread by the oral—faecal route, and so are diseases of poor hygiene. Hepatitis B is more commonly spread by serum contamination and can also be spread by saliva and semen. The virus attacks liver cells via the portal system and produces hepatocellular disease.

Incubation period

This varies, depending on the virus. Hepatitis A

has an incubation period of between 15 and 40 days. Hepatitis B has an incubation period of up to 90 days and non-A and non-B between 40 and 60 days.

Prodromal signs and symptoms

Most children develop anorexia, constipation and abdominal pain over a period of 3 to 4 days. The urine is noted to be 'dark' and then the full clinical picture develops.

Clinical course

After the prodromal phase hepatomegaly is palpated and splenomegaly may also occur. After the passage of dark urine for 1 or 2 days many children regain their appetite and slowly improve over the next few days, without clinically visible jaundice. Others develop jaundice and this may last for several weeks or even months before regressing. These cases (with jaundice lasting 2 to 3 months) are not cases of chronic hepatitis. When the jaundice occurs the appetite generally returns. Recovery is generally complete. Hepatitis B virus has a similar clinical picture but the onset tends to be slow and insidious.

Diagnosis

Specific IgM antibodies to HAV occur early in the disease, but the virus has not yet been isolated. Diagnosis is then by exclusion. The disease generally occurs in the epidemic form. Sporadic cases are rare.

Liver function tests are used to assess the severity of the infection and to monitor the progress of the disease. The important tests are the transaminase, serum bilirubin and serum albumin. Transaminase values may return to normal after 2−3 months but generally remain raised for several months. Leucopenia generally occurs.

Associated with HBV are three antigens HBsAG (HB surface antigen or Australian antigen) produced by the surface of the virus, HBcAG (HB core antigen) from the core of the virus and HBeAG (HBe antigen). Antibodies are produced to all three. HBsAG is present in the serum of the infected person at the onset of the illness and may remain in the serum for years. The patient is then a carrier. HBcAg is not present in the serum of an infected person but is detected in the hepatocytes during an acute infection. HBeAg presence in the serum is transitory in the early stage of an infection, possibly for 2 to 3 weeks. Its persistence in the serum after this period is indicative of the patient progressing to chronic hepatitis.

A patient carrying the HBsAg is a potential source of spread of the disease, but, apart from Taiwan and some other Far Eastern countries, the carrier rate is only 1 per cent of the population. In Taiwan it may be as high as 15 per cent. In Libya it is between 3 and 4 per cent.

Expectant mothers who are carriers may well infect their babies, particularly at birth where the baby is covered by maternal blood, and mild trauma might transmit HBV infection, causing hepatitis or making the baby a carrier.

Differential diagnosis

A hepatitis may also occur during the course of infections caused by other viruses.

This hepatitis is caused by a secondary infection of the liver. The viruses are CMV, Epstein−Barr (associated with infectious mononucleosis), varicella/zoster, herpes simplex and rubella. Wilson's disease may also present as a hepatitis.

Complications

The most frequent complication in hepatitis A, B, non-A and non-B is fulminant hepatic failure and incipient hepatic failure may occur at any stage of the illness. Early signs of this development are persistent anorexia, deepening of jaundice and ascites. Shrinking of liver size with persistent jaundice is a bad sign.

Bone marrow aplasia, myocarditis and pancreatitis occur but are rare complications. Chronic acute hepatitis may occur, particularly after a hepatitis B infection.

Chronicity is difficult to define but any hepatitis of more than 6 months duration is thought to be chronic, but diagnosis should be made by needle biopsy. The persistence of the antigen in a case of hepatitis B is significant.

Prognosis

In 90 per cent of cases of hepatitis A the prognosis is good, but complications always make this worse. This is particularly so in hepatitis B.

Management

There is no specific treatment and no restriction to activity or diet. Sedatives and diuretics must be avoided. Chronic active hepatitis responds well to steroids which should not be given in any other case.

Prevention

Immunization is important, but unfortunately only passive immunity by way of immune serum globulin (ISG) is available for HAV infections. It contains anti-HAV, which has a half-life of 25 days. Protection up to 6 months may be obtained with double the normal dose.

Passive immunity is also available for protection from HBV. However, active immunization based on HBsAg is now available for HBV and this will give protection to those at high risk from HBV, the laboratory worker and others.

Tetanus

Tetanus is an infectious disease caused by a Gram-positive rod bacillus (*Clostridium tetani*) producing a powerful exotocin. This attacks the central nervous system (neurotoxic). The disease occurs in man and animals and has a world-wide distribution. There is a high mortality rate in areas where medical facilities are poor. This is particularly so in tropical and subtropical countries. Outside the host the bacillus forms a spore which protects it and allows it to remain viable in the soil and water for some time. It also may remain in the alimentary tract of herbivores for some time and so can be spread in the faeces.

Mode of spread

The portal of entry in the human is via deep contaminated wounds where there is poor oxygen availability. Under these conditions the bacillus multiplies and produces its exotoxin. In the case of the neonate the portal of entry is commonly the umbilicus (Figure 5.15), but may be in circumcision wounds or other minor surgery carried out in poor hygienic conditions. Occasionally entry is made via cautery burns during traditional medical therapy.

The toxin attacks the central nervous system either via the blood stream or along the axon cylinders of the peripheral motor nerves. It becomes fixed in the ganglion cells of the anterior horn of the spinal and cranial nerves and produces the motor stimulation resulting in the typical spasms of tetanus. Damage is not permanent, however, and the effects of the toxin wears off in 3 to 4 weeks.

Incubation period

This is between 7 and 10 days. Shorter periods do occur and these indicate a very poor prognosis.

Prodromal signs and symptoms

After the incubation period the child develops a fever and this is accompanied by muscle spasm, generally involving those muscles supplied by the cranial nerves.

Clinical course

Those muscles most commonly involved are the masseters resulting in facial spasm and the inability to open the mouth. The pharyngeal muscles may also be involved and this could result in asphyxia. The spasms only last for a few seconds, but they may recur frequently and spread down the whole body, chiefly involving the extensor muscles. This

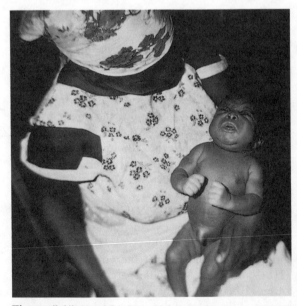

Figure 5.15 An eight-day-old baby with neonatal tetanus, the source of the infection was the umbilicus and the earliest sign was failure to suck — the baby survived

results often in opisthotonos, the more frequent the spasms the worse the prognosis. The muscle spasms are extremely painful. As the disease is self-limiting, the spasms become less frequent in 3 to 4 weeks. The mortality rate is high and is generally due to complications. Any outside stimulus may produce a spasm, and these should be kept to a minimum. However, a darkened room is not advisable as it may mask important physical signs such as cyanosis.

Diagnosis

This is on clinical grounds only. Once the condition is in mind diagnosis is not difficult. The presence of trismus (masseter spasm) and generalized spasm that is aggravated by external stimuli may be diagnostic.

Differential diagnosis

In older children and adults severe abdominal muscle spasm may be diagnostic but has to be differentiated from the acute abdomen. In modified cases the child may present with severe muscle cramps accompanied by very tender muscles. This may be thought to be some form of muscular rheumatism. The only differential diagnosis in the neo-natal period might be that of hypocalcaemic tetany. In neo-natal tetany there are long periods of remission (as compared with the steady progress of neo-natal tetanus), the feet and hands only are usually affected and the condition responds to the giving of calcium.

Complications

Respiratory complications
Death may occur in the first day or so from asphyxia, due to spasm of the larynx.

Pneumonia, probably as a result of aspiration of the contents of the stomach during a spasm, occurs quite commonly in neonates and may be fatal. Pneumonia may also occur in the third or fourth week of the illness, possibly as a result of general debility. This may also be fatal.

Cardiovascular complications
After about 10 days of severe spasms, hypertension develops and the child or infant may die of heart failure or a stroke.

Gastro-enteritis
This is a severe form and may be a cause of death. Its relationship to tetanus is obscure. Constipation and retention of urine are also quite common. Aspiration pneumonia and laryngeal spasm resulting in asphyxia are causes of death in the early part of the illness.

Renal complications
Children and infants have developed acute renal failure in about the third week. This probably is related to the development of hypertension.

Prognosis

This is not good in small babies and the shorter the incubation period the worse the prognosis.

Management

As the disease is self-limiting the principles of treatment are to keep the convulsions down to a minimum to prevent complications. The treatment of tetanus in most industrial countries is now in the hands of the anaesthetists. The patient is curarized and put on to artificial respiration until the disease has run its course. Complications still occur but the mortality rate has been reduced considerably.

When the diagnosis has been made, the source of the entry of the bacillus is sought. This is generally a deep contaminated wound. In the case of neonatal tetanus this is generally the umbilicus. This has to be cleaned extensively, and should be carried out under heavy sedation. Intravenous or intramuscular diazepam is the drug of choice. The bacillus is sensitive to penicillin and this together with 20 000 units of anti-toxin should be given at the same time. Penicillin should be continued for 10 days, but most people think that one dose of anti-toxin only should be given, and an even smaller dose, 10 000 units, is all that is necessary. While the child is still sedated a nasogastric tube should be passed into the stomach to aspirate the contents. The tube should be left in position, for future medication and feeding. Anti-toxin should be given intravenously.

It is very important that a spasm chart is kept accurately. Sedation is very important but over-sedation will kill. Most people try to contain the spasms to two to three per day. This is why a spasm chart is so important. The smaller the infant the more easy it is to oversedate.

Many drugs have been used and advocated, but it is probably best to use a short-acting one every 4 hours, and diazepam is probably the drug of choice. Chlorpromazine has been used but has many side effects and can cause hypothermia. Phenobarbitone has too long a half-life to be controllable. However, you have to use what is available. Diazepam may be given 4-hourly. Rectal paraldehyde may also be used.

Nutrition and hydration

In the worry to control the spasms it is often easy to forget nutrition and hydration. If possible fluid should not be given intravenously at any time, as overhydration is another cause of death. Fluid should be given by the nasogastric route. This route should also be used for nutrition. For the first 2 weeks at least food should be given in the form of milk mixed with corn oil.

In older children pain from muscle spasm may be a problem, and this can persist for some months after recovery. In the early stages pethidine can be very helpful, used alternately in therapy with diazepam. However, later this should be discontinued and soluble aspirin can be effective.

Prevention

Immunization for tetanus is covered in Chapter 8. Active immunization is important and passive immunization is achieved with human tetanus immunoglobulin. If a child has a deeply infected wound and the possibility of tetanus is considered, then a good surgical toilet together with an intramuscular injection of long-acting penicillin is the best form of prophylaxis.

It is important to realize that a child who recovers from an attack of tetanus is not immune from another attack and should immediately have a full course of active immunization.

Infectious mononucleosis

This is an infection caused by the Epstein–Barr virus. It is mainly a disease of children and young adults with low infectivity. Cases tend to be sporadic but epidemics in closed communities have been reported.

Mode of spread

Droplet infection via the nasopharyngeal route.

The virus multiplies in regional lymphoid tissue, and enters the blood stream this way, to most parts of the body.

Incubation period

This is between 4 and 21 days.

Prodromal signs and symptoms

The onset is gradual with malaise, fever and anorexia. Many cases have acute sore throat while others have only slight discomfort in the fauces area.

Clinical course

Fever may last for up to 3 weeks and can be quite high. The tonsils may become acutely inflamed and produce a membrane. Generalized lymphadenopathy occurs after the first week and may last for several months. Splenic enlargement occurs in 50 per cent of cases and hepatomegaly with jaundice may occur. A widespread papulomacular oedematous rash occurs in about 20 per cent of cases. In the majority of cases the disease subsides after about 3 to 4 weeks and most children have a fairly quick convalescent period unlike adults who may have a protracted convalescence.

Diagnosis

This is made on clinical grounds combined with haematological and serological changes.

Haematological changes

Atypical mononuclear cells appear in the peripheral blood film. These are large and vacuolated and have an irregular nucleus. A leucocytosis may also be present. In some cases (see complications) leucopenia occurs, but more seriously a profound thrombocytopenia is present. A transient antoimmune haemolytic anaemia may also be present.

Serological tests

By the second week of the illness agglutions to sheep red cells are present and can be detected by the Paul–Bunnel reaction. This is not, however, a specific test.

Agglutination of horse red cells also occurs and is the basis of the rapid 'monospot' slide test.

Specific EB IgM antibodies may be present, indicating a recent infection of the EB virus. EB IgM antibodies are of little value in diagnosis as they only indicate a past infection. There are therefore four major diagnostic criteria which must be present before a diagnosis is made:

1. clinical picture
2. typical changes in the peripheral blood
3. positive agglutination test
4. raised titre of EB IgM antibodies

Differential diagnosis

The disease is diagnosed too frequently, as it mimics most viral infections including measles. The early stages of typhoid fever may also be mistaken for glandular fever. Cytomegalic virus infection and toxoplasmosis may also present in a very similar manner. The diagnosis should not be made unless the case satisfies the four diagnostic criteria.

Complications

Neurological complications in the form of polyneuritis, transverse myelitis, cranial nerve palsies, aseptic meningitis and encephalomyelitis occur but are rare. A myocarditis may also develop. Haemolytic anaemia (auto-immune), thrombocytopenic purpura rupture of the spleen and orchitis have been reported. Hepatitis does occur but is not common.

Prognosis

This is generally good, and recovery in children is rapid. Death is rare but may occur from rupture of the spleen.

Management

There is no specific treatment so management is largely supportive. Steroids may help in thrombocytopenic purpura and severe neurological complications. They should not be used otherwise.

Prevention

There is no available preventive treatment.

Special notes

It has been found that some cases of infective mononucleosis, particularly those with a rash, react very severely to ampicillin and an anaphylactoid reaction may occur.

Intra-uterine infection

The fetus can acquire many infections in utero from the transplacental route but only the four commonest will be dealt with in this chapter:

1. rubella
2. toxoplasmosis
3. cytomegalic virus
4. congenital syphilis

All may cause damage to the fetus, depending on the stage of the pregnancy. The earlier the infection is acquired, the more likely the fetus is to be damaged. If the mother is infected in the first 2 to 3 months of pregnancy the fetus is 90 per cent sure of being infected, although the disease may be mild or even symptomless.

Rubella

Thanks to immunization of girls in the premenarche period, the rubella syndrome is now becoming rare.

Clinical
- low birth weight (due to placental insufficiency)
- cataract, microphthalmosia and hypoplasia of iris, glaucoma and retinopathy
- lymphadenopathy with splenomegaly
- deafness
- congenital heart disease
- hepatitis
- thrombocytopenia and haemolytic anaemia
- microcephaly

The severity of the syndrome depends on the stage of the pregnancy but it is possible for a fetus not to be affected. Multiple congenital abnormalities may be present or only one or two. The severity of the maternal infection is no indication of the outcome to the fetus.

Diagnosis
This depends upon the laboratory. Antibody tests for rubella are positive as soon as the rash appears in the mother. Rubella specific IgM remains positive for 2 months and is indicative of a recent infection.

Management

If a mother develops rubella (diagnosis confirmed by laboratory tests) in the first 3 months of pregnancy, this is an indication for abortion in many countries. It must be remembered, however, that it is possible that the fetus is not affected.

Prophylaxis

This is carried out by innoculating all girls in the premenarche period with the attenuated live virus. This practice is now widespread and the disease is becoming rare.

Toxoplasmosis

Severe disease *in utero* only occurs if the mother acquires the disease in the first 3 months of pregnancy.

Clinical

- low birth weight (due to prematurity)
- hepatosplenomegaly
- jaundice
- thrombocytopenia
- choroidoretinitis and microphthalmia
- intracranial calcification
- hydrocephaly and microcephaly
- epilepsy

Diagnosis

Serological diagnosis based on toxoplasmosis dye test. Specific toxoplasma IgM.

Treatment

1. exchange transfusion if hyperbilirubin severe
2. pyrimethamine 0.5 mg/kg/day for 2−3 weeks and sulphadiazine 150 mg/kg/day for 2−3 weeks.

Treatment can be prolonged for some weeks.

Cytomegalic virus

The cytomegalic virus (CMV) causes little damage to mature cells but can destroy fetal cells. It is secreted in the urine, breast milk and saliva.

Clinical

- low birth weight (placental insufficiency)
- hepatosplenomegaly
- jaundice
- thrombocytopenia
- choreoretinitis
- intracranial calcification
- microcephaly

Diagnosis

Virus isolated in urine or saliva. Specific IgM.

Treatment

If hyperbilirubinaemia present, exchange transfusion − little else.

Syphilis

This disease has been eradicated from many countries but is still present in others. Congenital syphilis is caused by a septicaemia of the spirochaete *Treponema pallidum*.

Signs and symptoms may present early or late. Late manifestations will not be dealt with here.

Clinical

Early manifestations:

- hepatosplenomegaly
- jaundice
- snuffles − mucopurulent rhinitis with later destruction of the nasal cartilage and bridge
- papulomacular skin eruptions, particularly on the soles of the feet.
- pemphigous
- alopecia
- condylomata
- mucocutaneous condylomata
- osteochondritis at end of long bones
- periostitis → painful → pseudoparalysis
- deformed teeth 'Hutchinson's teeth'

All the features occur within the first few months.

Diagnosis

Organisms isolated from infected organs and diagnosed by dark-ground illumination. Serological tests:

- Wasserman complement fixation
- VDRL flocculation
- FTA indirect immunofluorescent
- TPI immobilization test

Treatment

Drug of choice − benzathine penicillin, 100 000 units/kg/body weight. Three injections at weekly intervals.

AIDS

Acquired immunodeficiency disease was first recognized as a disease in 1981 when it predominantly affected homosexual men. The thymus dependent lymphocytes are chiefly involved (T cells). Death occurs from invasion of opportunist pathogens.

Aetiology

A retrovirus is responsible for the disease but this may not be the only factor. Inhabitants of Central Africa have a very high incidence of the disease and there may be a genetic predisposition in certain races or other infections common in this area may predispose people to infection with the AIDS virus.

The virus has been called the lymphadenopathy virus (LAV) and the human lymphotrophic virus type III (HTLV III). It is now known as human immunodeficiency virus (HIV). Tests have been devised for antibodies to HIV. The presence of antibodies indicates previous exposure to the virus but does not confer protection.

Mode of spread

The virus occurs in most body fluids but the disease is not very contagious. Infection is produced by either a large initial infecting dose or multiple exposure. Infection in adults may occur from the following:

- anal intercourse
- contaminated needles (especially common in drug addicts)
- sexual intercourse between bisexual males and their wives (the 'at risk' group of females)
- blood transfusion from the blood of infected donors

  Babies acquire the disease from the following:

- 'at risk' mothers
- drug addicted mothers
- promiscuous mothers in areas of high incidence of HIV
- blood transfusion (especially haemophiliac and leukaemia children)

Babies are infected *in utero* or during the birth process. Most babies are carriers but they may develop the disease and they may present with the stigmata of other intra-uterine infection.

Incubation period

This is long and may range from 2 to 3 months to over 5 years. Children who are HIV-positive (have anti-bodies to HIV) may not develop the disease and to date only between 5 and 10 per cent have been known to develop it.

Clinical course

The disease in older children at onset may be insidious. Early symptoms may be as follows:

- fatigue
- anorexia
- intermittent fever and night sweats
- persistent cough
- diarrhoea and weight loss

Early clinical signs may be as follows:

- generalized painless lymphadenopathy
- persistent candidiasis (oral and anal)
- lesions of Kaposi's sarcoma
- hepatosplenomegaly

  Later opportunistic infections may occur. The commonest are as follows:

- *Pneumocystis carinii*
- oral and systemic *Candida albicans*
- herpes simplex infection
- cytomegalic virus infection
- *Toxoplasma gondii* infection

Diagnosis

This is made by the clinical picture of an immune deficiency disease and the presence of antibodies to HIV in the serum.

Differential diagnosis

Any immune deficiency starts in childhood, particularly severe combined immunodeficiency (SCID), Wiskott—Aldrich syndrome, ataxia, telangiectasia, Di George syndrome and many viral infections that suppress cell-mediated immunity, such as measles.

Complications

Any opportunist infection will develop in a child with AIDS.

Prognosis

This is at present difficult to assess. To date, 8 years after the recognition of the disease only between 5 and 10 per cent of HIV antibody positive children develop the disease. All these children are obviously susceptible, but some trigger mechanism such as a severe systemic infection or severe malnutrition may be needed for the disease to develop.

Management

No live vaccines should be given to children with AIDS or who are HIV antibody positive.

As the disease is neurotropic, pertussis vaccine also must not be given. Killed polio virus immunization may be given intramuscularly, as may immunization for tetanus and diphtheria. Measles, rubella, mumps and influenza immunizations are from live attenuated viruses and should not be given.

A child with HIV antibody positive serum or with AIDS must be given intramuscular specific zoster immune globulin if exposed to varicella.

As yet there is no effective treatment. Opportunist infections should be treated vigorously in children at risk. The nutrition of children at risk must be maintained at a high level.

Fevers in children

Situations in which the response to infection is altered

The new-born infant
The infant cannot control his temperature well. If placed in a hot room he becomes febrile, and in a cold room he becomes chilled. His response to infection is very poor. The fever may be irregular. In severe infections it may even be subnormal.

The malnourished child (including marasmus and kwashiorkor)
The response to infection results in a normal or subnormal temperature. No rise in temperature is a bad prognostic sign. All cases of kwashiorkor should be suspected of having an infection.

Fever without physical signs

Malaria
If no response to anti-malarials in 48 hours, the fever must be due to some other cause.

Ear and throat infections
Fever may be high and associated with convulsions and delirium. N.B. Always look into the ears and throat of all febrile children.

Measles
In the prodromal stage, before the rash develops, look for Koplik spots.

Typhoid fever
The child is toxic and looks ill. He may have severe abdominal pain. Older children may also have severe headaches.

Urinary tract infection
Always suspect it, especially in girls. Always examine a fresh specimen of urine in the laboratory if possible, and if the laboratory is closed and a refrigerator is available, keep the specimen there until the laboratory is open.

Miliary tuberculosis
This often occurs in an infant or young child. The child will be feverish but may not appear very ill in the early stages. A cough is not a significant symptom.

Pyogenic meningitis
In toddlers and children under the age of 18 months, classical signs are often absent. Always carry out a lumbar puncture if in doubt.

Non-specific fevers
These are often due to virus infections and associated with upper respiratory tract infections, rashes and even diarrhoea.

Complications of fevers

'Febrile convulsions'
Usually occur at the onset of the fever and a lumbar puncture is generally necessary in any child under the age of two years to exclude meningitis.

Dehydration
Dehydration may develop and should be managed appropriately (see page 31).

Kwashiorkor
This develops rapidly if the child's nutritional state is poor at the onset of the illness. Fever depresses the appetite.

6

Tuberculosis and Leprosy

Childhood tuberculosis

Tuberculosis, caused by *Mycobacterium tuberculosis*, remains one of the ten leading causes of death in the world. The disease takes a heavy toll in childhood years, particularly in the developing world.

General considerations

Mycobacteria are obligate aerobes. The organism contains polysaccharide, lipid (which gives acid-fastness) and protein which is responsible for the delayed hypersensitivity in the host.

Antibodies play a minor role in host immunity. The bacterial antigens sensitize T-lymphocytes which produce lymphokines that stimulate the macrophages, thereby increasing intracellular killing of the tubercle bacilli. This is accompanied by a delayed type hypersensitivity skin reaction to tubercular protein. This reaction develops in 4 to 8 weeks following infection.

Epidemiology

Infants and children are infected by adults in the household or at school, sputum-positive adults carry the highest risk for them. A casual exposure is less likely to cause infection and repeated exposures in thickly populated areas is the usual cause of infection. Pulmonary disease is caused by droplet infection. Ingested tubercle bacilli may cause infection in the mouth, tonsil or in the intestines. Skin and conjunctiva may be infected by direct contact. Transplacental infection of the fetus is extremely uncommon.

Infants and adolescents tend to have more severe disease. Infections such as measles and whooping cough lower host immunity and predispose to severe disease. Malnutrition and diabetes also increase the risk of infection.

Pathology

A primary complex is a parenchymatous lesion along with involvement of draining lymphatics and regional lymph nodes. First contact with tubercle bacilli results in a primary complex. The lung is the most common site (Figure 6.1). The other sites of primary infection include the tonsil, the intestine and the skin.

Infection stimulates an inflammatory reaction in which the leukocytes are replaced by macrophages on the second day. These macrophages transform into elongated epitheloid cells which surround a central necrotic area of caseation. Multi-nucleated foreign body giant cells in the lesion complete the characteristic histological picture.

The lesion may completely resolve or heal by fibrosis or calcification. Primary lesions are more likely to calcify.

If the infecting dose is overwhelming or the host immunity compromised, (e.g., malnutrition, measles, whooping cough, diabetes, corticosteroid therapy) the lesion spreads (Figure 6.2). Progression of the parenchymal lesion gives rise to a progressive primary complex. The caseating material erodes into a bronchus causing a bronchogenic spread with pneumonia and cavitation. The lymph node may erode into a bronchus, blood vessel, adjoining pericardium or the oesophagus. An enlarged lymph node may compress a bronchus leading to collapse. (Figure 6.3)

When caseating material is discharged into a blood vessel it leads to haematogenous spread. This occurs early in the course of primary infection. The haematogenous spread may be minimal when the tubercle bacilli settle in various organs or massive when acute miliary tuberculosis results. Repeated disseminations also take place from the primary focus during the course of the disease. The apex of the lung, spleen, liver, superficial lymph nodes, kidney, bone and the central nervous system

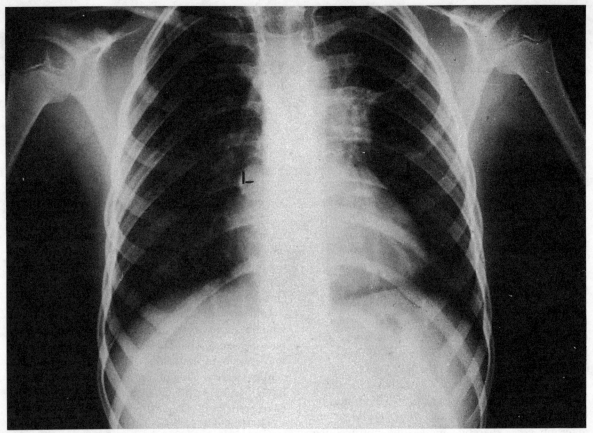

Figure 6.1 X-ray of a seven-year-old with a primary tubercular infection of the left lung, the enlarged hilar gland is well demonstrated

are some of the important sites of haematogenous spread.

Pleural infection may occur by direct spread from the lung or by the haematogenous route. Tuberculous pleurisy is uncommon below 6 years of age.

Clinical presentations

Primary complex

It may be totally asymptomatic and may only be detected on chest X-ray or by recent tuberculin conversion. Generally the symptoms are mild and non-specific. Irregular fever, failure to thrive and malaise are the usual features.

Progressive primary complex

When the parenchymal lesion causes an intense local inflammatory reaction, the child presents with toxaemia, fever, cough, night sweats, weight loss

and physical signs of consolidation.

Bronchial compression

It may lead to a collapse that may be asymptomatic. More commonly the patient presents with a brassy cough and a localized wheeze. Bronchiectasis may develop.

Acute miliary tuberculosis

This usually develops 3 to 6 months after infection and is more common in infants and young children. The onset may be acute or insidious. High fever, anorexia and weight loss are the usual presenting symptoms. There are often no respiratory symptoms in the early stages but progressive dyspnoea and cyanosis develop as the disease advances. Liver, spleen and lymph nodes are enlarged in the majority of cases. Meningeal involvement occurs in one-third of cases. Miliary tuberculosis may exist with a negative tuberculin test.

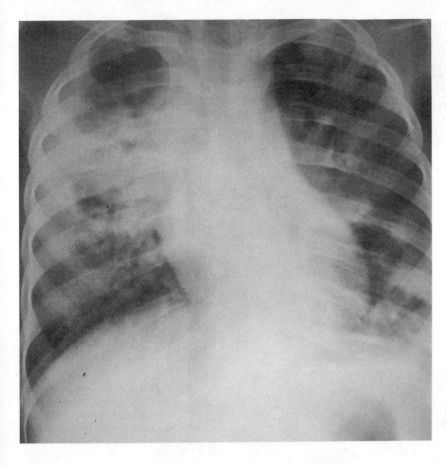

Figure 6.2 X-ray of a malnourished 12-year-old child with adult type tuberculosis. There is a tuberculous bronchopneumonia chiefly involving the right lung and a large cavitation in the right upper lobe

Pleurisy

Generally it develops insidiously and the symptoms are mild in the form of fever, cough, malaise and weight loss. It may start acutely with chest pain aggravated by deep inspiration and coughing. As fluid accumulates, respiratory embarrassment develops.

Chronic/reactivation tuberculosis

There is a high risk of chronic pulmonary tuberculosis developing with localized cavity formation in adolescents. It is more common if primary infection occurs in late childhood.

It presents with cough, fever, malaise, expectoration, haemoptysis and weight loss. Physical signs of cavitation may be present. These cases are generally sputum positive and are responsible for the spread.

Tuberculous lymphadenitis

Superficial lymph nodes are generally affected by haematogenous spread. Lymph nodes of the draining area are also involved as part of the primary complex if the primary lesion is in the skin, mouth or tonsil. Tuberculous lymphadenopathy is a complication of early haematogenous spread. The groups of glands involved frequently include the cervical, axillary and inguinal. The lymph nodes enlarge gradually, are painless and discrete at first, with progression of the disease, the glands become matted together and become adherent to the overlying skin and underlying tissues. If untreated the glands may soften and rupture resulting in chronic sinus formation. Tuberculous lymph nodes have to be differentiated from Hodgkin's disease.

Skeletal tuberculosis

This is another manifestation of early haematogenous spread. Clinical disease involving bones and joints generally starts within a year of the primary infection. The thoracic spine is the most common site of bone tuberculosis. Tuberculosis of the hip, the knee and small bones of hands and feet are other sites of infection.

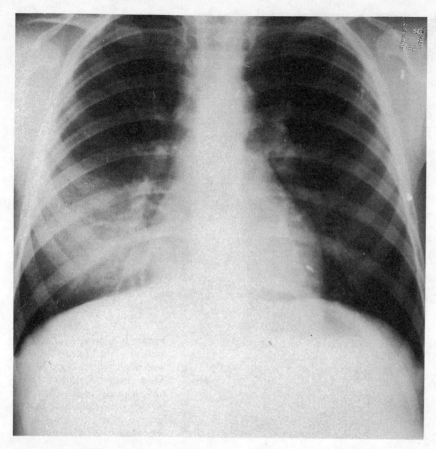

Figure 6.3 X-ray of a 10-year-old child with middle lobe collapse due to compression of the middle lobe bronchus by enlarged hilar glands

Most bone lesions are located in the metaphyseal end of the epiphysis because of the rich blood supply.

Spinal tuberculosis causes destruction of the vertebral body which collapses causing an angular kyphosis (gibbus). Cold abscess formation, radiculitis and cord compression are generally responsible for the symptoms. Severe pains, more commonly at night, referred pains due to irritation of nerve roots and compression paraplegia are some of the presenting features.

Skin tuberculosis

Skin disease more commonly follows direct contact and clinically presents as a localized chronic inflammatory lesion. Haematogenous infection causes multiple lesions.

A primary complex presents as a skin ulcer with painless swelling of the regional lymph glands. The most common form of skin lesion is the one that follows rupture of a tuberculous lymph node or a cold abscess. This form is known as scrofuloderma.

Miliary involvement of the skin presents with various forms of lesions including vesicles, pustules and umbilicated lesions.

Erythema nodosum

Tuberculosis is one of the most common causes of erythema nodosum (Figure 6.4). The lesions in the form of red papules are located over the shins and the forearms and are devoid of tubercle bacilli. These lesions represent a hypersensitivity reaction to tubercular proteins.

Abdominal tuberculosis

Involvement of the gastrointestinal tract may be in the form of a primary complex with ulcerative lesions in the small intestine and regional adenitis of the mesenteric glands. Intestinal ulceration may also occur due to swallowed infected material from a pulmonary lesion or as haematogenous spread to abdominal organs including the liver, spleen, kidney, lymph nodes and the peritoneum.

Peritonitis may be in the form of serous ascites or as a plastic, adhesive peritonitis adjacent to caseating mesenteric lymph nodes. The lymph nodes and

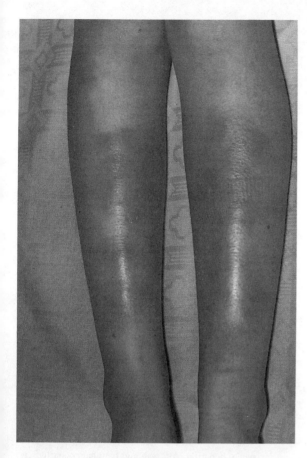

Figure 6.4 Erythema nodosum in a child with tuberculosis

the involved part of the peritoneum may present as an abdominal mass. The infected omentum may become rolled up into a transverse mass across the upper abdomen.

Diagnosis

In an endemic area any child presenting with failure to thrive, weight loss, anorexia, fatigue, chronic cough or fever of unknown cause should be suspected to have tuberculosis. A history of tuberculosis in a family contact is helpful.

Tuberculin test

This is one of the most useful aids in the diagnosis of primary tuberculosis. The test generally becomes positive in 4 to 8 weeks after infection. An induration of 10 mm or more constitutes a positive reaction. A mild hypersensitivity to tuberculin also follows successful BCG vaccination but the indu-

ration rarely exceeds 9 mm. A recent tuberculin conversion from negative to positive (irrespective of the size of induration) is definite evidence of recent infection.

The tuberculin test may be negative in the presence of active infection in the following conditions:

- patient receiving corticosteroids
- patient on immunosuppresant therapy
- presence of severe malnutrition
- acute miliary tuberculosis
- for 6 to 8 weeks following measles

Routine haematology
The total leukocyte count is generally raised with a lymphocytic response. The ESR is always high.

Radiology
X-ray of the chest must always be done in a suspected case of tuberculosis. Other radiological investigations depend upon the clinical presentation.

Isolation of the organism
Ziehl—Nielsen stained smears and cultures should always be done from the body fluids (gastric lavage, sputum, laryngeal or tracheal aspirate, pleural or ascitic fluid, CSF, etc.) in an effort to identify the tubercle bacillus.

Management

Chemotherapy is the mainstay of treatment. Several effective drugs are now available (Table 6.1). A single agent must never be used alone in the management of active disease. Two drugs are used in uncomplicated cases and three in severe forms of tuberculosis. Isoniazid (INH) and rifampicin is the ideal combination. However, rifampicin is too expensive for routine use in many developing countries where the disease is widespread and resources limited. A combination of INH and ethambutol has been found to be very effective and a satisfactory alternative. Thiacetazone should not be used in the management of childhood tuberculosis. Treatment schedules for various forms of tuberculosis are given in Table 6.2. Corticosteroids (prednisolone 1−2 mg/kg/day) as an adjunct are indicated in endobronchial tuberculosis, in tuberculous meningitis and miliary tuberculosis. It should be given for the initial 4 to 8 weeks only.

General supportive measures, and more import-

Table 6.1 *Anti-tuberculous drugs (first line)*

Drug	Dosage	Comments
Isoniazid (INH)	10–20 mg/kg/day orally Max: 500 mg/day	May cause peripheral neuropathy or hepatitis. Transient rise in liver enzymes may occur without significant hepatotoxicity. Pyridoxine supplementation 10 mg/100 mg INH given if daily INH dosage exceeds 300 mg. Effective penetration in CSF even without meningeal irritation.
Ethambutol	Initial: 25 mg/kg/day orally 1–2 months Thereafter: 15 mg/kg/day	Mild gastrointestinal symptoms; albuminuria. Reversible papillitis is a serious complication. Should be used with caution in young children.
Rifampicin	20 mg/kg/day orally Max: 600 mg/day	Stains body fluids red. May cause gastrointestinal symptoms, skin rash, rise in liver enzymes, hepatitis and reversible leukopenia.
Streptomycin	40 mg/kg/day i.m.	Resistance develops rapidly. It may cause permanent 8th nerve damage. It is not recommended for prolonged use. The only indication is tuberculous meningitis.
Para-aminosalicylic acid (PAS)	300 mg/kg/day orally	Delays bacterial resistance when combined with INH. May cause severe gastrointestinal symptoms, leukopenia, hepatitis, skin rash and lymphadenopathy. Now seldom used in management of childhood tuberculosis.

Note: PAS has to be given in 3–4 divided doses to minimize gastrointestinal side effects. All other drugs can be given as single daily dose.

antly nutritional care, are equally important for a good therapeutic response.

Prevention

Immunization with BCG provides partial protection. The main advantage of BCG lies in the fact that it minimizes the risk of disseminated disease even if the child develops a primary infection.

Detection and treatment of adults with tuberculosis constitutes the best means of disease control.

Chemoprophylaxis

Isoniazid in a dose of 10 mg/kg/day (max. 300 mg daily) is used for chemoprophylaxis in the following situations:

1. Household contacts of a patient. All tuberculin positive contacts are given 1 year's prophylaxis. The tuberculin negative contacts are given chemoprophylaxis for 3 months after which the tuberculin test is repeated, and if positive, treatment is continued for another 9 months.
2. Asymptomatic primary complex. Isoniazid is given for a period of 1 year.
3. Recent Mantoux conversion in a child up to 6 years.
4. When using corticosteroids or immunosuppressants in a tuberculin positive patient.
5. Newborn babies born to a sputum positive mother. The baby is treated with INH and given INH-resistant BCG (if available). Prophylaxis is continued for 3 to 6 months. If INH-resistant

Table 6.2 *Treatment schedule for various types of tuberculosis*

Type	Drugs recommended	Duration of therapy	Comments
Primary complex	Isoniazid and ethambutol or Isoniazid and rifampicin or Isoniazid and PAS	12 months	• INH is used in a dose of 10 mg/kg/day • Nine months therapy is adequate if rifampicin is used • Ethambutol should be used with caution in infants and small children under 2 years of age
Endobronchial tuberculosis	As above	12—18 months	
Pleural effusion	As above	As above	
Skeletal tuberculosis	INH, rifampicin and ethambutol/PAS	24 months	• Rifampicin is used for initial 6 months only • INH is given in dose of 20 mg/kg/day for the first three months and then reduced to 10 mg/kg/day
Miliary tuberculosis	As above	As above	
Tuberculous meningitis	As above or INH, streptomycin and ethambutol	As above	• Streptomycin is used in dose of 40 mg/kg/day i.m. for 1—3 months • INH is given in dose of 20 mg/kg/day for first 3 months and then reduced.

BCG is not available, INH is given for 3 months and a tuberculin test done. If the test is positive, INH is continued for another 9 months. Tuberculin negative babies are given BCG.

Tuberculous meningitis

Occurs most commonly in infancy and early childhood and usually develops within 6 months of the primary infection. Untreated it is fatal. Delayed diagnosis and late treatment will not prevent cure but will inevitably lead to permanent neurological and intellectual damage. Early diagnosis and adequate treatment will allow the majority to survive without permanent damage.

Although the classical signs of an acute bacterial meningitis are generally present, the clinical picture is not an acute one and in untreated cases the interval between early, vague symptoms and death may be more than 1 month.

Symptoms and signs

Early symptoms are generally vague, with anorexia, vomiting and constipation. After the first week photophobia may be present. At the same time the child becomes consistently drowsy and focal neurological signs, particularly sixth nerve palsy, and squints are common. Older children may develop ataxia.

Neck stiffness and opisthotonos are late signs.

In the first week of the illness feeding problems in young babies are often diagnosed and treated. In older children a diagnosis of cerebral tumour may be made. Convulsions are a late sign but they may be focal. Fever occurs in the early stages but is generally low grade.

Papilloedema is a late sign.

Diagnosis

A high index of suspicion should always be present

in the doctor's mind in areas where tuberculosis is prevalent. It is probably better to carry out a lumbar puncture when there is any doubt, than to wait.

Lumbar puncture

Tuberculin tests are often negative in the early stages and diagnosis is made from the CSF findings. The bacilli can only be isolated from the CSF but they are scarce. A sample of 20 ml of CSF should be left to stand in a test tube. A spider web clot will form after 1−2 hours (due to the high globulin levels in the CSF) and the bacillus may be found in the clot. CSF findings are summarized in Table 6.3.

Table 6.3 *CSF findings in tuberculous meningitis*

Colour		Cells	Protein	Glucose
Early cases	Clear	Raised, chiefly polymorphs	Raised slightly	Low
Later cases	Clear	Raised but now chiefly lymphocytes	Very high	Very low

Chest X-ray

This must always be carried out in all suspected cases. Choroidal tubercles are very common and can be diagnosed by CAT scan, if available. With the high protein content in the CSF, fibrosis can occur in the basal area and there may be a block in the CSF. The CSF would then have to be obtained from a cisternal tap. In young infants CSF can more easily be obtained from the ventricles.

Management

This is by chemotherapy and a schedule is shown on page 69.

Leprosy

Leprosy is caused by *Mycobacterium leprae* and is a very slowly developing disease, more so than tuberculosis, and there may be several years between the onset of infection and the appearance of signs and symptoms. Human cases are probably the only primary source of infection, although recently it has been suggested that some animals may be reservoirs.

Infection appears to spread mainly from the nasal discharge of infected persons. Spread from skin to skin is only a minor method of spread. Breast milk of an infected mother also contains a large number of bacilli. The disease involves the skin, peripheral nerves and underlying cartilage in the nose.

Clinical features

The disease is classified into the following three groups:

1. full tuberculoid − TT
2. borderline − BB
3. full lepromatous − LL

Not all patients, however, fall into these three main groups because the clinical spectrum is so varied and features of more than one type may be present in any individual patient. Each borderline classification is unstable and may pass on to the next classification.

Tuberculoid leprosy (TT)

Leprosy is a disease involving mainly the skin, subcutaneous vessels and peripheral nerves. The skin lesions in TT are large reddish plaques with raised and well marked outer edges. Occasionally they are depigmented and they are always hairless and anaesthetic. (Figure 6.6)

The plaques are few in number and do not appear in the groin or axilla. Only one or two peripheral nerves are involved and these are visibly swollen. The commonest nerves involved are those behind the ear (great auricular), in the leg (peroneal) and the elbow (ulnar).

Borderline leprosy (BB)

The skin lesions are more numerous and there may be small 'satellite' lesions at the edge of the large areas. The edges are irregular and difficult to define and some lesions may just be circles of raised reddened skin. There are also numerous nodules in the skin. Anaesthesia is not so marked as in TT and LL and the peripheral nerve thickening not so obvious. (Figure 6.7)

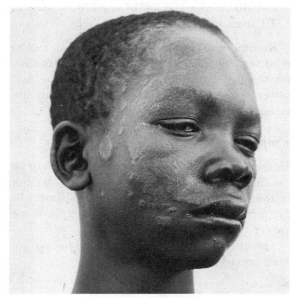

Figure 6.5 A tuberculoid leprosy showing scattered areas of hypopigmentation with anaesthesia (Reproduced courtesy of Lepra)

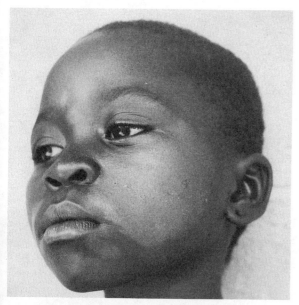

Figure 6.6 Borderline leprosy showing areas of depigmentation and anaesthesia (Reproduced courtesy of Lepra)

Lepromatous leprosy (LL)

In these cases the skin is extensively involved symetrically with macules and nodules which may run into each other forming large 'succulent' areas, in the ear and face, resulting in the so-called 'lion face' (Figure 6.8). In some areas the infiltration is so marked that the skin has a smooth, shiny appearance and does not at first appear involved. In the face the naso-maxillary bone and cartilage becomes destroyed. The lower legs and feet may appear oedematous.

Complications

Bony destruction

Apart from the direct damage to the bones of the nose and face due to the disease, the bones of the digits (hands and feet) become destroyed due to trauma as a result of loss of sensation from peripheral nerve damage.

Erythema nodusum

This occurs as an allergic manifestation as in tuberculosis, but may occur on the face as well as the arms and legs.

Ophthalmic complications

Leprosy can cause primary conjunctivitis, keratitis and iridocyclitis, cataract and eventually phthisis bulbae. Secondary infection of the eye can also result from damage to the fifth nerve, resulting in an anaesthetic eyeball.

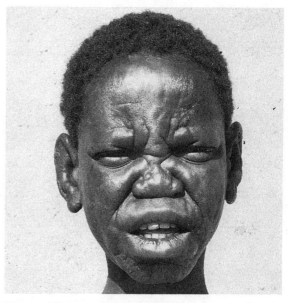

Figure 6.7 Lepromatous leprosy in a 12-year-old boy (Reproduced courtesy of Lepra)

Diagnosis

This is carried out by skin biopsy of one of the lesions and the organism is detected by staining the biopsy. *Mycobacterium leprae* is present also in nasal secretions in LL type.

Active treatment

Dapsone has been the standard form of treatment for some years. Dose:

    25 mg per week for a month orally
    25 mg twice weekly for a month
    50 mg twice weekly for a month
   100 mg twice weekly for a month
   100 mg thrice weekly thereafter for life in LL

and BB disease and for 10 years in the case of TT disease.

Resistance to dapsone is now occurring and to minimize this rifampicin may be given additionally for the first 6 months. Dose: 300–500 mg/day. Other drugs which have been used recently are clofazimine and ethionamide.

Prophylaxis

Household contacts for all cases of leprosy must be examined regularly in the case of TT and BT but in the case of BB, BL and LL children should be given prophylactic doses of dapsone for at least one year.

The use of BCG in giving protection has not yet been proved satisfactory.

7

Meningitis

Meningitis is essentially a disease of childhood, and remains a major problem in developing countries. Fifty per cent of cases are under a year of age, and 80 per cent under 5 years. The high vascularity of the brain and the low immunity of infants are probably important factors.

Aetiology

Organisms

The 'big three' are:

Haemophilus influenzae — commonest under three years of age
Diplococcus pneumoniae
Neisseria meningitidis

In a considerable proportion of cases — up to 50 per cent in some series — no organism can be identified, even when no antibiotics had been given prior to admission.

In neonates the predominant organisms are Gram negative — *Escherichia coli, Pseudomonas, Klebsiella, Salmonella* etc., though occasionally *Staphylococcus* is found.

Gram negative organisms are also commonly found in debilitated and malnourished children, e.g. with kwashiorkor, who develop meningitis. *Salmonella* species are relatively common at all ages in the tropics, and especially in children with sickle cell anaemia.

Infection is generally through the bloodstream, organisms gaining entry through the upper respiratory tract following an apparently trivial or unrecognized infection.

Much less commonly meningitis may be secondary to:

1. direct injury to the head, especially if there is a compound fracture, or fracture of the base of the skull, ethmoid plate or frontal area
2. otitis media (+/− mastoiditis); especially with chronic suppurative otitis media
3. cerebral abscess — there is a special association with cyanotic congenital heart disease
4. open myelomeningocoele or encephalocoele
5. infected valves inserted for management of hydrocephalus

Other factors predisposing to meningitis

1. poor social and economic circumstances — poverty, overcrowding and poor nutrition
2. males are affected more often than females — for reasons unknown
3. depressed or altered immunity — in relation to poor nutrition and low birth weight; the immuno-suppressed on drugs e.g. steroids; and in immune deficiency diseases
4. removal or absence of the spleen increases sus-ceptibility especially to pneumococcal infection, e.g. after trauma or in asplenia — the increased susceptibility of patients with sickle cell anaemia and the nephrotic syndrome to pneumococcal infection is well known

Clinical features and presentation

Although the onset is sudden, the early symptoms of meningitis in young children are often vague and ill-defined, in general the younger the child the more non-specific are the symptoms. In infants it is almost impossible to detect early neck stiffness or a positive Kernig's sign and no reliance should be placed on trying to obtain these signs. The main symptoms are fever, with or without vomiting and an alteration in behaviour, the infant becoming lethargic, uninterested in feeds, drowsy and unre-sponsive, wanting to sleep all the time. When disturbed, the child is irritable and may have a high-pitched cry. Recognition of this change in sensorium — 'leave me alone' is probably the most important alerting sign. The anterior fontanelle may be full or tense. Convulsion may be due to the fever *per se* (in the early stages) or to the meningitis, and *lumbar puncture is essential* to distinguish between the two.

In children over 3 years of age, the classical signs of meningeal irritation are more likely to be present — headache, photophobia, delirium, irritability, neck stiffness and a positive Kernig's sign. Papilloedema is uncommon in the acute stage. Neck stiffness can be detected by asking an older child to sit up. If present, the hands will be placed on the bed on either side of the trunk, forming a 'tripod', the arms extending as the child sits up to keep the head and neck in extension and protect the neck from flexing forwards. Alternatively the child can be asked to flex the knees, bend forwards and kiss them.

Partially treated meningitis

This is most likely to be either a *Haemophilus* or pneumococcal infection, and generally follows an upper respiratory tract infection which has been present for some days and treated with antibiotics, usually penicillin or ampicillin. Following an initial improvement, the child becomes ill again (or sometimes fails to improve) with an insidious slow deterioration, antibiotics masking the typical features.

Meningococcal septicaemia and meningitis

This may sometimes present with dramatic suddenness and overwhelming infection. The onset is abrupt with fever, shock, peripheral circulatory failure and petechial haemorrhages appearing in the skin as one looks at the child. These rapidly coalesce, producing widespread areas of purpura and necrosis, the result of a vasculitis and disseminated intravascular coagulation (DIC). Internal bleeding may occur in any organ, in particular the adrenal glands, and death occurring within a few hours from shock, toxaemia and DIC, the Waterhouse—Friedrichsen syndrome. Meningococci can be cultured from the purpuric areas of the skin, as well as blood and CSF. The rapid development of petechia and purpura are so characteristic that diagnosis is not difficult. Once it is suspected, treatment is urgent and must be started immediately, without waiting for blood culture and other investigations

unless these can be done at once. An intravenous drip must be set up at once and penicillin given in full doses (see Treatment, below). Plasma, plasma expander or saline are required to combat shock. The role of corticosteroids (hydrocortisone, prednisolone, or dexamethasone) is still controversial, especially in established DIC though many paediatricians use them. Heparin may be required in the management of DIC.

Meningococcal meningitis in Africa

Large scale, devastating epidemics of meningococcal meningitis — mainly group A — sweep across the African 'meningitis belt' in the Sahel extending from Sudan in the east to Mali in the west, in a cyclical pattern about every 10 years or so, although in some areas recently, e.g. Northern Nigeria, it has become almost an annual event. There is a clear seasonal incidence, with peaks in the dry months, February to April, epidemics subsiding sharply with the onset of the rainy season. Routine vaccination is impractical, because of the high cost, uncertainties about the duration of immunity produced by the vaccine (though antibodies have been found up to 5 years after vaccination), and the irregular occurence of epidemics. There is, however, increasing evidence that mass vaccination programmes, instituted at the start of an epidemic, appear to be successful in controlling and to some extent aborting epidemics. In Northern Nigeria, 0.5 ml of a polyvalent (Group A and C) vaccine (Institut Merieux, France) was given in the deltoid area using a Ped-O-Jet injector with no significant side effects. As the vaccine is relatively expensive, only those at greatest risk — children between 3 and 15 years — were vaccinated. A satisfactory cold-chain is essential if the vaccine is to retain its potency. Unfortunately, resistance to sulphonamides (approaching 100 per cent in some areas) has now made mass chemoprophylaxis with this drug of uncertain or doubtful value. During a recent epidemic in Mali, treatment of established cases of meningitis with a single dose of chloramphenicol in oil (1—3 g depending on age) is reported to have been successful, patients being observed in hospital for 5 to 8 days.

Diagnosis

Diagnosis depends on:

1. all doctors working in the tropics having a high

index of suspicion about meningitis in infants and children, and

2. always doing a lumbar puncture whenever the diagnosis is considered — meningitis cannot be diagnosed in any other way.

Lumbar puncture is safe, even if pressure is considered high, provided that:

1. the spinal fluid is obtained slowly in a controlled way using a stillette, and
2. small volumes of 1 to 2 ml are obtained for diagnostic purposes.

If lumbar spinal fluid cannot be obtained in small infants, a ventricular tap should be considered.

Send the cerebro-spinal fluid (CSF) for:

1. cell count, Gram film and culture
2. protein
3. glucose
4. chloride if tuberculous meningitis is suspected.

A blood culture should always be done, and a blood sugar at the same time as the lumbar puncture.

Up to 50 cells may be present in CSF before it becomes turbid. If in doubt, compare the CSF with a tube of distilled water. Table 7.1 shows the interpretation of CSF results.

Treatment

If complications are to be avoided, treatment must be prompt and adequate. The combination of benzyl penicillin and chloramphenicol still remains unsurpassed for treatment of bacterial meningitis before the causative organism has been identified. Many strains of pneumococci and meningococci

Table 7.1 *Interpretation of CSF results*

	Cells	Appearance	Glucose*	Protein	Gram film[†]
Bacterial meningitis	Predominant polymorphs 100–10 000/mm^3	Turbid → frank pus	Reduced — may be undetectable. Range 0–30 mg/100 ml Average 10–15 mg/100 ml Normal about 35 mg/100 ml	Increased. 100–200 mg/100 ml	Bacteria usually seen. Gram film may be misinterpreted, so always give full antibiotic treatment until cultures available.
Partially treated bacterial meningitis	Total cell count generally raised. Mixed polymorphs and lymphocytes. May be >1000 cells/mm^3	Clear or turbid	Normal or slightly reduced.	Slightly increased.	Cultures often sterile (sub-cultures may be positive). If in doubt give full antibiotic treatment.
Viral meningitis	0 → 300 mainly lymphocytes	Clear (unless very high cell count)	Normal (unless severe vomiting)	Slightly increased 20–100 mg%.	Cell count increased and pleomorphic in mumps.
Tuberculous meningitis	200 → 500 mainly lymphocytes	Opalescent	Reduced — may be none	Increased up to 500 mg — clot may develop on standing.	ZN film essential. Polymorphs may predominate in early or acute onset TBM. Skin tests negative in fulminant cases.

Notes * Always do a blood glucose at the same time, and compare. CSF glucose is usually slightly lower.
  [†] Film of centrifuged deposit stained with Gram's stain.

are now resistant to sulphonamides, and these are no longer used. Recently, reports have appeared of successful treatment of meningitis using some of the new third generation cephalosporins, but these drugs are very expensive and unlikely to be available in most developing countries for a long time yet.

Drugs

- benzyl penicillin 200 000 units (120 mg)/kg/24 hours − 4 hourly bolus injections
- chloramphenicol 100 mg/kg/24 hours − 6 hourly bolus injections

In rare event of penicillin hypersensitivity, give cephaloridine 100−150 mg/kg/24 hours − 6 hourly bolus injections.

All drugs should be given intravenously through a drip or indwelling intravenous cannula for a minimum of 3−4 days and much longer if there has been any delay in starting treatment. If *Haemophilus influenzae* is cultured, then penicillin can be stopped and treatment continued with chloramphericol alone; likewise if a *Pneumococcus* or *Meningococcus* is cultured, chloramphenicol can be stopped after 3−4 days and treatment continued with penicillin alone.

If a child with *Haemophilus* meningitis is well, afebrile and alert by 5 to 6 days, intravenous therapy may be stopped and treatment continued with oral chloramphericol in a reduced dosage of 50−75 mg/kg/24 hours divided into 6 hourly doses.

Treatment should normally be given for at least 10 days though the duration will depend to some extent on the severity and course of the illness; in meningococcal infection 7 days treatment is often adequate.

Repeat lumbar puncture is probably unnecessary if progress has been satisfactory, the child has clinically recovered and antibiotics stopped after 10 to 14 days. After stopping antibiotics, the child should be observed in hospital for a further two days before discharge.

A repeat lumbar puncture is indicated if:

1. fever persists or response to treatment appears unsatisfactory or
2. there is a recrudescence of fever and apparent relapse after initial improvement.

Occasionally persistence of fever in an otherwise clinically well child is due to the drugs and subsides when antibiotics are stopped.

Intrathecal drugs

Antibiotics for intrathecal use have to be specially prepared, free of preservatives, and are not always readily available. There is some doubt as to whether antibiotics given by the lumbar route achieve adequate levels in the central nervous system, and in most cases intrathecal therapy is unnecessary.

Culture negative, or suspected partially treated meningitis

This is often more difficult to treat effectively than a new, untreated case, and should be treated with benzyl penicillin and chloramphenicol in full dosage for at least 10 days.

Ampicillin has proved disappointing in the treatment of bacterial meningitis and its use is not advised. To obtain satisfactory CSF levels, particularly as meningeal inflammation subsides, it is necessary to give doses of 400 mg/kg/day *intravenously* for at least 2 weeks to sterilize the CSF. Problems with fluid balance, the siting of i.v. drips and thrombophlebitis, as well as discomfort for the child, all make this difficult to achieve in practice, and failure of successful treatment is reflected in a high incidence of complications. Finally, ampicillin-resistant strains of *H. influenzae* are now common in many parts of the world.

Supportive treatment

Intravenous fluids

As well as providing a route for antibiotic therapy (and so avoiding the necessity of frequent, painful intra-muscular injections), i.v. fluids may be necessary to maintain an adequate fluid intake in the early days of treatment. In some cases of meningitis there may be an inappropriate secretion of anti-diuretic hormone (see Complications). If so, intravenous fluids should be restricted to between 50 and 60 ml/kg/day.

If it is impossible to establish an i.v. drip, then a 'cut-down' should be done. If this is not successful, then antibiotics must be given intramuscularly, and a nasogastric tube inserted to give fluids.

Observations and care

Whilst the child is unconscious or drowsy, appropriate neurological observations should be charted regularly along with pulse, respiration, temperature and blood pressure. Head circumference should be measured daily to detect early onset of hydrocephalus. The child should be kept quiet and disturbed as little as possible. Milk feeds can be continued through a nasogastric tube.

Anticonvulsants

Are probably only necessary if the child has convulsed or is very irritable. Immediate control of convulsion is by either diazepam (0.25 mg/kg) given slowly i.v., or paraldehyde by i.m. injection (0.2 ml/kg). Both can also be given rectally. For prolonged management give phenobarbitone 5 to 8 mg/kg/day in two or three divided doses orally or intramuscularly.

Steroids

These have *no* place in the management of acute purulent meningitis.

Complications

Convulsions

Persistence of these beyond 72 hours after admission suggests underlying brain damage or severe infection responding only poorly to treatment.

Inappropriate secretion of antidiuretic hormone (ADH)

This causes retention of both intracellular and extracellular fluid, resulting in a low serum osmolality, low serum sodium (< 130 mmol/l), a low urinary output of high specific gravity and cerebral oedema. The latter, with the associated rise in intracranial pressure produces clinical deterioration, with progressive drowsiness, unconsciousness, irregular respirations, papilloedema, pin point pupils and finally cardiorespiratory arrest. Fluid intake must be restricted to 50 to 60 ml/kg/day intravenously, checking urine specific gravity and serum sodium levels. Urgent treatment is an i.v. mannitol infusion (2 g/kg over 30 mins), dexamethasone 2 mg/kg/day and frusemide (1 mg/kg/dose as required); alternatively saline 3 per cent infusion can be given in an emergency.

Subdural effusion

This is most commonly associated with *H. influenzae* infections, though may also occur after pneumococcal infections. It is often bilateral and usually appears during the second week of treatment. After an initial improvement, there is clinical deterioration with recurrence of fever, vomiting, drowsiness, convulsions and focal neurological signs. Fontanelle tension is increased, and there may be increase in head circumference if the effusion is large. Diagnosis is made by performing subdural taps. The fluid — from 2 to 20 ml — is usually sterile and xanthochromic with a high protein content. Subdural taps should be performed daily or on alternate days until the effusion subsides, usually within 2 to 3 weeks. Not more than 30 ml of fluid should be removed at any one time. Excessive aspiration may, in fact, prolong the presence of the effusion. Small effusions often subside spontaneously without treatment. Craniotomy is only very seldom indicated.

Hydrocephalus

Is secondary to inflammatory adhesions especially around the base of the brain and choroid plexuses, interfering with the circulation of CSF. It may be suspected if:

1. there is failure to obtain CSF from a lumbar puncture — a 'dry tap'
2. persistence of low CSF sugar and
3. increasing head circumference, bulging anterior fontanelle and suture separation — Established hydrocephalus requires drainage through insertion of a ventriculo-atrial or ventriculo-peritoneal shunt.

Long-term neurological sequelae

These may be as high as 15 to 25 per cent in survivors and are directly related to the severity of the infection; delay in starting treatment, and adequacy of treatment. Many cases are still diagnosed far too late, because lumbar puncture is delayed, or else undertreated with disastrous results. It is the author's opinion that meningitis can never be overtreated.

Sequelae which may be transient or permanent include Cranial nerve palsies especially III, IV and VI; hemiplegia, monoplegia, deafness, (usually permanent) blindness (which may be cortical), mental retardation and epilepsy. Later problems, such as behaviour disorders, learning disorders, hyperactivity and epilepsy may only manifest themselves when the child is older.

8
Immunization

Immunization is an essential part of infectious disease control. It has played a major role in the control of these diseases in industrialized countries and has had a dramatic impact on both morbidity and mortality, resulting in their virtual disappearance. Unfortunately there are still many countries where this has yet to be achieved. WHO estimated that in 1984 four million children were affected with a physical or mental disability due to one of six infectious diseases — tuberculosis, diphtheria, tetanus, whooping cough (pertussis), polio and measles. It is against this background that WHO and UNICEF launched the Expanded Programme on Immunization (EPI) in 1977 with the object of having all the children in the world fully immunized against these six common infectious diseases by the year 1990. The EPI is an ongoing permanent programme, since each year a new generation of infants has to be vaccinated at the proper time; it is an important component of primary health care. Failure to maintain high immunization rates results in the reappearance of diseases, often in epidemic proportions, as happened in the late 1970s in Britain with whooping cough.

The following abbreviations are used:

BCG	bacillus Calmette-Guérin
DNA	deoxyribonucleic acid
DPT	diphtheria, pertussis and tetanus toxoid
DT	diphtheria and tetanus toxoid
EPI	expanded programme on immunization
HBsAg	hepatitis B surface antigen
HBIg	hepatitis B immunoglobulin
HIV	human immunodeficiency virus
Ig	immunoglobulin
IgA, IgG, IgM	immunoglobulin classes
IPV	inactivated polio vaccine (Salk)
MMR	measles, mumps, rubella vaccine
IU	international units
OPV	oral polio vaccine (Sabin) (trivalent)
TIg	tetanus immunoglobulin
TT	tetanus toxoid.
UNICEF	United Nations Children's Fund
WHO	World Health Organization
ZIg	varicella—zoster immune globulin

The terms 'vaccination' and 'immunization' have the same meaning and are interchangeable.

Active immunity

Active immunity produces lasting protection. Modified, or attenuated, forms of live micro-organisms, killed organisms or their products are used to stimulate antibody production in the host.

Live vaccines:

Viral	Bacterial
measles	BCG
mumps	typhoid (oral)
rubella	
Sabin (live polio-myelitis, oral OPV)	
yellow fever	

Killed vaccines:

Viral	Bacterial
Salk (killed poliomyelitis, injectable, IPV)	pertussis
	cholera
	typhoid,
influenza	paratyphoid
hepatitis B	A and B
rabies	(injectable,
typhus	conventional)

Toxoids

Bacterial
diphtheria
tetanus

Other vaccines

Meningococcal

Monovalent and bivalent, derived from capsular polysaccharide. The monovalent vaccines are groups A and C. The bivalent is A + C. Unfortunately group B is not immunogenic in man.

Pneumococcal

Polyvalent consisting of up to 23 purified polysaccharide antigens from the most prevalent serotypes.

A number of vaccines are now being manufactured by recombinant DNA technology and other biosynthetic processes. These techniques enable specific antigenic components or toxins of the organism to be produced in a highly purified form, making for a much safer and less toxic vaccine without many of the unwanted and potentially dangerous side effects often from other components. Vaccines currently being produced, or about to be produced, in this way include hepatitis B, cholera, pertussis and typhoid.

Active immunization and immunization schedules

The basic schedule is similar in most countries although there are slight variations depending on local circumstances such as the prevalence of a disease in the community, the age at which it presents and the need to protect susceptible children (Tables 8.1, 8.2). Examples are measles and polio.

In many countries where measles is a disease of infancy and the first year of life, immunization is given at 9 months; in Western Europe it is a disease of older children and immunization can be delayed until 13 to 15 months. In large epidemics, on the recommendation of the Ministry of Health, measles vaccine may be given at 6 months. A second dose should then be given at 12 months.

In countries where polio is not controlled, OPV can be given at birth with BCG, then at 6 weeks, with two additional doses 4 weeks apart with DPT. Completion before 6 months will help to reduce the incidence of provocation paralysis from infections in the second half of infancy. The minimum interval between doses for DPT and OPV is 1 month. There is no maximum interval. If a course of immunizations is interrupted, it should be continued where it was left off. Do not start all over again.

The timing of immunization in premature babies is the same as for full-term infants, and should not be delayed on account of prematurity.

Table 8.1   *Typical immunization schedule for Western Europe*

Age	Vaccine	Dose and site	Remarks
Birth or at first contact	BCG	0.05 ml intradermal	Must *not* be given subcutaneously. Dose 0.1 ml over 1 year. May be given later with DPT and OPV. Can be repeated after 5 years.
Birth	BCG(+ OPV)		OPV optional
3 months	DPT + OPV	0.5 ml deep s.c. or i.m. injection 3 drops (oral)	DPT can be given safely and effectively from 6 weeks if necessary
5 months	2nd DPT and OPV	Same	Minimum interval between first and second = 4 weeks. Preferred interval is 6 to 8 weeks.
8 to 11 months	3rd DPT and OPV	Same	Interval of 4 to 6 months preferred between second and third immunization
13 to 15 months	Measles or MMR	0.5 ml deep s.c. or i.m. injection	
5 to 6 years	DT and OPV		At school entry

Table 8.2 *Alternative immunization schedule for use in countries where rapid and full immunization is necessary*

Age	Vaccine	Dose and site	Remarks
Birth or first contact	BCG		
Birth	BCG and OPV		
6 weeks	DPT and OPV		
10 weeks	2nd DPT and OPV	As in Table 8.1	
14 weeks	3rd DPT and OPV		
9 months	Measles or MMR		Can be given with DPT and OPV
18 months	DPT and OPV		
5 to 6 years	DT and OPV		

The minimum vaccination requirements necessary to give basic protection are:

BCG — one dose
DPT — three doses
OPV — four doses
Measles (or MMR) — one dose after 9 months.

Tables 8.1 and 8.2 show two different schedules. That in Table 8.1 shows the timing of immunization as practised in many Western European countries, while Table 8.2 is based on WHO recommendations for countries where there is an urgent need to complete all immunizations as early as possible in infancy. The timing at which active immunization is given takes into account a number of theoretical as well as practical considerations:

1. Cell mediated immunity is present at birth and so BCG can be given at that time.
2. Humoral immunity develops more slowly and is only well established by 2 to 3 months of age, hence most immunizations are delayed until this time, (with the exception of hepatitis B to the newborn).
3. Polysaccharide vaccines (meningococcal, pneumococcal and *Haemophilus influenzae*) do not stimulate significant amount of antibody until 2 years of age.
4. The response to active immunization may be inhibited by maternal antibody transmitted across the placenta. Quite high titres of measles antibody may persist up to 9 months or even longer, resulting in the failure of active immunization if given too early.
5. The efficacy of soluble protein antigens (toxoids) can be considerably enhanced by the absorption on to a microbiologically inert adjuvent such as aluminium hydroxide gel. The gel-toxoid complex is insoluble and after injection forms a depot in the tissues from which antigen is slowly released giving a prolonged stimulus to the immune system. It also produces a foreign body inflammatory reaction attracting immunologically competent cells such as lymphocytes and macrophages to the site of injection.
6. The number of doses of vaccine and the interval between them depends upon the type of vaccine. Live vaccines and purified polysaccharides can be given as a single dose, with the exception of oral polio. Toxoids require two or three doses with an optimum interval of 8 weeks between first and second, and 6 to 12 months between second and third. Clearly, some compromise is necessary when infants must be protected at an early age against disease and immunization programmes must then be completed in a shorter time (see Table 8.2).

Complications and contra-indications

All injected vaccines may cause an anaphylactic reaction. Always have adrenaline 1:1000 solution readily available for immediate subcutaneous injection. Patients should remain in the clinic for half an hour after immunization.

Local reactions at the site of injection, especially after triple antigen (DPT) are common. Some redness and pain may occur up to 72 hours, especially after repeat immunizations.

Generalized reactions include fever, malaise, irritability and sometimes drowsiness and convulsions. Fever may begin within 2 to 3 hours, and most reactions occur within 24 to 48 hours. The most severe reactions are usually associated with pertussis and are related to the presence of whole killed bacteria. Studies from the UK suggest that the incidence of severe reactions resulting in permanent neurological damage is about 1:100 000 following a full course of three immunizations. Febrile reactions may be treated with paracetamol.

Contra-indications

No child should be denied the protection afforded by immunization unless there are sound medical contra-indications, or unless the risk of a severe reaction outweighs the risk of the disease.

General contra-indications to all immunizations

- any acute febrile illness — immunize when the child has recovered
- children whose immune response is impaired, e.g. with malignant disease, especially of the reticulo-endothelial system; on immunosuppresive therapy; on corticosteroids, or receiving deep X-ray treatment.
- children with congenital immune deficiency syndromes
- pregnancy should be avoided for 3 months after receiving any live vaccine

Contra-indications to pertussis immunization

- a history of cerebral irritation or brain damage in the neonatal period
- infants who have already suffered from seizures
- a history of a *severe* local or general reaction, including a neurological reaction to a preceding dose

The following are not absolute contra-indications but special consideration needs to be given to certain groups of children in whom the possible risk of a vaccine reaction has to balanced against the risk of developing whooping cough and its consequences. Such groups include:

- children whose parents or siblings have a history of idiopathic epilepsy
- children with developmental delay thought to be due to a neurological defect
- children with established non-progressive neurological disease

Note that even when pertussis immunization is contra-indicated, infants should still be immunized against diphtheria and tetanus, and given OPV.

Contra-indications to measles immunization

There are no absolute contra-indications, other than the general contra-indications to all live vaccines. Special consideration needs to be given to children with a *personal* history of convulsions, or whose parents or siblings have a history of epilepsy. Such children should be immunized but at the same time be given specially diluted immunoglobulin (see below) to attenuate any possible reactions. Allergies and sensitivities to eggs is not a contra-indication unless there is a history of severe hypersensitivity, e.g., anaphylaxis, laryngeal spasm or bronchospasm.

The following are not considered to be contra-indications to immunization, indeed some of these groups of children are especially in need of protection:

- allergy; asthma or eczema in patient or family
- convulsions or epilepsy in a distant relative
- chronic lung or heart disease
- mental retardation; Down's syndrome
- chronically discharging ear
- weight below 5 kg
- undernutrition (but not severe malnutrition)
- neonatal problems — jaundice; prematurity; breech delivery; respiratory distress
- mother pregnant

Simultaneous administration of vaccines

The following combinations of vaccines can be given together without interfering with antibody response or resulting in an increased risk of adverse reactions:

- DPT or DT and OPV
- OPV and measles or MMR
- DPT, OPV and MMR, provided that DPT and MMR are given at different injection sites
- hepatitis B vaccine, DPT and OPV provided that hepatitis B vaccine and DPT are given at different injection sites

Different live vaccines can be given at the same time, but must be given at different injection sites. They may not however be given at different times within the same month, since the first will interfere with the 'take' of the second one.

The cold chain

All vaccines, particularly live vaccines, must be stored under the correct conditions of temperature from the time of production to injection to remain active. One of the main reasons for the failure, or apparent failure, of immunization is a break in the cold chain, allowing the vaccine to become warm and resulting in a loss of potency. Major problems are usually due to:

- refrigeration and transportation difficulties between the place manufacture and storage centres, or storage centre and peripheral clinics
- failure or fluctuation in power supplies to storage centres
- lack of cold packs or cold storage facilities at immunization centres
- lack of understanding by personnel at all levels of the need to maintain the cold chain right until the time of immunization

Measles and polio vaccines are particularly expensive to store and deliver since they must be kept stored at $-20°C$ in a deep freeze after manufacture. In clinics they can be kept refrigerated at not more than 4°C for up to 3 months. After removal from the refrigerator and reconstitution, the vaccines should be kept in an ice-pack and used within 1 to 2 hours depending on the ambient temperature of the surroundings.

Vaccines should never be left open in the hot sun. DPT and tetanus toxoid should never be frozen. Diphtheria and tetanus toxoids, either singly or as components of DPT or DT are the most stable, followed by the pertussis component of DPT, inactivated polio vaccine, freeze dried BCG, freeze dried measles and the least stable being live polio vaccine.

Passive immunization

Passive immunization offers immediate protection, which may be complete or partial against a number of life threatening diseases. Serum containing high titres of the relevant antibody is derived from human or animal sources.

Human immunoglobulin (Ig)

Three types are available:

1. *Standard immunoglobulin*: normal Ig, polyvalent. It consists almost entirely of IgG, and contains 16.5 per cent of human plasma proteins.
2. *Specific immunoglobulins*. These contain antibody in a high titre to one specific disease. Specific Ig is obtained from pooled HBsAg negative plasma from convalescent or deliberately immunized donors by plasmapheresis and regular donors known to have high levels of a specific antibody.
3. *Intravenous immunoglobulin*. This is similar to standard Ig but is modified to make it suitable for intravenous use. It consists almost entirely of IgG but only in about one-third concentration of standard Ig.

Standard immunoglobulin is manufactured from a pool of at least 1000 units of human venous plasma negative for HBsAg and HIV negative, and is given by deep intramuscular injection. Peak blood levels are reached 2 to 4 days later and followed by a slow decline, so that the recommended dose results in protection for about a month. The duration is dose dependent, and the clinical effects depend on the antibody content. Immunoglobulin offers protection only when given before or within a few days of exposure, early in the incubation period. When clinical symptoms have appeared, immunoglobulin is of no value in modifying the disease.

Indications for the use of immunoglobulin

Standard and special Ig must be given by deep intramuscular injection and not more than 1 to 3 ml should be given in any one site, depending on the size of the child. Standard and special Ig must never be given intravenously because of the risk of an immediate anaphylactic reaction. Standard Ig is of value only in the following three conditions:

1. *Measles.*
- to prevent an attack in unvaccinated children at special risk – immunosuppressed, debilitated or malnourished, with chronic chest or heart conditions, or a history of convulsions
- to allow an attenuated attack
- to reduce a reaction to measles vaccine
- give no later than 5 days after exposure

- dosage: to prevent an attack: under 1 year 250 mg, 1–2 years 500 mg, 3 years and over 750 mg
- to attenuate an attack give half the above doses
- to reduce the reaction to measles vaccine give 25 mg only (0.5 ml/kg)

2. *Hepatitis A*. Give not later than 6 to 7 days after exposure. Dosage = 250 mg. For travellers, give 0.02 to 0.05 ml/kg and repeat if necessary every 3–4 months.

3. *Agammaglobulinaemia*. Give as long-term antibody replacement therapy, dosage 0.5 ml/kg monthly. Local pain and long-term injections make intravenous Ig now preferable.

Specific immunoglobulins

Specific immunoglobulins are available for protection against the following infections:

Hepatitis B

HBIg is given after mucosal exposure to HBsAg positive blood, and newborn infants of mothers who are seropositive. Two injections of HBIg at 1-monthly intervals offer up to 75 per cent protection. By combining HB vaccine with HBIg prolonged protection can be obtained. For the protection of newborn infants of antigen positive mothers give:

1. HBIg 0.5 ml within 12–24 hours at birth, and *not* later than 48 hours
2. hepatitis B vaccine 10 µg (0.5 ml) at the same time as HBIg but at a separate injection site, or within 1 week of birth – repeat the same dose of vaccine at 1 month and 6 months of age

Varicella-Zoster immunoglobulin (ZIg)

This is given for the prevention of varicella (or zoster) in contacts who are either immunosuppressed or have serious debilitating disease, and in newborn infants of mothers who develop chickenpox 6 days or less before delivery or shortly afterwards. ZIg should be given not more than 4 days after exposure; it may modify an attack but cannot be relied on entirely to prevent an attack. Dosage:

Neonates and under 1 year	100 mg
1–5 years	250 mg
6–10 years	500 mg

Double dosage may be given to immunosuppressed children.

Tetanus immunoglobulin (TIg)

This is given for the prevention of tetanus after injury or exposure in unimmunized or only partially protected individuals, and for immediate treatment on diagnosis. For prophylaxis of neonatal tetanus and tetanus after injury, give 25–500 units. Permanent protection is afforded by combining TIg with the first of three doses of tetanus toxoid. For the initial treatment of clinical tetanus give 5000 iu of TIg.

Rabies immunoglobulin

Rabies immunoglobulin should be given once only, immediately at the beginning of treatment along with the first dose of human diploid rabies vaccine.

Animal sera

Only a small number of antisera of animal origin are now used because of the very real risks associated with the injection of foreign proteins and anaphylaxis. The important ones still in use are diphtheria antitoxin, some anti-snake venoms and botulin antitoxin. Tetanus and rabies antitoxins of animal origin are no longer used.

Before giving any animal antisera, obtain a history of any previous injections or exposure, and of asthma and other allergic symptoms, and perform sensitivity tests. If both are negative, then the appropriate dose of serum may be given, but negative tests do not preclude the risk of anaphylaxis or serum sickness 6 to 10 days later. Adrenaline 1:1000 solution and hydrocortisone must be available for immediate use in case of anaphylaxis.

A skin test is performed by placing a drop of serum diluted to 1:100 on a superficial scratch. A positive reaction, wheal or erythema, develops within 30 minutes. Alternatively an intradermal injection of 0.1 ml serum diluted to 1:100 will give a positive wheal within 30 minutes.

Further reading

Campbell A.G.M. (1986). Immunisation – complications and contra-indications: true and false. *Maternal and Child Health*, **11** (8), 254.

Department of Health and Social Security (1984). *Immunisation Against Infectious Disease*, Her Majesty's Stationery Office, London.

Pontecorvo M. (1985). *Vaccines Sera Immunoglobulins*. Minerva Medica, Turin.

9

Renal Disease

Congenital abnormalities of the renal tract

Congenital abnormalities of the renal tract are common. There is a strong association between congenital abnormalities of the heart and kidney, greater than would be expected by chance, and between the renal tract, the lower alimentary tract and lower spine and legs, suggesting a common genetic or environmental factor operating at a critical stage of development. They may only be discovered during the investigation of urinary tract infections, renal failure, hypertension or an abdominal mass.

The effect of most congenital abnormalities is to produce either dysfunction of the urinary tract or obstruction to the flow of urine. Both result in stasis of urine followed by infection, while obstructive lesions also produce back pressure up the urinary tract. The end result is hypertension and renal failure.

Dysplastic kidney

Nephrons are abnormal in structure and renal function is poor. The kidney may be enlarged or hypoplastic, being small and shrunken, with a reduction in number and size of nephrons and calyces.

Hydronephrosis (dilatation of the renal pelvis)

This may be unilateral or bilateral. The commonest causes are an obstruction at the pelvi-ureteric junction or vesico-ureteric junction, a duplex kidney with reflux and urethral valves.

Duplex kidney with bifid collecting system

One or both kidneys may be affected (Figure 9.1).

Many different variations are found, ranging from two completely separate renal pelves equal in size and each with its own ureter, or a large moeity and a small one with separate or a single ureter or ureters fusing. Reduplications may be silent and symptomless, discovered by accident or found during the investigation of urinary infections. The ureter from the lower pole is often the abnormal one, reflux is common and it enters the bladder above the ureter from the upper pole. Occasionally the ureter may have an ectopic opening elsewhere, or end as a ureterocele at the distal end in the bladder.

Renal agenesis

The absence of both kidneys is incompatible with survival and affected infants die shortly after birth. They have a characteristic facial appearance, low set ears, micrognathia and hyperteleorism, and there is associated oligohydramnios and hypoplasia of the lungs (Potter's syndrome).

Absence of a single kidney is commoner and compatible with normal life if normal in structure.

Fusion of the kidneys (horseshoe kidney)

The kidneys may fuse in the mid-line, resulting in a single kidney. One or both ureters may be present.

Ectopic kidney

This is due to failure to migrate to the normal position (as in horseshoe kidney), and remains within the pelvis. Abnormalities of the ureter are common. It is more susceptible to trauma in the pelvis.

Cystic disease of the kidney

A simplified aetiological classification is:

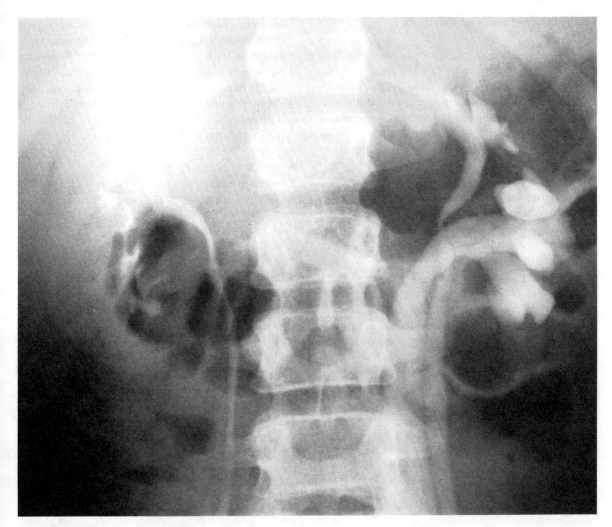

Figure 9.1 Duplex left kidney with hydronephrosis

1. *An infantile form with multiple cysts*, usually fatal within a few months of birth. Cystic disease of the liver is often present. Some forms may have an autosomal recessive inheritance.
2. *An adult form*, which may be present from infancy. There is a family history with autosomal dominant inheritance. Cysts may be large enough at birth to obstruct the delivery.
3. *Cysts* due to a dysplastic kidney. These may unilateral or bilateral, and are not inherited.

Pelvi-ureteric junction obstruction

Congenital narrowing results in hydronephrosis Occasionally it may be due to aberrant renal vessels pressing on the ureter.

Abnormalities of the ureter

Abnormalities of the ureter, at the insertion into the bladder may result in either obstruction and subsequent dilation of the lower end and ureterocoele formation, or vesico-ureteric reflux.

Abnormalities of the bladder

These are not common. Diverticuli sometimes occur. Abnormalities of innervation of the bladder from second, third and fourth sacral nerves result in a neurogenic bladder, the commonest causes being spina bifida, sacral agenesis or spinal dysraphism.

Posterior urethral valves

These are seen almost exclusively in boys and are due to folds of mucosa in the proximal urethra obstructing the flow of urine. Affected boys pass a poor stream of urine which may just dribble out, the bladder is distended and hydronephrosis results from back pressure. Renal failure may be present at birth. Urgent surgical treatment is essential.

Infections of the urinary tract (UTI) and vesico-ureteric reflux (VUR)

Predisposing factors

- Any congenital abnormality of the renal tract resulting in obstruction and stasis of urine which then becomes infected
- vesico-ureteric reflux — about one in four children with a UTI will have some degree of reflux (Figure 9.2)
- in the first year of life the incidence between boys and girls is equal, possibly because of infection with organisms under the prepuce, thereafter infection is about four times commoner in girls, probably because the short female urethra makes ascending infection much more likely; recurrent infection in boys always requires investigation.
- infection with fimbriated or 'sticky' *Escherichia coli* which bind specifically to epithelial cells of the urinary tract — these strains of *E. coli* form the predominant gut flora in a number of children with otherwise unexplained recurrent infections, pyelonephritis and renal scarring
- constipation
- infrequent or incomplete micturition
- neurogenic bladder
- renal calculi

Clinical features

The younger the child the more vague and ill defined are the symptoms and signs, and the classical symptoms of loin pain, frequency, dysuria and fever may be absent, especially in children under 4 or 5 years old. Symptoms may include:
- an offensive smelly nappy with fish-like odour
- abdominal pains
- malaise and anorexia
- unexplained malaise and fever in infants without other physical signs
- sudden onset of enuresis (day or night) in a previously dry child

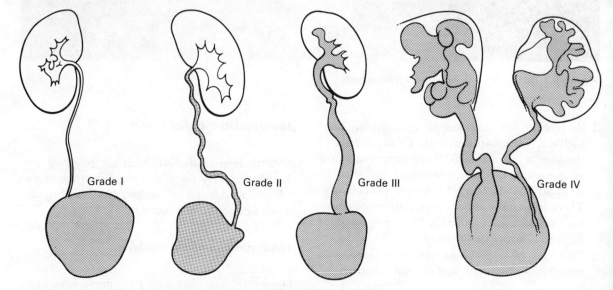

Grade I – Reflux does not reach renal pelvis. No dilatation of ureter.
Grade II – Reflux into renal pelvis. No dilatation of ureter or renal pelvis.
Grade III – Slight dilatation and distension of ureter and pelvi-calyceal system.
Grade IV – Gross distension of whole ureter and pelvi-calyceal system with hydronephrosis.

Figure 9.2 Diagram showing the four grades of vesicoureteric reflux

- acute retention of urine
- haematuria
- failure to thrive in infancy

Diagnosis

One of the main problems in making a diagnosis is the difficulty in obtaining a satisfactory specimen of urine. Ideally all urine specimens should be refrigerated or kept cool after collection and cultured within 2 hours of collection. Urine is a good culture medium for bacterial growth and at room temperature in warm climates the number of organisms may double within 20 minutes. Methods of collection include:

- *bag urine*, this is frequently contaminated by perineal organisms and may give a false positive.
- *mid-stream specimen* from older children who can be asked to void on request.
- *clean catch specimen*, in a sterile container, from infants − it is tedious because of the need to wait but more reliable.
- *suprapubic bladder puncture* is very useful and reliable in infants as the shallow pelvis makes the bladder readily accessible but is difficult over one year of age.
- *catheterization* is not recommended for routine use, though can be used in difficult or urgent situations.
- *nitrite test* − this depends on the ability of bacteria (mainly Gram negative) to convert nitrates to nitrite, it is useful as a screening test, but may give false negatives, false positives are rare.
- *dip slide cultures* may give a provisional diagnosis within 12 to 24 hours, but correct reading is important

Urine microscopy (with both a quantitative white cell and red cell count) is essential. A mixed growth of organisms in the absence of pyuria suggests contamination and culture should be repeated; if pus cells are present with a mixed growth in a 'first' infection, an abnormality of the urinary tract should be suspected. A pure growth of an organism in numbers greater than 10^5 per ml in the presence of pyuria indicates infection. The presence of red cells indicates inflammation.

E. coli is the commonest infecting organism but a wide variety of bacteria, both Gram negative and Gram positive including *Proteus* spp., *Streptococcus faecalis* and *Staphylococcus albus* can be found. A mixed growth of bacteria including *Pseudomonas* with pyuria strongly suggests a congenital abnormality in the urinary tract.

Investigations

Any child who has had more than one UTI should be fully investigated since about 5 per cent will have some radiological abnormality of the urinary tract. As there is no way of knowing with certainty that the presenting infection is, in fact, the first one, this means that in practice every child requires investigation. This includes:

- basic biochemistry − electrolytes, blood urea, calcium, phosphate, creatinine
- measurement of blood pressure
- an ultrasound examination of the renal tract with plain X-ray of the abdomen to exclude a renal calculus) or intravenous urography (i.v.u.)
- micturating cysto-urethrogram − this is an unpleasant examination for young children; it need not be done routinely on every child with a UTI and should be reserved for those with some evidence suggestive of reflux on the ultrasound or i.v.u., or recurrent infections with a normal i.v.u. or ultrasound since the latter may not exclude a mild degree of reflux; in spite of these reservations, a micturating cystogram is a valuable investigation in the children under five
- radionucleide studies may also detect reflux when an MCU cannot be done
- a ^{99m}technetium DTPA scan indicates the function of each kidney and ^{99m}technetium DMSA scan provides an indication of tubular function

Vesico-ureteric reflux (VUR)

VUR is the retrograde passage of urine from the bladder into the ureters and kidney during micturition. Urine then drains back into the bladder forming a stagnant residue until the child next voids urine. Reflux thus provides a mechanism for infection to pass upwards into the kidney. In the majority of children the cause is uncertain; it may be due to a congenital abnormality of the vesico-ureteric junction, dysfunction with an atonic ureter, and exaggerated by the nearly 90° insertion of the ureter and thinness of the bladder wall in infancy. Reflux diminishes as children grow older, the insertion of the ureters is at a more acute angle and the increasing thickness of the bladder wall forms a more effective valve mechanism.

Vesico-ureteric reflux, when associated with reflux into the kidneys and UTIs causes permanent renal damage through scarring and occurs sufficiently often that it makes routine radiological investigations mandatory. Large scale studies have shown that the risk of renal scarring is greatest in the first year of life, especially for boys, and that many children investigated after the age of 1 year for what is thought to be a first infection already have renal scarring suggesting that they have had previous unrecognized (and untreated) infections. In schoolgirls with asymptomatic bacteriuria the incidence of scarring is the same at 12 years of age as at 5 years. Scarring thus appears to occur mainly in early infancy, emphasizing the vulnerability of the infant kidney and is uncommon after the age of five. It is essential, therefore, to examine the urine of any infant with unexplained fever. Prompt treatment of a UTI in infancy will not only prevent renal damage from occurring but continuous prophylactic antibiotic therapy will control further infection, prevent further renal scarring and enable normal renal growth to take place. Progressive scarring will result in destruction of nephrons, chronic renal failure and hypertension. Prophylactic antibiotic treatment should probably be continued until all reflux has stopped, in some cases this may be until adolescence.

Treatment

Initial acute or occasional acute infection
Treat for 7 days to 10 days with ampicillin (amoxycillin, or amoxycillin with clavulanic acid), co-trimoxazole, cephalexin, nalidixic acid or trimethoprim. Avoid co-trimoxazole and nalidixic acid in infancy and G-6-PD deficient patients. An adequate fluid intake should be given. Culture the urine after completing treatment and investigate if it is the initial attack.

Prophylaxis
Co-trimoxazole and nitrofurantoin (once daily) and nalidixic acid (twice daily) are all suitable for long-term prophylaxis. When a breakthrough infection occurs the sensitivity of the organism should be determined before starting treatment. After an adequate course of treatment, i.e. 7−10 days, recul-ture the urine and revert to prophylactic treatment again if the infection has been eradicated. Amoxycillin, cephalexin and trimethoprim are not recommended for long-term prophylactic treatment.

Simple measures of treatment include:

- double micturition − the child voids and then waits up to 1 minute and then voids again urine which has refluxed and drained back into the bladder. This is especially important on waking and last thing at night.
- encourage the child to drink freely with a high fluid intake during the day.
- treat any constipation.

Surgery for VUR
Surgery should be avoided if at all possible, and especially in the first year of life. Even in the presence of severe reflux, normal renal growth will take place if infection can be prevented. After several months of freedom from infection some improvement in the degree of reflux may be seen. The indicators for surgery are:

- relief of obstruction, e.g. at vesico-ureteric junction
- increasing reflux and progressive dilatation of upper urinary tract in spite of prophylactic antibiotics
- recurrent infections in spite of prophylactic antibiotics, and progressive renal changes − reimplantation of the ureters may then be considered
- nephrectomy in children with total or nearly total loss of function in one kidney or with hypertension

Prognosis

This depends directly on the extent of renal damage (scarring), the presence of obstruction and reflux, and hypertension.

Urinary calculi (urolithiasis)

Urinary calculi are endemic in children even under the age of 5 years in Mediterranean countries, the Middle East and Far East, varying in size from pieces of gravel to large stones in the kidney or bladder.

Calculi result from the precipitation and crystallization of substances of low solubility, e.g. calcium salts (phosphate, carbonate and oxalate), uric acid and urates and occasionally cystine, when urine becomes supersaturated. Stone formation is aided by increased urinary concentration and excretion of these salts and changes in the pH which diminish solubility.

Four types of stone are seen:

1. triple phosphate calculi (magnesium ammonium phosphate and calcium phosphate) secondary to urinary tract infection with urea-splitting bacteria
2. uric acid stones — these have been found to be relatively common in young children in developing countries and the Middle East
3. Calcium stones, oxalate or phosphate or both, these are commonly found in concentrated urine in hot climates
4. cystine stones are uncommon but occur in cystinuria, an inborn error of metabolism

Aetiology

In the majority of children (except for cystine stones) the aetiology remains unknown as no underlying metabolic or urological abnormality can be identified and recognized causes of renal calculi are seldom found. Disorders known to predispose to stone formation include paraplegia, poliomyelitis and other conditions associated with prolonged immobilization; schistosomiasis; a foreign body in the urinary tract and congenital abnormalities which promote stasis and infection.

Postulated causes of urinary calculi in young children are:

1. Frequent attacks of infantile gastro-enteritis or high fevers resulting in dehydration and concentrated urine in which salts and uric acid become supersaturated and are precipitated forming a nidus for stone formation.
2. A cereal diet with a high calcium content. The virtual disappearance of childhood urolithiasis in western countries during the past 100 years has been attributed to a change from a predominantly cereal diet to one with much more meat and dairy produce.

Epidemiological and clinical features of urinary calculi in childhood:

- common under the age of 5 years

- higher incidence in boys
- frequent in the lower urinary tract
- uric acid stones are relatively common
- commoner in rural populations and lower socio-economic families.

Clinically, renal calculi present with loin pain, renal colic, haematuria or recurrent urinary infections. The diagnosis is confirmed by plain abdominal X-ray. Stones causing infections or other symptoms should be removed surgically. Patients known to have stones should be encouraged to maintain a high fluid intake.

Proteinuria

A small amount of protein is normally excreted in the urine each day. There are many confusing definitions of what constitutes 'significant proteinuria' but an excretion of more than 200 mg daily should be considered abnormal, the upper limit being normally about 150 mg. Girls and adolescents have a slightly higher excretion than boys. About two thirds of protein excreted in children is albumin, and one third is globulin plus Tamm—Horsfall protein (mucoprotein of tubular origin).

Urinary dip sticks which measure proteinuria are relatively imprecise and cover a range of values; accurate measurements should be made on timed 24 hour collections.

Dipstick reading	1+	2+	3+	4+
Protein mg/dl	30—99	100—299	300—999	>1000

More reliable methods of measuring the significance and degree of proteinuria are:

1. Semi-quantitative

   Measure $\dfrac{\text{Urinary protein mg/dl}}{\text{Urinary creatinine mg/dl}}$

   normal values are less than 0.2 in an early morning specimen
2. Quantitative

   normal urinary protein is $< 4\,mg/m^2/hour$ in a timed 12 to 24 hour collection

   significant proteinuria is $4—40\,mg/m^2/hour$

   nephrotic values are $> 40\,mg/m^2/hour$

Common causes of proteinuria in childhood

Benign orthostatic proteinuria

This accounts for about 75 per cent of all cases of childhood proteinuria. It may be transient, intermittent or permanent and is commoner in girls than boys. The cause is unknown but is probably related to changes in renal blood flow, the filtration fraction or the renin–angistensin system. Proteinuria is absent or minimal on waking and increases during the day, especially after standing for long periods.

Transient proteinuria

In association with:

- exercise
- fever
- dehydration and gastroenteritis

Glomerular disease
- acute glomerular nephritis
- chronic glomerular nephritis
- hereditary nephritis
- IgA nephropathy
- nephrotic syndrome

Tubular disease
- reflux nephropathy
- renal hypoplasia
- acute interstitial nephritis
- renal tubular acidosis

Investigation of proteinuria

Examine the early morning speciment of urine. A good deposit can be obtained from this for microscopy.

For orthostatic proteinuria, test the early morning specimen and serial specimens during the day. The early morning specimen should contain no more than a trace of protein, during the day proteinuria increases to 1+ or more. Drinking plenty of fluids during the day should ensure a good urine output. More than 200 mg protein in an overnight specimen is abnormal.

Further investigations will be directed towards the suspected underlying cause.

Haematuria

Up to five red blood cells per microlitre are normally present in freshly voided uncentrifuged urine. The cells are of glomerular origin and vary considerably in size and shape.

The commonly used dipsticks are much more sensitive to free haemoglobin than to intact red cells and will detect as little as 0.2 mg/dl of haemoglobin or myoglobin, approximately equivalent to between 5 and 20 r.b.c. per microlitre. A clinically significant number would be more than 50 r.b.c. per microlitre in a random urine specimen.

Macroscopic haematuria is one of the commonest symptoms of renal disease. The colour will vary from bright red to brown, depending on the site of origin of the blood, and the pH, concentration and age of the urine specimen. It must be distinguished from:

- haemoglobinuria and myoglobinuria
- a heavy deposit of amorphous urates which vary from salmon-pink to brick red in colour
- dyes in foodstuffs and drugs – these include beetroot, senna, phenolphthalein in alkaline urine and rifampicin
- porphyria (congenital erythropoietic type) or poisoning causing excessive porphyria production

Blue urine is seen in infants with abnormal tryptophan metabolism.

Black urine occurs in alcaptonuria, tyrosinosis, melanuria and during treatment with methyldopa.

Source of haematuria

It is seldom possible to be absolutely certain of the origin of the bleeding but the following guidelines are helpful:

Kidney and upper urinary tract
- urine is brownish coloured or 'smokey', resembling Coca-Cola or beer in colour
- proteinuria greater than 2+ on a dipstick
- red cell and white cell casts and granular casts almost always indicate glomerular disease
- red cells are deformed and variable in shape, often lacking haemoglobin
- renal tubular cells may be identified in the urinary sediment

Lower urinary tract
- terminal haematuria (urethral lesions however may cause bleeding at onset of micturition)
- blood clots in urine

- red cells are normal in shape, not distorted and have a normal haemoglobin content, though in acid urine this may be lost

Common causes of haematuria in childhood

- urinary tract infection − this is the commonest cause of gross haematuria, +/− fever, lower abdominal pain, frequency, dysuria, acute retention
- other infections
    - tuberculosis − usually microscopic haematuria
    - bacterial endocarditis
    - schistosomiasis − red, terminal haematuria in endemic areas
    - shunt nephritis
- trauma − may be renal or local to urethra or bladder − a foreign body in the urethra or vagina may cause unexplained haematuria
- acute glomerular nephritis − there is a typical history, brown urine, mild oedema and hypertension, casts and loin pain
- other forms of glomerular nephritis
- IgA nephropathy
- Henoch−Schönlein purpura
- benign focal glomerular nephritis
- hereditary nephritis − e.g. Alport's
- chronic glomerular nephritis − haematuria is uncommon, there is always significant proteinuria and casts.
- urinary calculi
- tumours of the renal tract
    - Wilms' tumour − the usual presentation is an abdominal mass but about 5 per cent present with haematuria +/− hypertension.
    - rhabdomyosarcoma of bladder
- bleeding disorders − haemophilia; leukaemia; idiopathic thrombocytopaenic purpura; sickle cell disease
- acute G-6-PD deficiency and autoimmune haemolytic anaemia tend to produce haemoglobinuria
- rare causes − hydronephrosis, polycystic disease, renal haemangioma, polyarteritis nodosa, systemic lupus erythematosus (SLE).

Investigation of haematuria

The cause is often obvious because of associated clinical features. If the diagnosis is not clear, and urine culture and clinical examination normal in the presence of microscopic haematuria, then an idiopathic or benign form of nephritis is most likely; acute nephritis is always accompanied by significant proteinuria. Appropriate investigation should exclude tuberculosis, bacterial endocarditis and other causes.

Acute glomerulonephritis

Aetiology

Acute glomerulonephritis is an immune complex disease associated with the consumption of complement, probably resulting from a preceding infection. Classically, nephritogenic strains of group A β haemolytic streptococci are the commonest infection, the evidence being culture of the organism from throat or skin swabs, and an acute rise in the anti-streptolysin O (ASO) titre, but hepatitis B virus has also been implicated in some cases, and it is thought that other viruses may be responsible in cases where there is no clear evidence of streptococcal involvement.

Clinical features

The peak incidence is in children of school age, but may occur from late infancy. Boys are affected slightly more often than girls. There may be a history of a sore throat or skin infection during the preceeding 2 to 3 weeks.

Acute nephritis is characterized by an acute onset with:

- oedema most noticeable around the eyes and face on waking, and, as it becomes more severe, around the ankles, legs and back of the hands
- haematuria − 'smoky urine', brownish in colour, with a progressive reduction in urinary output
- abdominal pain (probably due to oedema and stretching of the renal capsule)
- hypertension and headache − advanced cases may present with hypertensive encephalopathy, fits and anuria

Fluid retention results in hypervolaemia, some cardiomegaly and an apparent mild anaemia.

Laboratory findings

The principal biochemical changes are a raised

blood urea and serum creatinine indicating decreased glomerular filtration, diminished C3 serum complement, and a raised ESR. A rise in ASO titre and culture of β haemolytic streptococci from skin or throat swabs are helpful confirmatory evidence.

The urine contains red cells, protein and cellular casts of both red and white cells. The specific gravity is usually over 1020 and osmolality increased, over 500 mmol/l (mOsm/l).

Renal histology shows mesangial proliferation, deposits of IgG and C3, and polymorphonuclear leucocyte infiltration.

Clinical course

The majority of children will have an uncomplicated course with a diuresis within 1 to 2 weeks from presentation. During this time oliguria, haematuria and hypertension persist. A small number will progress to almost total anuria and require peritoneal dialysis, the indications being (1) severe fluid retention, (2) blood urea over 300 mg/dl (50 mmol/l), (3) severe electrolyte disturbance with serum potassium > 7 mmol/l, and bicarbonate persistently < 15 mmol/l. About 4 or 5 per cent may develop severe complications such as severe oliguria or anuria, hypertensive encephalopathy or severe fluid retention resulting in cardiac failure. After diuresis, microscopic haematuria and a trace of proteinuria may persist for several months before finally disappearing, the child remaining clinically well. Long-term prophylactic penicillin following acute nephritis is *not* necessary; relapses are rare and rheumatic heart disease is not associated with acute nephritis. A small number — not necessarily those with severe complications — progress at a variable rate into chronic renal failure with persistent proteinuria, with or without haematuria and elevated blood urea and creatinine, and hypertension. Others may progress into a nephrotic-like syndrome — about 5 per cent in some sub-tropical areas may go on to develop a nephrotic syndrome.

Principles of management

Restriction of fluid intake
This is to prevent pulmonary, cerebral and peripheral oedema.

Restrict fluid intake to 300 ml/m²/24 hours plus volume of urine output over previous 24 hours.

Careful measurement of fluid intake and output is essential.

Daily weighing provides an excellent assessment of fluid retention.

Restriction of sodium, potassium and protein intake
In acutely ill children restriction is not usually a problem because of accompanying anorexia. Electrolyte-free glucose drinks and carbohydrates should be freely given to spare protein breakdown. Sodium and potassium intake should be restricted to 20 mmol/day of each. Protein intake should not exceed 20 g/m²/day. Normal diet can be resumed after the diuresis.

Control of hypertension
Although hypertensive encephalopathy may occur with only modest elevations of blood pressure, the risk increases rapidly once diastolic pressure reaches 90−100 mm/Hg or systolic pressure exceeds 150−160 mm/Hg. Blood pressure should be measured twice daily or more often if indicated. Sedation with phenobarbitone may be required if blood pressure rises. Headache, dizziness or blurred vision denote impending encephalopathy. Acute encephalopathy must be treated in the usual way, with intravenous diazoxide or hydralazine, followed by oral hydralazine, propranolol or methyldopa.

Eradication of streptococci
A 10-day course of penicillin in full dosage should be given in all cases, whether or not streptococci are cultured from the throat swab. Organisms may be present in the tonsillar crypts and cannot always be isolated from surface swabs. In a small number of patients a full course of penicillin may fail to eradicate streptococci and a further course may be needed. Children who are sensitive to penicillin should be given erythromycin.

Note − It is not necessary to give long-term prophylactic penicillin after acute nephritis.

Bed rest
This is not necessary in mild cases, and often difficult to enforce, but excessive activity must be avoided. In the presence of increasing and severe hypertension, bed rest and sedation will be required.

Nephrotic syndrome (nephrosis)

Definition

The nephrotic syndrome (NS) is a clinical entity having multiple causes and characterized by:

- generalized oedema and ascites − the massive oedema (anasarca) may be accompanied by gross scrotal or vulval oedema, pulmonary oedema and pleural effusions (Figure 9.3)
- hypoalbuminaemia
- massive proteinuria $\geq 3.5\,g/1.73\,m^2/day$

Other features (not essential to the diagnosis) include hypercholesterolaemia and hyperlipidaemia, and disorders of coagulation.

Aetiology

The many causes of the nephrotic syndrome are summarized in Table 9.1. Minimal change NS is by far the commonest cause in childhood, though in some parts of the world other causes are important. In tropical Africa there is a strong association with quartan malaria, while in areas where bilharzia is endemic schistosomal NS is common. Renal involvement in sickle cell disease may result in nephrosis, as may amyloidosis of the kidney in familial Mediterranean fever. The recognition that mercury is highly toxic led to its withdrawal from use in teething powders in young children. Congenital nephrosis is uncommon outside of Scandinavia, but may occasionally be inherited.

Pathophysiology

The basic defect is an increase in glomerular permeability resulting in a massive leak of protein into the urine. This may be due to either deposition of immune (antigen-antibody) complexes on to the glomerular basement membrane or possibly the

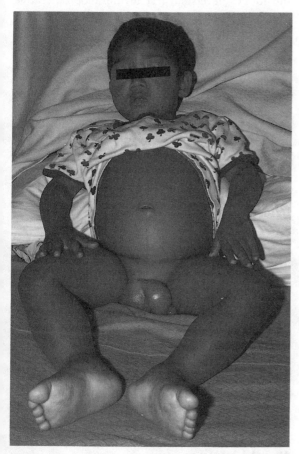

Figure 9.3 Nephrotic syndrome showing massive scrotal oedema

Table 9.1 *Aetiology of nephrotic syndrome*

Primary:

Minimal change nephrotic syndrome	Frequency 75%
Focal segmental glomerulosclerosis	10%
Membranoproliferative glomerulonephritis	10%
Miscellaneous, including congenital NS	5%

Secondary to generalized diseases − infections and immune complex diseases:

Post infections:	*Other:*
Group A β haemolytic streptococci	Henoch−Schönlein purpura
Hepatitis B	Systemic lupus erythematosus
Quartan malaria (*Plasmodium malariae*)	Polyarteritis
Schistosomiasis	Amyloidosis
Congenital syphilis	Renal vein thrombosis
Bacterial endocarditis	Sickle cell anaemia
HIV (AIDS)	Lymphoma
	Allergy−pollen and insect stings
	Chronic mercury intoxication
	Tropical nephropathy (S. Africa)
	Drugs − penicillamine, gold, mercury

basement membrane itself being the antigen involved. The exact mechanism of injury leading to an alteration of glomerular permeability is not known, but may involve an alteration of electrical charges.

Initially smaller protein molecules are lost in the urine, mainly albumin, resulting in a selective proteinuria. Non-selective proteinuria refers to the indiscriminate loss of all proteins. Hypoalbuminaemia develops when urinary losses exceed the rate of production of albumin by the liver. This leads to a reduction in intravascular colloidal osmotic pressure and permits the transudation of fluid into the interstitial tissues. The result is a fall in plasma volume and hypovolaemia. Urinary protein losses of > 4 g/day usually result in hypoalbuminaemia. Salt and water retention also contribute to the development of oedema, possibly due to intrarenal mechanisms rather than increased aldosterone secretion. Increased protein loss results in a compensatory hepatic protein synthesis of lipoproteins, mainly low density lipoprotein and hypercholesterolaemia. Protein may also be lost through the bowel wall from mucosal oedema causing a protein losing enteropathy.

Increased hypercoagulability of the blood may cause spontaneous thromboses in renal, pulmonary and systemic veins and is due to increased levels of factors V, VII, VIII and X, fibrinogen and platelets, though decreased levels of factors IX, XI and XII may develop.

Idiopathic nephrotic syndrome (minimal change NS)

The aetiology is unknown, glomerular damage presumably resulting from some immunological insult. The peak incidence is between 2 and 6 years of age with boys being affected slightly more often than girls. Relapses are commoner in the winter months. The onset is usually insidious with development of gradually increasing oedema, usually noticed first over the face, and becoming generalized over about a week. Apart from the gross oedema, which may close the eyes, and necessitate scrotal support, there are few other symptoms. In a few cases there may be a history of a preceeding respiratory infection.

Clinically, there is no haematuria on microscopy and blood pressure is normal. Urinary output is normal though reduced in hypovolaemia.

Diagnosis

The diagnosis is usually obvious, and is confirmed by the combination of gross oedema, gross proteinuria and hypoalbminaemia. The differential diagnosis is from angioneurotic oedema and other disorders with excessive protein loss − protein losing enteropathy, kwashiorkor and severe hookworm anaemia.

Laboratory findings

An increase in the haematocrit (PCV) indicates the onset of hypovolaemia. The blood count is otherwise normal.

Blood urea and creatinine are normal. The serum may appear fatty due to raised cholesterol and triglycerides. Serum albumin is almost invariably <30 g/l, and may fall as low as 15 g/l. IgG levels are also low; α_2 globulin is often raised.

Complement levels are normal in idiopathic NS, and low C_3 levels suggest membranoproliferative glomerulonephritis, with antigen−antibody complexes and the possibility of SLE.

The urine contains massive amounts of protein. Smaller proteins leak more readily than larger proteins and when protein consists mainly of albumin it is known as selective proteinuria. It may be determined by electrophoresis of urinary protein.

$$\text{Selectivity index} = \frac{\text{Urine : plasma ratio of low molecular weight protein}}{\text{urine : plasma ratio of high molecular weight protein}}$$

If:
   <0.1 indicates highly selective proteinuria − i.e. mainly albumin
   >0.2 indicates low or non-selective proteinuria, reflecting a general loss of protein or more severe glomerular damage.

Up to 15 or 20 g/day of protein may be lost ($\geqslant 50$ mg/kg/day) and albumin/globulin ratio is then reversed.

In severe cases tubular damage may result in aminoaciduria. Urinary sodium is low if there is hypovolaemia with salt and water retention.

Urine microscopy reveals fat bodies containing macrophages and granular casts.

Renal histology

The glomeruli appear normal on light microscopy,

but electron microscopy reveals loss of foot processes and swelling of podocytes on the glomerular basement membrane. These changes reverse on recovery.

Complications

1. Hypovolaemia and shock will develop as serum albumin falls progressively below 20 g/l. Symptoms indicative of hypovolaemia include cold peripheries and poor peripheral circulation, abdominal pain, low central venous pressure and low urinary sodium <10 mmol/l.
2. Infection, especially pneumococcal septicaemia and peritonitis and Gram-negative infections. These are due to loss of immunoglobulins, impaired opsonization and possibly impaired lymphocyte function. Urinary tract infections are especially common. High dosage steroid therapy also increases the risk of infection.
3. Thrombosis — arterial or venous. Elevated levels of clotting factors, hypovolaemia and hyperviscosity and increased platelet aggregation all contribute to an increased risk.
4. Acute renal failure. This is usually pre-renal due to hypovolaemia, sepsis or both, and may be complicated by acute tubular necrosis.
5. Malnutrition. Severe muscle wasting due to protein loss is evident once oedema disappears. The risk of sudden overwhelming sepsis is increased in these cases.
6. Hyperlipidaemia. This is mainly an increase in serum cholesterol, low density and very low density lipoproteins. High density lipoprotein levels are usually normal.

General management and treatment

The majority of children presenting with uncomplicated NS can be presumed to have idiopathic (minimal change) NS and this is steroid sensitive. Renal biopsy is now regarded as unnecessary.

General management
1. Weigh daily.
2. High protein diet — at least 3 g/kg/day with no added salt. In practice this is not always easily to achieve because of anorexia and malaise.
3. Accurate record of fluid intake and urinary output. If oliguric, restrict intake to previous day's output plus allowance for insensible losses (10 to 15 ml/kg/day).
4. Daily urine testing for protein and blood on the early morning specimen and random specimens during the day, using dipsticks (e.g. Albustix). A 24-hour urine collection is essential to measure total urinary protein losses.
5. Prevent hypovolaemia by monitoring serum albumin and haematocrit. Give salt-free albumin infusions, 1 g/kg as often as is necessary to maintain serum albumin above 20 g/l.
6. Treat vigorously any intercurrent infection or sepsis. If there is a risk of pneumococcal infection, give penicillin, but routine prophylactic penicillin in NS is not necessary. Chickenpox contacts in the acute stage or while on steroids should be given zoster immune globulin.
7. A careful explanation of the chronic nature of the illness and its natural history with tendency to relapses should be given to parents.

Treatment with steroids
The majority will respond to oral prednisolone, 2 mg/kg/day divided into two or three daily doses (maximum 80 mg/day), provided that there are no other general contra-indications to steroid therapy. An initial response in the form of diuresis and weight loss is usually seen within 2 weeks from the onset of treatment, but may occasionally be delayed for up to 6 weeks. After the initial diuresis and weight loss, and urine has been free of protein for about a week the dose can be gradually reduced. Further reductions in dosage can be made about every 4 or 5 days if the urine remains protein-free, until all treatment has been stopped by about 6 to 8 weeks.

Some children can only be kept free of proteinuria by a small dose of prednisolone daily, e.g. 5 or 10 mg. If long-term maintenance is necessary an alternate day regime for prednisolone is preferable, as this has less effect on growth. Prolonged use of steroids will result in all the usual complications including cushingoid appearance, and suppression of immune responses and growth.

About half of children with NS will either require maintenance treatment or relapse after stopping treatment, but will respond readily again to further short courses of oral prednisolone, the aim being to keep the urine totally free of protein or to show only a trace from time to time.

Parents and patients can be readily taught to test their urine at home with a dipstick test, and keep a diary of their daily tests.

Frequent relapsers often respond to higher doses of steroids and are probably best maintained on low dose alternate day prednisolone. Transient increases in proteinuria occur with any intercurrent infection and may require either a short course of prednisolone or an increase in maintenance treatment. Soluble prednisolone should be used whenever possible.

All children with NS should have their height plotted at regular intervals on growth charts to monitor the effect of steroids.

Diuretics

These should only be given if there is no response to steroids. Diuretics increase the risk of hypovolaemia unless salt-free albumen or protein has been given first. Potassium supplements may be required.

Renal biopsy

Renal biopsy is indicated only in patients not responding to steroids; in those who relapse very frequently or in those presenting with abnormal or unusual features such as haematuria or hypertension; or with progressive deterioration or evidence of multisystem disease.

Cytotoxic agents

These are reserved for treatment of frequent relapsers or if there is failure to respond to adequate doses of prednisolone. The long-term effects of such treatment are not known, thus both cyclophosphamide and chlorambucil inhibit spermatogenesis and may impair fertility if given for prolonged periods.

Regimes:

cyclophosphamide 2 to
  3 mg/kg/day
or   plus low dose
chlorambucil   prednisolone for
  0.15 mg/kg/day   8–12 weeks

If there is no improvement by 12 weeks, then stop treatment.
Azathioprine has been shown to be ineffective.

Prognosis

The majority of children with idiopathic NS will eventually go into remission though sometimes only after a series of relapses, often over several years.

During this time they may require many courses of prednisolone. Patients may be regarded as cured if the urine has been protein-free, with no relapses for 1 to 2 years. The major threats to life are from intercurrent infections, the complications of steroid therapy and development of progressive renal failure.

Other types of nephritis

Focal segmental glomerulosclerosis

This describes a histological picture in which only occasional glomeruli, or segments of a glomerulus are affected. Microscopically there are large intracapillary deposits of hyaline material, degeneration of podocytes, which frequently become separated from the basement membrane, and deposits of IgM and C3 within the hyaline material.

The patchy distribution of the lesions does not correlate well with the clinical features which are variable. There is microscopic haematuria, a raised blood urea and raised blood pressure. Only about 10 per cent of patients are steroid responsive. Some undergo spontaneous remission but the long-term prognosis is poor with variable progression to end stage renal failure.

Membranoproliferative (mesangiocapillary) glomerulonephritis

This accounts for about 10 per cent of childhood nephrosis. The onset may be insidious or rapid, presenting with a mixed picture of both nephritis and nephrotic symptoms, i.e. macroscopic haematuria, hypertension, raised blood urea and low C3 with generalized oedema. There is no response to steroids or immunosuppressive agents. The course of the disease is variable, some patients remaining in apparent remission or stable for several years before progressing into renal failure.

The histological picture is one of mesangial hypercellularity, with an increase in the mesangial matrix and splitting or reduplication of the basement membrane, in which dense deposits can be seen on electron microscopy.

Nephritis of Henoch-Schönlein purpura

Although the kidney is almost always involved in

the acute stage of Henoch-Schönlein purpura, with transient proteinuria and microscopic haematuria, only a small number go on to develop a frank nephritis or nephrotic syndrome. The long-term prognosis is good with about 75 per cent recovering over 5-year period. The histological picture, of hypercellularity and crescent formation, appears to correlate well with the clinical picture, but even those with large numbers of crescents may eventually recover. Steroids and immunosuppressive drugs alone or in combination do not appear to influence the prognosis or course of the disease. Children who present with a combined picture of acute nephritis and a nephrotic syndrome and have a large number of crescents in the renal biopsy generally have a poor outcome, eventually going into renal failure.

Quartan malarial nephrosis

A high incidence of NS associated with *Plasmodium malariae* infection occurs throughout West, Central and East Africa. The age of onset is somewhat later than in most parts of the world — between 5 and 7 years. Patients are generally resistant to steroid therapy, immunosuppressive agents and antimalarials, and the prognosis is poor with slow progression to renal failure and hypertension. Renal biopsy shows a varying degree of membranous glomerulonephritis and glomerulosclerosis with capsular adhesions and thickening of capillary walls. Deposits of *Plasmodium malariae* antibody complexes are found in the glomeruli.

Membranous glomerulonephritis

This is the commonest cause of NS in Southern Africa but has also been reported in children from places as widely divergent as Poland and Japan, with a tentative association with hepatitis B. The histological picture is one of diffuse thickening of the basement membrane on light microscopy. Fine granular immune complex deposits with immunoglobulin on the epithelial surface of the basement membrane are seen on immunofluorescence.

Hereditary nephritis

Several different forms of hereditary nephritis have been described. The best known is Alport's syndrome, probably due to a defect in the glomerular basement membrane. Inheritance is autosomal dominant in most families, though with variable penetrance, and other modes of inheritance have been described. Girls and women are generally less severely affected than boys, most of whom have progressed to renal failure by early adult life.

The disorder presents usually with progressive microscopic haematuria and proteinuria, later macroscopic haematuria may appear, and hypertension and chronic renal failure develop. Nephrosis is rare. Sensineural deafness is a frequent associated finding; hearing loss may be subclinical in early childhood, detectable only on audiometry, but becomes progressively more severe. Some 15 per cent of patients also develop abnormalities of the eye and lens. There is no effective treatment, other than that of chronic renal failure, the prognosis being generally worse for boys. Family members should be screened both for renal disease and deafness.

Renal tubular disorders

Fanconi's Syndrome

This refers to a number of disorders with multiple proximal tubular defects, characterized by glycosuria, aminoaciduria, phosphaturia and tubular acidosis due to bicarbonate wasting.

The commonest form is cystinosis, a recessively inherited inborn error of cystine metabolism in which cystine crystals are widely deposited throughout the body tissues. Affected infants present with failure to thrive, recurrent vomiting and dehydration, polyuria and polydipsia and rickets. In addition to the above features, there is a metabolic acidosis, hypokalaemia and low plasma phosphate. Diagnosis is confirmed by demonstrating cystine crystals in the bone marrow, lymph nodes, skin or by slit-lamp examination of the cornea and conjunctiva. Progressive renal failure occurs by the age of 10 years, requiring haemodialysis or renal transplantation.

A secondary Fanconi syndrome develops in a number of disorders in which renal tubular damage occurs. These include poisoning with heavy metals (lead, mercury), other chemicals and drugs including outdated preparations of tetracycline, Wilson's disease and galactosaemia.

Renal tubular acidosis (RTA)

This develops as a result of an inability of the tubules to acidify urine and excrete acid. The classical form is distal (type I) tubular acidosis. Most cases are inherited but secondary forms occur in hyperparathyroidism, excessive vitamin D administration and hypercalciuria; amphotericin toxicity; malnutrition; systemic lupus erythematosus and other disorders causing tubular damage.

It presents around 2 years of age with failure to thrive, polyuria and polydipsia, constipation, renal calculi and rickets. Potassium deficiency may cause weakness. Diagnosis is confirmed by finding a hyperchloraemic metabolic acidosis, a urine pH greater than six and failure to acidify urine after a standard ammonium chloride load. Treatment is with alkali, equivalent to daily endogenous acid production, as oral sodium and potassium citrate (Shohl's solution), 1 to 3 mmol/kg/day, the dose being adjusted to keep plasma bicarbonate within the normal range and urinary calcium below 2 mg/kg/day to avoid development of nephrocalcinosis. Proximal tubular acidosis is very rare.

Haemolytic uraemic syndrome

The haemolytic uraemic syndrome (HUS) is characterized by uraemia, thrombocytopenia and a microangiopathic haemolytic anaemia. It is an important cause of acute renal failure in infancy and childhood.

Aetiology
The HUS is now believed to result from a gastro-intestinal infection with verocytotoxin producing *Escherichia coli* of several different serotypes, especially O157:H7. At least two verocytotoxins (VT) have been identified, very similar in structure and antigenicity to shiga toxin, the virulent toxin of *Shigella dysenteriae* type I. The source of the *E. coli* is probably from contaminated food, especially of animal origin.

Pathophysiology
VT has a marked cytopathic effect on endothelial cells producing swelling of capillary endothelial cells and widening of the subendothial space. These microangiopathic changes are seen throughout the body but especially in the kidney. There is also a reduction in the platelet count, increased platelet aggregation and production of abnormal forms of factor VIII from endothelial cells, resulting in increased anticoagulant activity.

Clinical features
The syndrome may occur sporadically or in epidemics, especially in the summer and early autumn, and may be preceded by a mild gastrointestinal or respiratory illness. It can vary from a mild diarrhoeal illness to haemorrhagic colitis and the HUS. Symptoms include abdominal pain, pallor and oedema. Haemorrhagic symptoms may include haematuria, gastrointestinal bleeding and purpura. The anaemia may become rapidly severe and jaundice appears within 1 to 2 days. The blood urea rises, sometimes rapidly, to 300 mg/dl (50 µmol/l) or more with hypertension and encephalopathy.

Blood picture
A peripheral blood film shows many distorted and fragmented red blood cells − 'burr cells' − a leucocytosis and, as haemolysis increases, a reticulocytosis. The platelet count is reduced, as low as 50 000 per µl in severe cases. Fibrin degradation products are present in the plasma. C3 levels are normal. Coombs' test is negative.

Management
This is essentially supportive, and consists of measures to control acute renal failure (see page 99) and the management of hypertension which can be difficult to control. Peritoneal dialysis may be necessary. Treatment with heparin has not been shown to be effective as it is usually given after the microangiopathic process is already well established, too late to have much effect.

Anaemia must be corrected by small frequent blood transfusions, maintaining Hb at 8−10 g/dl if there is progressive haemolysis. Small transfusions are less likely to result in a significant rise in blood pressure. A transfusion with fresh platelets may be necessary if there is profound thrombocytopenia.

Prognosis
This depends on the severity of the renal lesions and complications including hypertension, mortality may be as high as 30 per cent, though children under 2 years of age tend to have a better prognosis.

Viral haemorrhagic fever with renal syndrome

Viral haemorrhagic fever with renal syndrome (HFRS) is a viral nephropathy caused by several different RNA viruses of the Hantaviridiae family. They are widely distributed across Europe and Asia, from Scandinavia across Europe and Russia to China and Japan, extending southwards to the Balkans and Mediterranean areas, and are responsible for a number of disorders previously known under different names, e.g. nephropathia epidemica in Scandinavia, Korean haemorrhagic fever and Hantaan virus fever. In China, HFRS is one of the most important viral infections with a mortality of up to 5 per cent but milder forms occur in Scandinavia, the Balkans and European Russia. Serological differences can be demonstrated between patients in the Far East and in Europe.

HFRS is essentially a zoonosis and a natural infection of rodents, humans acquiring the disease accidentally by contact with infected rodent urine, although human to human transmission can occur following exposure to infected secretions or blood.

Clinical features

The disease occurs in sporadic and epidemic forms. Symptoms include fever, headache and eye pain, lumbar pain and tenderness, conjunctivitis, periorbital oedema and petechial haemorrhages, especially on the palate and in the axillae. The clinical picture is very variable, from a mild, almost silent infection with proteinuria and mild renal dysfunction without haemorrhagic disease, to one with a severe haemorrhagic diathesis, fever, shock, and oliguria and anuria. A period of oliguria develops in the majority and is followed by polyuria as renal function recovers.

Laboratory findings include thrombocytopenia, associated with abnormal platelet function, haemoconcentration, proteinuria and uraemia in severe cases. Diagnosis is based on the finding of specific viral antibodies and isolation of the virus from blood or urine. Commoner disorders, including haemolytic uraemic syndrome, should first be excluded.

Management

As the virus is highly infectious, it is essential to prevent transmission in hospital and exposure of staff to infected materials. Suspected or diagnosed cases should be isolated and nursed with properly applied standard barrier nursing techniques.

The disease is usually self-limiting and management is supportive, with careful attention to fluid balance to avoid circulatory overload, and to treatment of renal failure. Small frequent transfusions of blood or platelets may be necessary.

Acute renal failure

Definition

Acute renal failure (ARF) is the sudden failure of the kidneys to excrete urine sufficient in amount or correct composition to maintain normal body fluid and electrolyte composition.

Although oliguria is a common feature ($<180-250 \, ml/m^2/day$), it is not an essential component of ARF, which can be observed with a urine output within the normal range — non-oliguric ARF. Other features include a metabolic acidosis, hyperkalaemia and a raised blood urea, serum creatinine and phosphate.

The normal urinary output ranges from 1.5 to 3 ml/kg/hour. Oliguria is defined as an output of less than 0.8 ml/kg/hour.

Aetiology

The many causes of ARF can conveniently be divided into three groups depending on the underlying mechanism:

1. *Pre-renal*
   This is due to decreased perfusion of the kidney caused by hypovolaemia, dehydration and gastroenteritis, haemorrhage, burns, shock, cardiac failure, hypotension, trauma, etc. It is probably the commonest cause of ARF in children.
2. *Intrinsic renal disease*
   This includes acute glomerulonephritis, renal infections, renal vein thrombosis, haemolytic–uraemic syndrome, nephrotoxins and disseminated intravascular coagulation, as well as untreated pre-renal failure.
3. *Post-renal*
   Obstructive uropathy from any lesion in the lower urinary tract is the major cause. These include congenital disorders such as obstruction at the pelvi-ureteric junction or vesico-ureteric

junction, posterior urethral valves, acquired conditions such as tumours, strictures, haematomas and trauma, calculi, deposition of crystals (sulphonamides and uric acid) and neurogenic bladder, resulting from spina bifida or trauma to the spinal cord.

Pathogenesis of ARF

This is complex and often the end result of several interrelated or separate pathological events rather than a single process, however three major factors contribute to the development of ARF:

1. renal haemodynamics − alterations in renal blood flow result in renal vasoconstriction through a number of still ill-understood mechanisms.
2. ischaemic damage and necrosis of tubular epithelial cells − as long as tubular cells remain damaged, the maintenance phase of ARF continues.
3. a disturbance of cellular and metabolic mechanisms

The common factor in all causes of pre-renal ARF is the decrease in intravascular volume with a reduction in renal blood flow and perfusion of the kidney, i.e., reduced glomerular filtration rate. There is increased tubular reabsorption of sodium and water. Urinary urea and osmolality are increased and sodium excretion decreased.

In intrinsic renal failure, the pathogenesis varies according to the aetiology, thus the glomerular filtration rate may be reduced in acute glomerulonephritis while other mechanisms include blockage of renal tubules by epithelial debris and casts, interstitial oedema or back diffusion of filtrate through damaged renal tubules. In intrinsic ARF urinary urea and osmolality are reduced, and sodium excretion increased. A series of tests on blood and urine are helpful in differentiating between pre-renal and intrinsic ARF (Table 9.2). However, if pre-renal failure is not corrected, it slowly passes into renal failure and so do the tests. The tubules begin to lose their ability to conserve sodium and exchange it for potassium, so urinary sodium begins to rise. As the concentrating capacity of the kidney fails serum creatinine and blood urea begin to rise and the urine/plasma ratio falls.

There are no specific tests for obstructive uropathy with ARF, though appropriate history, clinical investigations and X-rays are helpful. Acute tubular necrosis does not usually produce complete anuria and an output of 30 to 100 ml/day is usual. An output of less than this suggests obstruction, or acute glomerulonephritis, cortical necrosis or a vascular catastrophe with total necrosis of the kidneys. Complete and total anuria should raise the suspicion of obstructive uropathy.

Clinical features of ARF

Features of ARF *per se* include:

- oliguria

Table 9.2   *Pre-renal and intrinsic renal failure − laboratory differentiation*

Test	Pre-renal failure	Intrinsic renal failure
Urine specific gravity	>1.018	⩽1.010
Urine osmolality	>600 mmol/l (mOsm/l)	<400 mmol/l (mOsm/l)
	Exceeds plasma osmolality	Equal to or below plasma osmolality
Urine microscopy	Normal	Casts
Urine creatinine	>100 mg/dl	<70 mg/dl
	>8 mmol/l	<6 mmol/l
Creatinine urine/plasma ratio	>30	<20
Urine urea	>2000 mg/dl	<400 mg/dl
	>330 mmol/l	<66 mmol/l
Urea urine/plasma ratio	>14	<10
Urine sodium	<20 mmol/l	>30 mmol/l
Urine potassium	30−80 mmol/l	24−>30 mmol/l
Urine Na^+/K^+ ratio	<1	0.8−>1.0
	Usually 0.2	
Response to frusemide	Fair	None

- oedema and circulatory overload, including pulmonary oedema and congestive heart failure
- hypertension
- hyperkalaemia
- metabolic acidosis
- uraemia — irritability, drowsiness, coma and convulsions

There are three phases of ARF:

1. the initial sequence of events resulting in tubular damage
2. maintenance phase with low glomerular filtration rate
3. phase of recovery

Management of ARF

This is essentially one of supportive care until there is recovery of kidney function.

- identify the underlying cause and treat as appropriate
- catheterize the bladder to obtain urine samples, and determine the rate of urine flow (<0.5 ml/kg/hour = severe oliguria)
- put in an intravenous line for fluids, and measure central venous pressure
- investigation:
  - electrolytes, calcium, magnesium, uric acid
  - blood urea and creatinine
  - acid-base balance — pH, PCO_2, HCO_3
  - full blood count — film for fragmented RBC
  - urine: urea, creatinine, sodium, potassium, chloride; specific gravity, osmolality, pH, glucose; microscopy and culture

Induction of diuresis

Although a diuresis induced with frusemide or mannitol usually indicates pre-renal azotaemia, occasionally even in intrinsic renal disease an abnormal or higher urinary output may be induced without much effect on the course of the azotaemia. The use of diuretics may alter the composition of urine so that interpretation of tests may become difficult.

Use mannitol only when there is no circulatory overload. Infuse $0.2-0.5$ g/kg over 10 to 30 minutes ($1.0-2.5$ ml/kg of 20 per cent solution).

Frusemide is used when there is circulatory overload, and after correction of hypovolaemia; dosage is 1 mg/kg intravenously. Allow 2 hours for a diuretic effect. If urinary output increases by $5-10$ ml/kg during this period, the diagnosis is likely to be pre-renal failure. If output remains low, frusemide may be repeated once in the same dosage. In the absence of any response, the child is treated for intrinsic renal failure.

Note: If there is a reduction in ECF (dehydration), this must be restored irrespective of whether the patient has intrinsic renal failure. Caution is needed, however, to avoid circulatory overload.

Oliguric phase

General
During this phase:

- weigh the child daily or twice daily
- fluid intake and urinary output must be accurately recorded
- blood pressure measured four- or six-hourly
- blood and urine monitored daily for electrolytes, acid/base status, blood urea and creatinine and haemotological status
- a daily reduction in weight of 0.5 per cent is desirable

Fluid restriction.
Daily water intake is reduced to replenish insensible losses ($300-400$ ml/m^2) plus urine output plus any other losses. Insensible losses account for about one-third maintenance requirements and should be electrolyte free.

Electrolytes
Sodium intake — serum levels give a guide to requirements. In ARF hyponatraemia may be dilutional and sodium administration may further expand extracellular fluid space resulting in cardiac failure. Unless the child is vomiting or there is definite evidence of sodium deficit, it should be restricted.

Potassium — no potassium should be given during this phase.

Nutrition
Children with ARF are usually in a severe catabolic state. To minimize endogenous catabolism, a minimum of 1680 kJ/m^2/day (400 kcal/m^2/day) must be provided. Adequate nutrition can result in a positive nitrogen balance, aid recovery and wound

healing, and control of infection. Depending on the cause, many children can maintain an adequate oral intake of food. Glucose polymers and fats are especially useful as a source of energy. A central venous pressure line or cannulation of a large vein is preferable for parenteral dextrose infusions. Amino acid infusions should be used with care in the acute phase since they may aggravate renal failure, though small amounts of essential amino acids may hasten recovery. Multivitamin supplements should also be given. As renal function improves high class protein is gradually introduced.

Hyperkalaemia

This is a major metabolic abnormality and demands urgent attention. Urine is the main route of potassium excretion. In acidosis, potassium leaves the cells as H^+ ions enter and hence hyperkalaemia must be interpreted in relation to the degree of acidosis.

Urgent reduction of serum potassium is achieved by:

- Infusing 10 per cent calcium gluconate, (0.5 ml/kg) over 5 to 10 minutes; stop if heart rate falls below 100/minute
- Give 5 ml/kg intravenously of 25 g dextrose in 100 ml water containing soluble insulin 0.5 units/kg

These measures reduce serum potassium by shifting it back into the cells though they do not reduce total body potassium. This can be done by giving an ion-exchange resin, calcium resonium 1 g/kg, orally or by enema. It is effective within 12 hours.

Hypocalcaemia

This is secondary to the hyperphosphataemia when plasma phosphate is above 9.3 mg/dl (3 mmol/1). Serum calcium may fall below 8 mg/dl (2 mmol/1) and can be corrected by giving intravenous calcium gluconate. Hypocalcaemia may however be aggravated by the rapid correction of a metabolic acidosis, causing tetany or convulsions.

Metabolic acidosis

Treatment is directed towards correcting situations conducive to metabolic acidosis − e.g. shock, infection, hypoxia and inadequate calorie intake. It is however also partly due to the retention of H^+ ions, sulphate and phosphate. Active treatment is indicated if severe acidosis is present (pH < 7.10), by infusing sodium bicarbonate 8.3 per cent (1 ml/kg) slowly to avoid CNS complications.

Hypertension

If diastolic BP exceeds 100 mm/Hg (or is 3 SD above the age appropriate norm) it should be treated as a hypertensive crisis. A rapid rise in BP is more likely to result in symptoms and signs (headache, irritability and convulsions) than a slow rise. Antihypertensive drugs with rapid onset of action should be used − e.g. diazoxide, hydralazine, methyldopa and frusemide. Phlebotomy or dialysis or both may be required if hypertension is severe and unresponsive to antihypertensive drugs.

Circulatory overload

This may pose serious problems. Preventive measures include fluid and sodium restriction and treatment of hypertension. Anuric patients are unresponsive to diuretics. Digitalization, if necessary, must be done slowly and cautiously, maintenance doses must be adjusted depending on the status of renal function. Dialysis is necessary in refractory cases.

Infection control

Bacterial infections are responsible for about one-third of deaths in the acute phase. Prophylactic use of antibiotics is not recommended but any infection must be promptly treated. Dosage of drugs especially those excreted by the kidney, needs to be adjusted and appropriately reduced.

Indications for peritoneal dialysis

1. severe hyperkalaemia, unresponsive to medical management, levels above 7.5 mmol/1 usually require dialysis
2. severe metabolic acidosis which cannot be corrected with $NaHCO_3$, or when administration of sodium is undesirable such as fluid overload
3. severe fluid overload with heart failure, severe hypertension and pulmonary oedema
4. severe hypo- or hypernatraemia
5. uraemia − rigid criteria based on blood urea levels are not desirable, generally levels above 250 mg/dl are taken as an indication for dialysis; the rate of rise of blood urea and creatinine is more reliable, rapid rises indicating a need for dialysis; CNS symptoms are an indication.

Diuretic or recovery phase

This follows the oliguric phase and requires special attention.

1. *Acute glomerulonephritis*. In spite of the diuresis, renal tubular function is quite adequate to maintain homeostasis. The excess loss of fluids and electrolytes represents the excretion of those products accumulated during the oliguric phase. The loss is not sufficient to jeopardize renal function.
2. *Acute tubular necrosis*. Here, the excess diuresis is due to immaturity of the regenerating tubular epithelium which is not able to regulate the excretion of sodium, potassium and water. Hence it is important to replace fluids and electrolytes lost to prevent hypovolaemia recurring and possible reversion to the oligaemic phase.

Prognosis

This depends on the underlying cause of the ARF.

Chronic renal failure

Chronic renal failure (CRF) develops when progressive destruction and loss of functioning nephrons results in an inability of the kidney to concentrate and excrete normal nitrogenous waste products and maintain normal acid–base balance. In terms of glomerular filtration, CRF develops when glomerular filtration falls below about 15 ml/minute and severe renal failure when glomerular filtration is $\leqslant$ 5 ml/minute.

Presentation

In many cases the cause is clearly the end stage of known progressive disease – for example congenital abnormalities of the renal tract and kidney (such as dysplastic kidneys): hereditary disorders (nephritis and metabolic defects); glomerulonephritis, nephrotic syndrome and other forms of nephritis; recurrent urinary infections, pyelonephritis and reflux nephropathy, and cortical or tubular necrosis.

In other instances, the diagnosis is not clear and affected children present with failure to thrive, unexplained anaemia, unresponsive to treatment with iron, polyuria and polydipsia or enuresis,

hypertension or renal rickets. As renal failure progresses, there is increasing anorexia, vomiting and anaemia. Polyuria and polydipsia pass into oliguria and oedema. Biochemical changes become more pronounced with an increasing metabolic acidosis, hyperkalaemia, hyponatraemia, a fall in serum calcium and ionized calcium, a rise in serum phosphate and alkaline phosphatase and development of secondary hyperparathyroidism with generalized osteoporosis and renal osteodystrophy (renal rickets).

Management

The general principles of management are similar to those of acute renal failure.

Nutrition

An adequate diet is essential to maintain general health. The accompanying anorexia frequently results in an inadequate calorie intake; the aim should be to ensure at least 336 and preferably up to 420 kJ/kg/day (80–100 kcal/kg/day) using glucose polymers or other carbohydrate supplements together with vitamins and minerals. It is important that the diet is palatable and one which the child will eat and enjoy. In early CRF an adequate protein intake is essential to maintain growth and nutrition and should be of high biological value (first-class protein), but will have to be restricted to around 0.5 g/kg/day when serum creatinine exceeds 4 mg/dl (360 μ mol/l). Symptomatic treatment of vomiting with metaclopramide may be required.

Sodium

Intake should be restricted to about 2 mg/kg/day unless there is excessive salt loss in the urine. More severe salt restriction is necessary when hypertension and oedema are present. Sodium intake may be significantly increased during treatment with sodium bicarbonate, and sodium salts of drugs and antibiotics.

Potassium

Intake should not exceed 1 mmol/day. Food and drinks with a high potassium content should be avoided. Treatment with an ion-exchange resin (Resonium) may be necessary.

Water

Any restriction of fluid intake is contra-indicated

while there is polyuria and polydipsia; it may have to be increased in the presence of fever or very hot weather. When urinary output diminishes, or oedema appears, fluid intake must then be restricted.

Hypocalcaemia, hyperphosphataemia and renal osteodystrophy

Renal osteodystrophy begins when alkaline phosphatase exceeds 130 iu/l before the classical radiological changes develop. Calcium supplements, as calcium carbonate, may be necessary to maintain a daily intake of 1 g/day and adequate serum calcium levels, this also has the advantage of helping to control the metabolic acidosis.

Serum calcium can also be maintained within normal levels by giving vitamin D analogues (e.g. 1-α-hydroxycholecalciferol). Regular monitoring of serum calcium is essential as hypercalcaemia may develop, resulting in a further decrease in renal function and nephrocalcinosis. Vitamin D itself is not now used since its activity is poor and large doses are necessary.

Metabolic acidosis

This may contribute to a rise in serum potassium. Control with sodium bicarbonate will become necessary when serum bicarbonate falls below 15 mmol/l but it will however increase the sodium load and the risk of tetany from hypocalcaemia.

Hypertension

The onset is often insidious and the degree of hypertension variable; it is aggravated by sodium and fluid retention, including sodium bicarbonate given therapeutically. Treatment is with diuretics — frusemide and spironolactone — and hydralazine, propranolol or methyldopa. Angiotensin converting enzyme inhibitors should not be used as they may cause a further deterioration in renal function.

Anaemia

The anaemia of renal failure is due to defective erythropoietin production by the damaged kidney and is unresponsive to iron. It can be corrected by small transfusions of packed cells, care being taken to avoid circulatory overload. Any effect, however, is only temporary.

Long-term management

As renal failure progresses, a decision must be made on future management — namely, long-term haemodialysis and/or renal transplantation. This decision must be made sooner rather than later, and will be governed by the availability of facilities for haemodialysis and transplantation, as well as the wishes of the parents, and should be a joint decision with them, as far as is possible. Long-term peritoneal dialysis is not practical in young children. If neither dialysis nor transplantation is possible, then a sensitive and sympathetic approach to management in the terminal stages is essential; the aim being to relieve any suffering and make the child as comfortable as possible, avoiding aggressive treatment which will result in only transient improvement without increasing the quality of life or life expectancy. There should be a full discussion with the family to decide whether terminal care should be at home or in hospital, this will obviously depend on the family's ability to cope and their wishes.

10

Diseases of the Respiratory Tract

Respiratory infections, together with malnutrition and gastroenteritis, are the 'Big 3' diseases of infancy and childhood in the tropics/developing world.

Infection may be located at various levels in the respiratory tract:

1. *Upper respiratory tract*
   - nose — colds
   - pharynx (throat) — pharyngitis: sore throats: tonsillitis
   - middle ear — otitis media
   - larynx and trachea — laryngitis: laryngo-tracheitis (croup)
2. *Lower respiratory tract*
   - bronchi — bronchitis
   - bronchioles — bronchiolitis
   - lung — pneumonia and bronchopneumonia

Infants and preschool children will have between six and nine respiratory infections each year; although many of these will be relatively minor, they may be accompanied by considerable constitutional disturbances including febrile convulsions. About a quarter will involve the lower respiratory tract and tend to be more severe and prolonged, and about 20 per cent will result in a hospital admission in children under a year old.

Studies from the UK show that acute respiratory infections account for half the illnesses in preschool children and one third in school children, and are probably the commonest cause of acute medical admissions to hospital under the age of one year, while in India and Central America they are only exceeded by gastroenteritis. They are thus a major cause of morbidity and mortality. The presence of anaemia or malnutrition will significantly influence the outcome of any respiratory illness.

About 80 per cent of childhood respiratory infections are due to viruses or mycoplasma, the remaining are bacterial. There are about 200 known respiratory viruses including various serotypes and subtypes. It is generally impossible to say clinically which particular virus is responsible for a given infection as different viruses often produce a similar clinical picture, although certain viruses do tend to be predominantly associated with specific illnesses (Table 10.1). For example the respiratory syncitial virus (RS virus), although classically associated with acute bronchiolitis, may simply cause a cold or upper respiratory illness with a febrile convulsion, while adenoviruses can also cause acute bronchiolitis clinically indistinguishable from that due to RS virus infection.

Table 10.2 summarizes antibiotic treatment of respiratory infection.

Some general points about respiratory infections

1. Although the distinction between upper and lower respiratory infections is useful and clinically valid in adults and older children, it becomes much more blurred in infants and young children in whom a mild upper respiratory infection may quickly progress into a severe lower respiratory tract infection.
2. Spread is from person to person via droplet infection through close contact, sneezing and coughing.
3. Infections often appear in epidemics or mild epidemics, especially in 'closed' communities (schools, hostels, nurses' homes, etc.). Overcrowding and poor ventilation favours rapid spread. Epidemics tend to be seasonal and are more prevalent in cold, wet rainy seasons and winter; fewer epidemics occur in mild winters.
4. Boys tend to be affected more often than girls in ratio of 60/40.
5. The incubation period is usually short, a matter

Table 10.1 *Acute respiratory infections and common causal organisms*

Clinical syndrome	Common causal organism	
	Viral	*Bacterial*
Non-specific upper respiratory tract infection, Common cold	Rhinovirus +++ (more than 70 serotypes) Also adenovirus, RS virus ++ Parainfluenza ++ Enteroviruses (+/− gastrointestinal symptoms) ++	*Haemophilus influenzae, Streptococcus pneumoniae Branhamella catarrhalis* all as secondary invaders
Acute pharyngitis Tonsillitis	Adenovirus +++ (many different strains). Enteroviruses (Coxsackie A and B, ECHO) ++ Rhinoviruses ++	β-haemolytic streptococci *Corynebacterium. diphtheriae*
with ulcerative stomatitis	EB virus (glandular fever) + (older children) Herpesvirus Hominis ++ Coxsackie A	Vincent's organisms
Epidemic conjunctivitis with pharyngitis	Adenovirus	
Acute laryngo-tracheo-bronchitis (Croup)	Parainfluenza +++ Also adenovirus + RS virus + Measles +	*H. influenzae* esp. type b *C. diphtheriae*
Acute epiglottitis		*H. influenzae* type b
Acute bronchiolitis	RS virus ++++ Also adenovirus ++ parainfluenza +	
Acute pneumonias	Adenovirus ++ RS virus ++ Influenza ++ Parainfluenza + Measles ++	*Strept. pneumoniae* *H. influenzae* *Bordetella pertussis* *Staphylococcus, Klebsiella* Less commonly: *Escherichia coli*, haemolytic streptococci
Non-bacterial 'atypical pneumonia'.		*Mycoplasma pneumoniae* *Coxiella. burnetti*

Table 10.2 *Antibiotic treatment of respiratory infections*

Infection	Antibiotic	
	1st choice	2nd choice
Common cold	None	
Bronchiolitis	None	
Pharyngitis, tonsillitis	Penicillin	Erythromycin
Diphtheria	Erythromycin	Penicillin
Otitis media	Penicillin or ampicillin (amoxycillin)	Co-trimoxazole or erythromycin
Acute laryngo-tracheo-bronchitis (croup)	None or (ampicillin or amoxycillin)	
Acute epiglottitis	Chloramphenicol	Cefuroxime
Lobar pneumonia	Penicillin or chloramphenicol or ampicillin/amoxycillin	Erythromycin
Bronchopneumonia	Ampicillin/amoxycillin +/− flucloxacillin or chloramphenicol	Cefachlor or cefuroxime
Severe pneumonia (uncertain aetiology)	Ampicillin/amoxycillin + gentamicin	Cefuroxime or chloramphenicol
Staphylococcal pneumonia	Flucloxacillin + gentamicin	Fusidic acid
Mycoplasma pneumoniae	Erythromycin	Tetracycline

of days or a week at the most, and the onset sudden.

6. Most are highly infectious — as infectious as gastroenteritis, if not more so — and where possible affected infants should be isolated. Whether it is possible or practical to segregate or isolate such children in busy outpatient clinics is questionable* though every effort should be made in hospital to isolate children with obvious infections in cubicles.

7. Certain groups of children are particularly vulnerable — the debilitated, malnourished, anaemic, or premature; those with congenital heart disease, congenital malformations, or physical or mental handicap all have a much higher morbidity and mortality.

8. Most children become non-infectious after a few days. The degree of resultant immunity is very variable and depends on the infecting organism, thus infection with the RS virus produces lasting immunity while rhinoviruses and coronaviruses produce only transient immunity.

9. Children with respiratory infections are usually anorexic, and infants with nasal obstruction may

* 35 per cent of children with measles in a Cameroon study caught the disease at a clinic or hospital consultation!

have difficulty in sucking. Mothers must be made aware of the need to maintain adequate fluid and food intake, by small frequent feeds.

Viral upper respiratory tract infections

Viral upper respiratory tract infections with only mild coryzal symptoms but with a high fever (temperature 39° or 40°C) and often sudden in onset are commonly seen in outpatient clinics, especially in children between 9 months and 3 years of age. There is a 24 or 48 hour history of malaise and anorexia, followed by sudden onset of high fever and often accompanied by febrile convulsions, frequently exacerbated by mistakenly wrapping the child up tightly with layers of clothing. In spite of the considerable constitutional disturbance, there are often remarkably few, if any, obvious physical signs except perhaps mild inflammation of the throat and/or ears. Tepid sponging and paracetamol are the only treatment necessary; the temperature often goes down within 24 to 48 hours, by which time the child is much better, although sometimes a definite pharyngitis or otitis media, or bronchitis may follow. In the absence of obvious physical signs, the possibility of malaria or a urinary infection may have to be considered.

The common cold

Most babies will have at least one cold by 6 months of age, although they are uncommon and tend to be mild in the first few weeks of life presumably because of some protection from maternal antibodies.

Secretions and oedema rapidly obstruct the narrow nasal passages of young infants who find nasal breathing difficult especially during feeds. Infants breathe through their nose and do not learn to breathe through the mouth until they are about 4 or 5 months old. A blocked nose can produce considerable breathing difficulties and even respiratory distress when feeding because of inability to co-ordinate breathing and sucking. There is also evidence that nasal obstruction in some babies may reduce their respiratory drive rather than accentuating it, and is a contributory factor in some 'cot deaths' (sudden unexpected infant deaths).

Treatment

There is no cure for the common cold. Symptomatic treatment, however, may relieve distressing symptoms, but will not shorten the illness.

Nasal decongestants
These are helpful in relieving obstruction and breathing difficulties. Excess mucus should be gently cleared from the nose and one drop of ½ per cent or 1 per cent ephedrine nasal drops in normal saline inserted into each nostril about 15 to 20 minutes before each feed. The drops should not be used for more than 3 or 4 days as rebound nasal congestion will develop. Long acting preparations of up to 12 hours duration – though more expensive – can also be used. These include xylometazoline or oxymetazoline.

To instil nasal drops the infant should be placed on the mother's knee with the head well back so that the drops pass into the nasal cavity and not directly into the back of the throat.

Oral decongestants
These drugs, e.g. pseudoephedrine, are *not* recommended for use in young children.

Analgesics
Soluble aspirin and paracetamol are the best drugs for symptomatic relief of the miserable, febrile irritable child. There is probably not much to choose between them, though paracetamol is safer as it does not cause gastric irritation and bleeding.

Compound proprietary preparations containing an antihistamine, decongestant and sometimes cough sedative should not be given to young children as overdosage can readily occur and the sedative action of antihistamines causes excessive drowsiness and even respiratory depression.

Antibiotics
These have no place in the treatment of the common cold and should never be used. However, young children with a long standing profuse purulent nasal discharge, the result of secondary bacterial infection, are commonly seen in outpatient clinics and a short course of an antibiotic – penicillin, erythromycin or amoxycillin – may be justified.

General

Children with colds are usually reluctant to feed. Maintain an adequate fluid intake by encouraging the child to drink small amounts. Milk is the preferred fluid but many children will only take their favourite drink, and much patience and persuasion may be needed.

As many of the common infectious diseases begin with symptoms of a cold, a careful examination is necessary to exclude these.

Sore throat, pharyngitis, tonsillitis

Sore throat is one of the commonest childhood infections, though young children seldom complain of a sore throat, even when it is very inflamed or the tonsils frankly purulent and so it is an essential part of the routine examination of every child to look into the throat and ears. Failure to do so amounts almost to criminal negligence.

Examination of the throat

Most children are frightened by having spatulas or swabs stuck into their mouth and down the throat. An explanation to older children is worth while and asking for their co-operation by assuring them that nothing need be put into the mouth. They are asked to extend the neck and put the head well back, opening the mouth as widely as possible. A torch can then be shone vertically down on to the posterior pharynx and the child asked to say 'ah' loudly, or else put out his tongue. This may be repeated several times to obtain a good view. Alternatively, the child may be told that a spatula will be gently introduced into the mouth and the tongue gently depressed when asked to say 'ah'. An extra minute spent obtaining the child's confidence and co-operation in this way is time well spent.

When a child is struggling or screaming and co-operation obviously impossible, sit the child on the mother's knee facing forwards, and with an assistant holding the head back, proceed as above. With careful timing, it is often possible to get a good view of the pharynx while taking a history if the child is crying or screaming.

Clinical features

High fever, to 40°C (or even 41°C) with malaise, loss of appetite for both food and fluids, and sometimes vomiting, of 24 to 48 hours duration is the common presentation. Enlarged and tender cervical and tonsillar glands may be prominent, sometimes more than the tonsillitis itself, and may not always subside fully after an attack. Indeed after several episodes of tonsillitis the glands may remain quite large but discrete and mobile, causing both doctor and parents to worry that the child has something more sinister such as leukaemia or tuberculous glands.

Quite marked neck stiffness due to muscle spasm from inflamed and painful tonsils and cervical glands may mimic meningitis especially if the child is irritable, has a high fever, and a febrile convulsion. In such circumstances a lumbar puncture is essential to exclude meningitis, since it may coexist sometimes with tonsillitis.

Abdominal pain is quite common in older children and may precede a sore throat by 24–48 hours. The pain may be sufficiently severe to suggest acute appendicitis, and is thought to be due to enlarged, inflamed mesenteric lymph nodes which are visible at laparotomy. Adenovirus has been cultured from such glands.

Differential diagnosis

It is impossible to say what the infecting organism is from the appearance of the tonsils, but in general, the less severe the inflammation and exudate, the more likely it is to be viral, with adenovirus predominating. Beta-haemolytic streptococcal infection is still the commonest bacterial cause, and is often associated with a purulent exudate and systemic 'flu-like symptoms', headache and limb pains.

An exudate is also a feature of both glandular fever and diphtheria, and in the much less common acute leukaemia and agranulocytosis. In glandular fever, (uncommon in young children) the exudate is generally a paler yellow, and there may be petechiae on the soft palate, whereas the diphtheria membrane is greyish in colour and may bleed on attempting to lift it off the tonsil. Less common bacterial causes are pneumococci, meningococci and *Staphylococcus aureus*.

Management

The main problem in everyday practice is to decide, 'Is this a viral sore throat or a β-haemolytic streptococcal infection?'. Bacteriological services are generally not readily available and in any case decisions on treatment often have to be made on the spot and cannot be deferred for 24 hours until the bacteriological results are available. If a decision is made to use antibiotics, then penicillin remains the drug of choice for streptococcal infections. In busy outpatient clinics, or where patient compliance is in doubt, treatment should be started with an initial injection of a long acting variety — procaine or benzathine penicillin to be followed by oral penicillin V. Where there is known hypersensitivity to penicillin, erythromycin 125 mg 6 hourly may be given.

Initially, penicillin should be given in full doses for 10 days to eradicate streptococci completely from the tonsillar crypts, especially where there is concern about rheumatic fever, but it is seldom possible to achieve this in practice.

If there is no clear indication for penicillin, then symptomatic treatment with analgesics (paracetamol or soluble aspirin) should suffice. An adequate fluid intake must be encouraged. If diphtheria is suspected, given antidiphtheritic serum immediately before waiting for laboratory results.

Complications

Acute otitis media
Spread along the eustachian tube to the middle ear frequently co-exists with tonsillitis. The ear-drum

may be only mildly inflamed, especially with a viral aetiology, but if it is acutely inflamed, it is wise to treat with antibiotics.

Peritonsillar abcess (quinsy)
May complicate severe tonsillitis. It is extremely painful, with much local swelling, and the child is quite toxic. Surgical drainage is required.

Rheumatic fever
In spite of the known association between β-haemolytic streptococcal infection, and rheumatic fever, it is not always possible to obtain a history of a preceeding sore throat, nor in established cases of rheumatic heart disease is there always a clear history of rheumatic fever. Because of the frequency of rheumatic heart disease, it is wise to err on the side of caution and give penicillin in adequate dosage when in doubt.

Otitis media

This is one of the commonest childhood infections and frequently coexists with pharyngitis. More than half are bacterial infections with *Haemophilus influenzae* being the commonest organism in infancy, and *Streptococcus pneumoniae* predominant in older children and adults. *Branhamella catarrhalis*, streptococci and staphylococci are less often involved.

Clinical features

Constitutional disturbance is often marked and affected infants and young children are febrile, irritable, and miserable, difficult to settle and refuse their feeds. They have frequently kept their worried and anxious parents awake all night, crying and restless, settling for a few moments when cuddled, only to start crying again a short time later. The story that a child has been 'pulling at his ears' is suggestive but by no means conclusive evidence of otitis media.

Examination of the ears

This is essential to confirm the diagnosis, but it is not always possible to see the ear drum in small infants or it may be obscured by wax, which can be difficult to remove. In such circumstances, if the

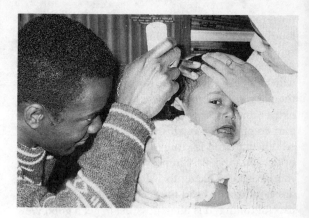

Figure 10.1 Examination of the ear

history is suggestive, it is justifiable to assume that the child has otitis media and treat accordingly.

Technique
Sit the child sideways on the mother's knee, pressing his inner arm against her chest. She is then able to steady his head with one hand, pressing it securely against her chest or shoulder, and with her other hand secure his shoulder and outer arm, and is this able to hold him firmly. The auroscope should be held as shown (Figure 10.1), in an inverted position against the side of the child's head, so that it will move with any sudden movements made by the child and the eardrum will not be damaged.

Treatment

The high frequency of bacterial infection and its complications makes antibiotic treatment essential. The predominance of *H. influenzae* and pneumococci makes ampicillin (or amoxycillin) the drug of choice. Unfortunately, the world-wide indisciminate use of ampicillin has resulted in an increasing number of resistant strains of *H. influenzae*, many of which are β-lactamase producing. Alternative antibiotics include co-trimoxazole, erythromycin and penicillin, or the newer, but more expensive preparations such as the combination of amoxycillin with the β-lactamase inhibitor clavulanic acid or cephaclor, one of the newer caphalosporins. It should be noted that many of the latter are inactive against *H. influenzae*. It is often useful in outpatient clinics to start treatment with an intramuscular injection of antibiotic and follow up with oral treatment for at least 5 to 7 days.

Decongestants

Nasal decongestants, e.g. ephedrine nose drops or one of the longer acting preparations (see common cold page 108) are thought to be helpful in reducing oedema and mucosal swelling of the eustachian tube, nasal mucosa and ostia of the sinuses and so promoting drainage of inflammatory exudate and fluids from the middle ear.

Ear drops

Ear drops with topical antibiotics are of no value in the treatment of otitis media.

Analgesics

Paracetamol or soluble aspirin are very helpful in relieving pain and general discomfort and should never be withheld.

Myringotomy

This is seldom necessary. The main indication is in the child with severe persistent pain, unrelieved by antibiotic treatment and in whom the ear drum is clearly bulging due to pus in the middle ear. Decompression will relieve the tension and pain, and drain off the pus.

Complications

With prompt and adequate treatment attacks of acute otitis media, mastoiditis, chronic purulent otitis media and the rarer venous sinus thrombosis and cerebral abscess are now becoming uncommon complications.

Remember, however, that occasionally acute bacterial meningitis may coexist with acute otitis media and in doubtful cases where there is neck stiffness or some clouding of consciousness, a lumbar puncture is essential.

Deafness

A conductive deafness of mild to moderate severity is, not surprisingly, common in children who suffer from recurrent attacks of acute otitis media, and if unrecognized may be responsible for learning difficulties and behaviour problems at school.

'Glue ear'

Recurrent attacks of otitis media may result in the accumulation of serous, mucoid or even purulent secretions within the middle ear with significant impairment of hearing. Such children should be referred to an ENT surgeon for drainage and possible insertion of grommets.

Laryngo-tracheo-bronchitis (LBT); croup: stridor: epiglottitis

Definitions

Stridor

Harsh noisy breathing due to obstruction at the larynx or just above or below it. It is almost always heard during inspiration.

Croup

Harsh barking dry cough.

The clinical picture of croup, associated with stridor, is usually due to acute laryngo-tracheo-bronchitis, or acute epiglottitis which is rarer, but much more dangerous. Most cases of croup are viral — due either to parainfluenza virus, or less often RS virus or adenovirus, though occasionally *Haemophilus influenzae* may be responsible, and diphtheria may present as croup

Pathology

The smaller the child, the greater is the likelihood of respiratory obstruction developing because of the very small size of the infant's larynx. Even a modest degree of mucosal oedema and inflammatory exudate may reduce the air flow by as much as 50 per cent. Moreover, because tracheal pressure is below atmospheric, inspiratory efforts tend to cause the trachea to collapse on itself and efforts to overcome this add to the work of breathing and frighten the child.

Clinical features

Although children of any age can be affected, it is most common between the ages of 6 months and 4 years. The onset is generally sudden, classically the child wakes up in the middle of the night with croup, or stridor, or both, having been quite well at bedtime, although some may have had symptoms of a mild upper respiratory tract infection for a day or two. Fever is not usually marked.

Although symptoms are alarming and frightening for parents, the illness runs a relatively mild course and is short lived in most children, symptoms subsiding with a minimum of treatment within 24 to 48 hours. In a few however, there is a rapid progression with increasing respiratory obstruction, the effort of breathing and inspiratory stridor is markedly increased, often out of all proportion to the modest increase in respiratory rate. Increasing drowsiness and restlessness are signs of cerebral hypoxia and CO_2 retention. Cyanosis is a late, pre-terminal event and demands urgent relief.

Acute epiglottitis

Is predominantly a bacterial infection with *Haemophilus influenzae* type b. Blood cultures are frequently positive. The epiglottis becomes acutely inflamed and oedematous, appearing as a cherry red swelling. There is considerable systemic disturbance with fever and toxicity, and the airway may be almost occluded causing severe respiratory distress. If acute epiglottitis is suspected, attempts should *not* be made to view the epiglottis with either torch and spatula or laryngoscope as this often results in spasm of the epiglottis or larynx with rapid deterioration and total obstruction.

Management

Croup should be managed in hospital under close observation for signs of early deterioration and respiratory obstruction once stridor is present. Pulse and respiratory rate should be recorded carefully and charted at half hourly intervals (or even quarter hourly in severe cases), together with the degree of recession and restlessness. Mild cases require no more than this close observation. *Sedation* should *not* be given. Although a young child may be restless and frightened by the effort of breathing and coming into hospital, sedatives may mask the restlessness of cerebral hypoxia – a most important sign – and depress respiration as well as making a child more confused. Relieving the tension and anxiety of parents is often sufficient to reassure the child.

Humidity

It has been customary in the past to nurse children with croup in oxygen tents or croupettes, surrounded by a sea of mist. There is however, very little firm evidence that it is of any benefit; tents are frightening for the child, prevent adequate observation by nurses and may become too hot or too cold. Humidity is best given via a nebulizer.

Oxygen

This is of course is essential to relieve hypoxia in severe obstructions, but it may also be of considerable benefit in moderate cases where a child is restless. Oxygen given directly from a cylinder is cold and dry and should never be delivered directly without first passing it through a warmed humidifier.

Antibiotics

As most cases of croup are viral, antibiotics are neither necessary nor beneficial. In some cases, with systemic symptoms:

- when a bacterial cause is suspected; or
- where there is doubt about the cause

ampicillin (or amoxycillin) should be given, preferably intravenously or intramuscularly initially. In cases where there is known to be a high incidence of ampicillin resistant or β-lactamase producing strains of *H. influenzae*, especially type b, chloramphenicol may justifiably be used instead. If *epiglottitis* is suspected (or proven), antibiotic therapy is mandatory and chloramphenicol, by intravenous or intramuscular injection, is the drug of choice.

Steroids

The place of corticosteroids in the treatment of acute LTB has never been clearly defined. The rationale of using steroids is that they may reduce the inflammatory swelling but the few clinical trials that have been done have failed to show any conclusive benefit.

General support

Insensible fluid losses through the respiratory tract may be high (especially in hot dry climates) and adequate hydration and fluid intake is essential. Intravenous fluids may be necessary as many children will be unable to maintain an adequate intake by mouth.

Tracheostomy

It is good policy to notify one's ENT surgeon and anaesthetic colleagues of the admission of every severe case of croup. It is always preferable to do a tracheostomy sooner, rather than later, in an unhurried manner by a skilled surgeon, under a general anaesthetic and in an operating theatre. Emergency tracheostomy, under less than ideal conditions, is a difficult and potentially hazardous operation, not to be undertaken lightly by the inexperienced, though sometimes it must to be done to save life. A useful temporary, emergency procedure is to take the widest bore needle available and puncture the trachea, introducing the tip of the needle through the midline of the neck anteriorly in the subglottic region, into the lumen of the trachea to act as a temporary tracheostomy tube.

Indications for tracheostomy

Increasing respiratory obstruction and the need for tracheostomy is indicated by:

1. a steadily rising pulse rate — over 160 per minute is significant
2. increasing restlessness — a sign of cerebral anoxia — and increasing respiratory effort in spite of treatment
3. increasing drowsiness
4. exhaustion
5. cyanosis — demands urgent relief.

Naso-tracheal intubation

An alternative to tracheostomy is naso-tracheal intubation. Specially made tubes with a cross arm over the nasal end are available for this purpose. The procedure requires some skill, and it may not always be possible to pass a tube through an oedematous narrow larynx, or laryngeal spasm may develop, so that facilities must be on hand for immediate tracheostomy if the procedure is unsuccessful. It should *never* be attempted in acute epiglottitis.

Precautions

After intubation, it is absolutely essential that the tube is securely tied in, the hand bandaged like a boxing glove, with elbows splinted, and the child heavily sedated to prevent him pulling out the tube. Light sedation merely makes the child more restless and liable to pull out the tube — with disastrous results. Warm humidified oxygen or air must be given down the tube. Close observation in an intensive care situation is essential after intu-

bation, and if these facilities are not available, then it is probably better not to undertake the procedure.

Extubation is often possible after 4 or 5 days- and usually by a week. It should be done by an experienced doctor, preferably under general anaesthesia, who must watch the child carefully for signs of obstruction over the next few hours and be prepared to re-intubate again if necessary, if signs of obstruction persist.

Respiratory obstruction

This is characterized by:

1. severe dyspnoea with intercostal, subcostal and sternal recession, and suprasternal recession also in severe upper respiratory tract obstruction — there is great inspiratory effort, with use of accessory muscles, the effort often being out of all proportion to the modest increase in respiratory rate.
2. stridor
3. signs of hypoxia and carbon dioxide retention — restlessness, tachycardia, rise in blood pressure and later drowsiness and cyanosis.

Causes

The history and timing may give important clues to the cause, as well as symptoms and signs relevant to the particular cause.

1. laryngo-tracheo-bronchitis — 'croup'
2. epiglottitis
3. inhalation of foreign body
4. diphtheria
5. pressure on the trachea — retropharyngeal abscess, or more rarely a congenital vascular ring encircling the trachea, or tuberculous glands
6. rarer congenital anomalies: cysts, papillomas, and congenital webs of the larynx, and congenital sybglottic stenosis; these may be symptomless until infected, with odema and inflammation developing

Inhalation of foreign body

Infants and young children are exploratory by nature and will put anything and everything into their mouth, and such objects may be accidentally inhaled. The list of objects recovered from the respiratory tract is almost endless, but the commonest are peanuts (groundnuts), beads, and small plastic objects. Inhalation may produce immediate choking, or symptoms and signs of obstruction resembling acute LTB with stridor, croup and a harsh brassy cough. The foreign body may lodge in the trachea, at the carina, or within a major bronchus with collapse of the lung beyond. Unless the obstruction is relieved the accumulation of secretions and secondary infection may be followed by the development of a lung abscess. Peanuts are particularly dangerous because they swell up after inhalation, causing further obstruction, become friable releasing further small particles and also release highly irritant oils causing intense local inflammation.

Symptoms and signs

Parents may be able to time the onset of stridor to within half an hour, and it is most likely to begin during the day. (Croup often starts at night.) Sometimes there may be a 'silent period' for a while after an initial period of coughing following inhalation. The child is afebrile until secondary infection develops, otherwise symptoms are identical to croup but without the expected improvement after 24–48 hours, or indeed may become progressively more severe.

If a major bronchus is occluded, it may be possible to detect diminished air entry in one lung, but this is not always possible. A foreign body lodged in a large bronchus may act as a 'ball valve' allowing air into the lung but closing on expiration, trapping air in the affected lung. A chest X-ray taken in full expiration may reveal translucency on the affected side due to air trapping in the expiratory film.

Diagnosis

Many foreign bodies are not radio-opaque and will not be seen on a plain chest X-ray, though this may reveal areas of atelectasis, pneumonia or even an abscess. A lateral film of the neck may be helpful to demonstrate the airway.

When a foreign body is suspected, bronchoscopy under general anaesthesia is always necessary.

Cough

Is second only to fever as a presenting symptom in infants and children. Recent onset of cough almost always signifies an acute respiratory infection.

Chronic cough requires investigation and may be indicative of any of the following:

1. *atelectasis of a lobe or part of a lobe* — following an acute lower respiratory infection or recurrent inhalation of feeds — and is the commonest cause of persistent cough
2. *residual cough following pertussis* — this may last for several months
3. *persistent post-nasal drip*
4. *inhalation of a foreign body* — always to be suspected
5. *bronchiectasis*
6. *tuberculosis* — persistent cough is uncommon in primary tuberculosis unless there are enlarged hilar glands pressing on a bronchus
7. *asthma* — a persistent cough often accompanies bronchospasm
8. *rarer congenital anomalies of the lung* — e.g. bronchial cysts, sequestered lobes, congenital emphysema, and also mediastinal tumours

A persistent dry cough suggests irritation of the respiratory tract rather than infection.

Cough medicines in children

Cough medicines should not be given to young children. Doctors and all health workers are often under intense pressure from parents to prescribe cough medicines, but this must be resisted. It is worth explaining to parents that cough is nature's mechanism for protecting the lungs against disease — preventing the entry of invading organisms and removing infected mucus and secretions from the lungs and respiratory tract. Suppression of cough may prolong the illness by causing further damage.

Most medicines which effectively suppress cough contain either codeine, or synthetic codeine derivatives, which can produce significant respiratory depression in young children, or antihistamines, which may have a quite marked sedative action; in either case with potentially dangerous consequences.

A simplified scheme for management of cough*

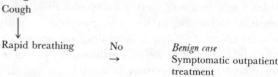

Cough

Rapid breathing   No →   Benign case
Symptomatic outpatient treatment

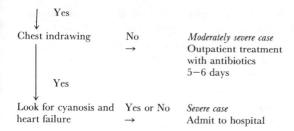

↓ Yes		
Chest indrawing	No →	*Moderately severe case* Outpatient treatment with antibiotics 5−6 days
↓ Yes		
Look for cyanosis and heart failure	Yes or No →	*Severe case* Admit to hospital

Indications for referral to a health centre or clinic*

- fever lasting more than 48 hours
- noisy or whistling breathing
- rapid breathing
  - respiratory rate > 50/min, for child under 1 year
  > 40/min, for child over 1 year
- Nasal flaring − movement of nostrils on breathing
- Cyanosis − lips and nails turn blue
- Chest indrawing − space between the ribs or at the bottom of the chest is drawn in while breathing in

Breathlessness in children

Tachypnoea (an increased respiratory rate), and dyspnoea (an increase in the effort needed to breathe) are not only common symptoms of respiratory disease but may be important symptoms of other disorders. The main causes are:

Respiratory diseases

1. diminished lung function:
commonly in
   - consolidation and/or collapse as in pneumonia
   - pleural effusion: empyema: pneumothorax rarer in
   - massive pericardial effusion: mediastinal tumours
   The degree of dyspnoea is proportional to the rapidity of onset rather than the degree of lung involvement.
2. respiratory obstruction

---

* Adapted from: Guerin, N. (1983). Acute childhood respiratory ailments. *Children in the Tropics*, **145**, 24−25. International Children's Centre, Paris.

Cardiac disease

Breathlessness is the commonest symptom of heart disease and is an invariable feature of cardiac failure.

Anaemia

By lowering the oxygen carrying capacity of the blood, anaemia will aggravate all forms of dyspnoea due to respiratory and cardiac causes.

Metabolic acidosis

Unlike CO_2, high levels of acid metabolites cannot be excreted from the lungs and the subsequent rise in $[H^+]$ concentration stimulates the respiratory centre.
Main causes:

- severe gastro-enteritis: hypernatraemic dehyration
- diabetic ketoacidosis
- salicylate poisoning
- 'Uraemia' and renal failure

There is often quite marked dyspnoea, breathing is deep and 'sighing' and sometimes appears slow although the respiratory rate may be increased, lung fields are remarkably clear on auscultation, with no signs of respiratory or cardiac disease.

Hysteria

Common in neurotic girls with an anxiety state. There is a sighing respiration and a desire for deeper breaths, and dyspnoea with mild effort. Other symptoms may include inability to breathe deeply, dizzyness and syncope, praecordial pain and palpitations.

Respiratory paralysis

The main causes are:

1. bulbar poliomyelitis − there may be little evidence of limb paresis
2. diphtheria − the acute infection may have passed unrecognized e.g. nasal diphtheria; myocarditis may also be present
3. polyneuritis − Guillain−Barré syndrome − following any acute viral illness
4. tetanus

5. drugs or toxic substances producing respiratory depression
6. encephalitis, cerebral malaria, meningitis, head injury etc.

There may be paralysis of the primary respiratory muscles, muscles of swallowing or both. Patients are restless and anxious, breaths are short and shallow with poor respiratory movements. The accessory muscles e.g. sternomastoids are used if they are not paralysed. Older children may be assessed by asking them to take a deep breath in and then count aloud as far as possible while holding their breath. If swallowing is paralysed as well, secretions will pool in the back of the pharynx with refusal to drink or eat for fear of choking.

Bronchiolitis

This is a highly infectious, acute viral infection, affecting mainly infants and young children, and often in epidemics especially in the cold and wet seasons. More than 80 per cent are due to the respiratory syncitial virus (RS virus). The distinctive features enable the diagnosis to be made on clinical grounds, affected infants becoming severely ill, sometimes in a matter of hours. There is an appreciable mortality in epidemics, and infants who have been premature seem particularly vulnerable.

Pathology

There is acute inflammation of the bronchioles, with secretions narrowing or completely blocking the terminal bronchioles and obstructing air entry into the alveoli. Patchy small areas of atelectasis and bronchopneumonia develop. The infant may 'drown' in his own secretions.

Clinical features

Bronchiolitis begins as a mild coryzal illness with a runny nose and fever for 24 to 48 hours, but there is then sudden deterioration with onset of a short harsh repetitive cough, rapid increase in respiratory rate, to 80 or 100/minute, an audible wheeze and signs of respiratory obstruction with intercostal, subcostal and sternal recession. Every breath is accompanied by considerable effort, with increasing difficulty in getting air in and out of the lungs. On auscultation there is a high pitched expiratory wheeze, with some fine crepitations throughout both lungs. As recovery begins, the wheeze lessens, is lower pitched and coarse crepitations appear. Cyanosis results partly from lower respiratory tract obstruction and partly from the accumulation of copious secretions in the nasopharynx.

Respiratory distress makes feeding impossible, and may be followed by right-sided heart failure and rapid exhaustion — sometimes in a matter of hours. An enlarged liver is commonly found, but it is sometimes difficult to say whether it is due to cardiac failure or simply due to airtrapping within the lungs pushing the diaphragm and liver down. A chest X-ray will show air trapping with translucent lung fields, lowering of the diaphragm and perhaps patchy areas of bronchopneumonia, and an enlarged heart if there is cardiac failure.

Recovery usually begins within 2 or 3 days with easing of the respiratory distress, a fall in respiratory rate and the wheeze becoming lower pitched. The wheeze, however, may persist and remain audible for up to 3 weeks or even longer, well after clinical recovery has taken place, causing much more distress to parents than the child, often described as a 'happy wheeze'. Some infants may continue to wheeze every time they develop another upper respiratory infection for up to a year or so after bronchiolitis. Subsequent immunity to the RS virus infection is usually permanent.

Management

Infants with bronchiolitis are highly infectious and should be isolated as far as is possible. They should be disturbed as little as possible, so as not to interfere with the work of breathing. Good nursing is the key to successful treatment. Infants should be sat in a chair or in the upright position to ease breathing, and *not* flat. Frequent suction is necessary to clear secretions from the nasopharynx and maintain a clear airway. Oxygen should always be warmed to 37°C and passed through a humidifier before administration, either through a head box or face mask loosely tied round the head. Feeding through a nasogastric tube is essential to maintain an adequate fluid intake and in severe cases, with frequent small milk feeds or preferably a continuous milk drip. Intravenous drips should be avoided because of the risks of overhydration especially if observation of drip rates and maintenance of accurate fluid records is suspect/unreliable. It is probably not necessary to nurse infants with bronchiolitis in large oxygen tents and high humidity which make observation and access difficult.

In clinically obvious bronchiolitis antibiotics are ineffective and unnecessary (because of the viral aetiology). They should however be used if a secondary bacterial bronchopneumonia develops during recovery, or when the diagnosis is uncertain and bronchopneumonia or staphylococcal pneumonia is suspected.

Antispasmodics (salbutamol and amimophylline derivatives) have no effect on the wheeze and should not be used.

Gentle physiotherapy followed by suction and clearance of the airways can be started in the recovery phase to assist in clearing secretions from the lungs, though care must be taken not to distress the infant further.

Cardiac failure is treated in the usual way and responds to frusemide.

The pneumonias

Bronchopneumonia

Patchy consolidation of alveoli throughout one or both lungs is much the commonest form of pneumonia in infants and young children, and also in older debilitated children. It may be a primary infection or quickly follow on from an apparently minor upper respiratory infection or bronchitis. Clinically, it is often impossible to distinguish between a viral and a bacterial cause. It is a common complication of both measles and whooping cough.

The onset may be gradual or rapid, with fever, rapid breathing, flaring of the alae nasae and cough. Vomiting is a frequent complication, due in part to the cough, but also from gastric irritation caused by swallowing the quite copious mucous secretions often produced. Signs in the chest include crepitations throughout both lung fields, and rhonchi. In severe cases cyanosis and cardiac failure may quickly develop. Patchy areas of pneumonic consolidation may be seen on chest X-ray but there is often a surprising discrepancy between the physical signs, which may be quite marked, and the X-ray findings which may be minimal or vice-versa.

Complications

A pleural effusion may develop initially as a sterile exudate, but later becoming secondarily infected with the development of an empyema, usually staphylococcal or pneumococcal.

Treatment

Infants and children should be nursed in a comfortable position, sitting up. Secretions may need to be cleared frequently from the nasopharynx, and oxygen — humidified and pre-warmed — give as necessary. Tube feeding may be necessary where there is marked respiratory distress or tachypnoea, though remember that an indwelling nasogastric tube does tend to block part of the nasal airway. Intravenous fluids are potentially dangerous and should only be given when dehydration is present, great care being taken not to overload the circulation. Physiotherapy is unnecessary in uncomplicated cases, but is helpful when recovery is slow with persistent signs of collapse or consolidation.

A broad spectrum antibiotic should be given as it is unlikely that the causative organism can be identified. Amoxycillin (or ampicillin) and flucloxacillin is a good combination; useful alternatives are (1) chloramphenicol, or in more severe cases (2) penicillin or amoxycillin (ampicillin) plus gentamicin, or (3) cefuroxime. The final choice will depend on a knowledge of local bacterial sensitivities.

Right middle lobe pneumonia

Right middle lobe pneumonia and consolidation often result from aspiration of mucus, secretions or feeds and may especially follow forced or hand feeding in debilitated and sick young children — a situation favoured by the anatomical arrangement of the bronchi in the right lung (Figure 10.2). Aspiration of feeds may also involve the right upper lobe in infants nursed flat. Foreign bodies commonly lodge in the right middle lobe bronchus, and should always be considered when resolution is slow. The middle lobe bronchus may also be compressed by enlarged right hilar glands, causing poor drainage and secondary infection.

Lobar (or lobular) pneumonia

This is consolidation of a lobe (or lobule) and is much more likely to be bacterial, *Streptococcus*

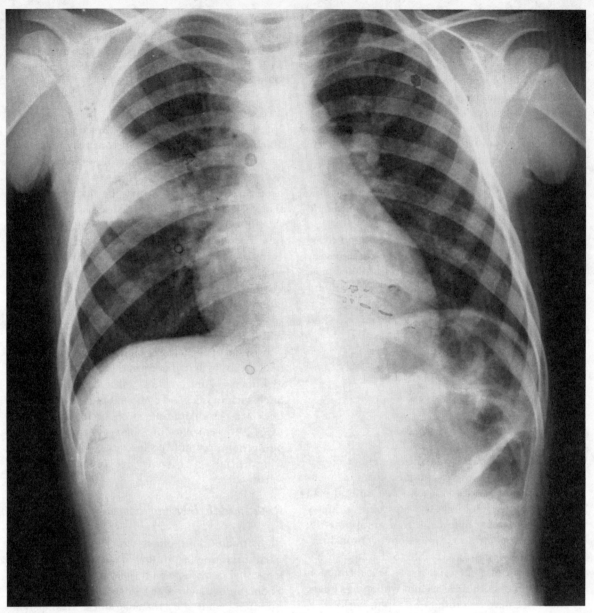

Figure 10.2 Right middle lobe pneumonia

pneumoniae being the commonest organism (Figure 10.3). Lobar pneumonia is rare below the age of 2 years (with the exception of right middle lobe pneumonia) but increases in frequency in older children.

The onset is usually sudden with high fever and dyspnoea, the child looks ill, toxic and flushed. Cough is variable, but if there is associated pleurisy may be painful. The classical signs of consolidation with diminished air entry into the affected lobe and bronchial breathing are present, though may be difficult to detect in small children and in the early stages. A pleural rub is sometimes present and diminished chest movements may be observed over the affected lung. Crepitations develop as resolution occurs. Abdominal pain may be a prominent symptom in the early stages of a lower lobe pneumonia, and meningism in an upper lobe pneumonia; both may be sufficiently severe to suggest either an acute abdomen or meningitis.

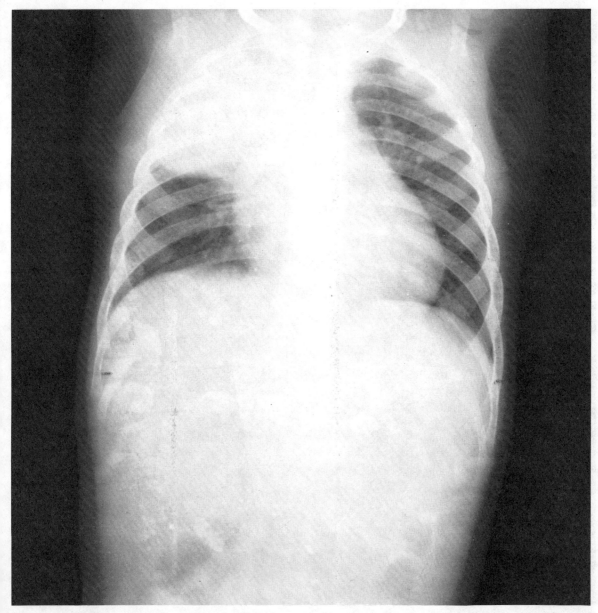

Figure 10.3 Lobar pneumonia — right upper lobe

Management

The response to benzyl penicillin is prompt and often dramatic. It is the drug of choice and should be given intramuscularly for the first 24 hours continuing with oral penicillin V for a further 4—5 days. General supportive measures must include an adequate fluid intake.

Complications

As in bronchopneumonia a sterile pleural effusion may develop and become secondarily infected with development of an empyema.

Staphylococcal pneumonia

This is commonest in the first year of life, and in older debilitated or malnourished children (Figure 10.4). In the early stages there is little to distinguish it from other pneumonias, but it rapidly becomes much more severe and should be suspected in any

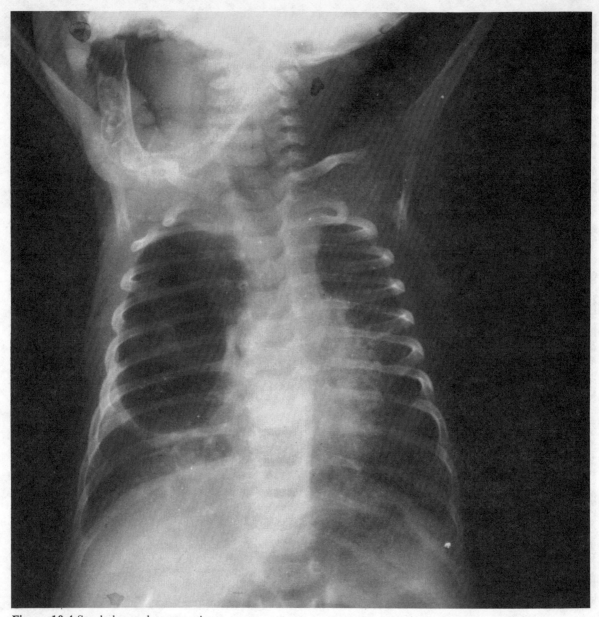

Figure 10.4 Staphylococcal pneumonia

very ill, toxic child with rapid respirations and obviously unresponsive to standard treatment.

Pathology
Small abscesses develop in the widespread patches of bronchopneumonia throughout the lungs (Figure 10.5). These abscesses develop into cysts with air above fluid levels, readily seen in chest X-rays. If the abscesses rupture into a bronchus, pus may be coughed up; if they rupture into the pleural cavity

a pneumothorax or pyopneumothorax develops. In extreme cases, cysts with air under tension may be as large as a whole lobe.

Diagnosis
Should be considered in any very ill, toxic child with pneumonia, or if there is a suggestion of cyst formation in the chest X-ray. Occasionally infection with *Klebsiella* pneumonia may give an almost identical clinical and radiological picture.

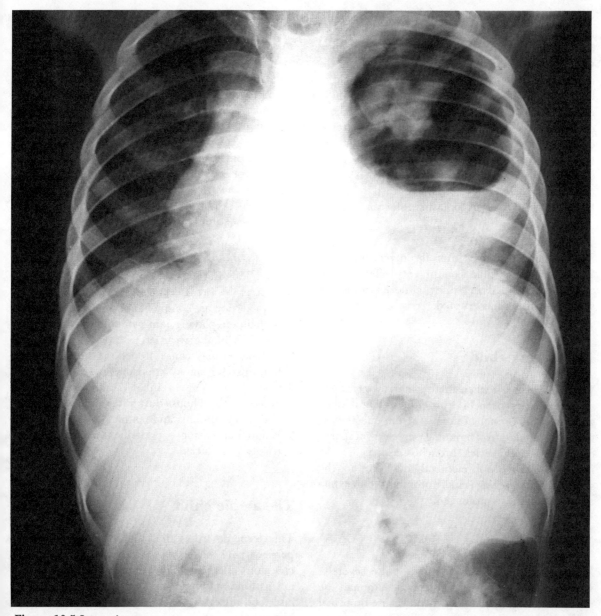

Figure 10.5 Lung abscess

Treatment

Treatment is with cloxacillin (or flucloxacillin), given initially by intravenous or intramuscular injection. Gentamicin or fusidic acid may be given in addition to cloxacillin.

Complications

Rupture of a cyst may occur at any time causing a pneumothorax, with sudden onset of severe and rapid dyspnoea. If the pneumothorax is under tension, urgent relief is necessary by inserting a needle into the pleural space and releasing the air through underwater drainage.

Mycoplasma pneumonia

(Formerly known as primary atypical pneumonia, Eaton agent pneumonia, or pleuropneumonia-like organism)
This is commoner in older children. It may be

suspected when symptoms and constitutional disturbance are more severe than the clinical signs — a high fever and dry persistent or spasmodic cough with scattered fine crepitations. Clinical diagnosis is not easy, but may be suggested by the radiological findings — small patchy, rather fluffy cotton-wool like areas of mottling rather than consolidation. Cold agglutinins may be demonstrated in the serum in about 50 per cent cases, though these also occur in other viral infections. Complications include muscle and joint pains, chest pain, and an erythema multiforme-like rash which is highly suggestive of mycoplasma infection.

Treatment

The infection responds to erythromycin given for 2 weeks. Tetracycline is also very effective but should be avoided in young children until the second dentition has erupted.

The wheezy child

Wheezing is heard when there is narrowing of the smaller airways (bronchi) from either inflammatory oedema of the bronchial mucosa (from infection or following inhalation of irritant gases) or from spasm of the bronchial muscles (bronchospasm as in asthma). Inhalation of a foreign body may produce the same effect. Wheezing is more pronounced in expiration which is also prolonged.

'Wheezy bronchitis'

Many infants wheeze, sometimes quite severely, with each respiratory viral infection, although the mechanism is not well understood because bronchial muscle is not well developed until about the age of 18 months, and the response to bronchodilators is poor. As infants get older this tendency to wheeze with respiratory infections disappears, though a few do go on to develop asthma. Wheezing is a marked feature of bronchiolitis and this tendency to wheeze with subsequent respiratory infections is quite marked in some infants. These attacks are often called 'wheezy bronchitis', which is a useful descriptive term, although it is not universally accepted.

Treatment is difficult because the response to bronchodilators is poor.

Asthma

The characteristic feature of asthma is wheeze due to narrowing of the airways from spasm of the bronchial muscles, and so it is also known as reversible airways obstruction. In addition there is oedema of the bronchial mucosa with increased secretions in the bronchi. As well as breathlessness, persistent cough is a prominent symptom and is due to bronchospasm. Children with asthma have airways (or bronchi) which appear to over-react or respond to a variety of stimuli by going into spasm; they often exhibit allergic symptoms as well. The commonest stimuli are:

1. Respiratory infections — especially viral. Many asthmatic children have a history of wheezy bronchitis in infancy.
2. Exercise — breathlessness and cough following any exertion are common, and such children find difficulty in playing games or doing PE at school. Changes in the weather — especially cold wet weather — may cause bronchospasm, as well as hot, dusty or smoky atmospheres.
3. Allergy — common inhaled allergens include house dust and house dust mites; pollens; moulds and fungi; animals and feathers.
4. Emotional tension — excitement or anxiety may trigger off attacks.

The atopic child

This term describes the child who develops hypersensitivity on exposure to a wide range of common allergens. The clinical manifestations are asthma, eczema, hay fever, perennial rhinitis and food allergies. There is often a strong family history.

Management

Unfortunately the concept of chronic disease and the need for continuous prophylactic treatment is ill understood by many patients in developing countries so that prevention of recurrent attacks is difficult. Many patients, moreover, may simply be unable to afford the prohibitive cost of continuous treatment in countries where drugs have to be paid for. Many of the newer, more effective drugs are also expensive and may not yet be available in some countries. A simple explanation of the nature and causes of asthma and avoidance of aggravating factors should be given where possible, in particular avoidance of smoky overcrowded rooms, cigarette smoke etc.

Prophylaxis of asthma — drug treatment

Table 10.3 summarizes the use of prophylactic drugs in asthma.

1. *Mild to moderately severe asthma.* Use a β-sympathomimetic drug alone or in combination with an aminophylline derivative. Long acting, slow release preparations of aminophylline are now available, given once or twice daily, and are a significant advance in treatment.
2. *More severe asthma.* Regular prophylactic inhalations, through pressurized aerosols, of either a topically active non-absorbed steroid e.g. betamethasone or beclomethasone, or sodium cromoglycate will reduce the frequency of attacks and can be combined with a β-sympathomimetic drug or aminophylline derivative, given as and when required to control more acute symptoms.

Various combinations of drugs can be used to suit the needs of the individual child but only one from each class of drug should be given. The β-sympathomimetics are all very similar in action and it is *not* necessary to give two different ones at the same time, otherwise there is a very real risk of an overdose. Likewise it is seldom necessary to combine an inhaled steroid with sodium cromoglycate, use either one or the other, but not both. Long-term treatment with oral steroids (prednisolone or prednisone) should be avoided because of the serious side effects, especially suppression of growth, osteoporsis, and adrenal suppression.

Table 10.3 *Drug treatment in the management of asthma*

Drug	Forms available
β-sympathomimetics	All available as syrup, tablets,
Salbutamol	subcutaneous injection, pressurized
Terbutaline	aerosol inhalation, nebulizer
Orciprenaline	solution.
Fenoterol	Pressurized aerosol inhaler only
Methyl xanthines	
Aminophylline	Syrup, tablets, suppositories, intravenous injection
Theophylline	Syrup, tablets
Steroids	
Beclomethasone	
Betamethasone	
Budesonide	Pressurised aerosol inhaler only
Rimiterol	
Prednisolone	Tablets (and injection)
Hydrocortisone	Injection (i.v., i.m.) (and tablets)
Sodium cromoglycate	Pressursed aerosol inhaler/insufflaton, nebulizer solution

Education of the child in the use of his drugs is important, e.g. the correct use of aerosol inhalers, or prophylactic value of salbutamol before games in exercise-induced asthma, to give the best results. Excessive use of salbutamol inhalers is common and the number of puffs allowed each day should be clearly stated. Emotional and educational problems may arise as severely affected children lose much time from school.

11

Heart Disorders and Acute Rheumatic Fever

Congenital heart disease

The incidence of congenital heart disease (CHD) seems to be remarkably uniform throughout the world at about 0.8 per cent of all live births. About a quarter will die in the first month of life because they have complex lesions either incompatible with survival or requiring major cardiac surgery, and another quarter will die by the age of one year. The more severe the lesion, the earlier will be the presentation.

Recognition of congenital heart disease

1. Difficulty with feeding and poor weight gain — feeding and sucking are the only forms of physical exertion that a baby undertakes. Infants may tire and become breathless and panting, unable to complete a feed, and so will fail to thrive. A tinge of cyanosis may be noted around the lips.
2. Sweating, especially after feeds. Sweating across the forehead may be profuse.
3. A heart murmur is usually, though not invariably, present. The heart may be clinically enlarged, with prominence of the left side of the chest, and a thrill palpable.
4. Cyanosis may be present — at rest or on feeding.
5. There is an increased liability to chest infections.
6. Cardiac failure may sometimes be the first presentation.

In older children

In older children with well compensated heart disease, recognition may be more difficult. Failure to thrive and growth failure are generally in proportion to the severity of the lesion. Other symptoms may include breathlessness on exertion and being more readily fatigued than children of the same age. Confirmation is by finding a heart murmur or abnormal heart sounds. Murmurs due to congenital heart disease must be distinguished from innocent (functional) murmurs and haemic murmurs in anaemic children with increased cardiac output. Haemic murmurs are seldom heard until the haemoglobin is below 7 g/dl.

Classification of congenital heart disease

In infants and young children it is seldom possible to make a precise diagnosis of the lesion, although a careful clinical examination, together with the additional information from a chest X-ray and ECG, if these are available, may suggest the most likely diagnosis. The final diagnosis can often only be made following specialized investigations such as 2D Echo cardiography, cardiac catheterization and angiography in specialized paediatric cardiac units. Precise diagnosis, however is probably irrelevant unless facilities for cardiac surgery are available.

Congenital heart lesions can be classified into one of the following groups: shunts, obstructive lesions, abnormal arrangements of vessels or complex lesions.

Shunts

These depend upon the presence of a communication between the pulmonary and systemic circulations, and are usually from left to right (L → R) because pressure in the systemic circulation is higher than that in the pulmonary circulation. L → R shunts do not produce cyanosis.

Examples:

ventricular septal defect (VSD)
atrial septal defect (ASD)
persistent patent ductus arteriosus (PDA)

All these defects result in an increased blood flow through the lungs.

In very large shunts, e.g. VSD or PDA, as much as a quarter or even a third of the output from the left ventricle may be shunted into the pulmonary circulation. There is both right and left ventricular enlargement and a thrill may be palpable over the site of the shunt. The increased blood flow through the lungs is seen on a chest X-ray as 'pulmonary plethora', due to congestion and prominence of the small blood vessels. There is an increased susceptibility to respiratory infections during which heart failure may develop.

Cyanotic heart disease

Right to left (R → L) shunts result in cyanosis because blood entering the right side of the heart is shunted to the left side and re-enters the systemic circulation without passing through the lungs. They are all characterized by some obstruction to pulmonary blood flow (e.g. pulmonary stenosis) and there is either an atrial or ventricular septal defect allowing R → L shunting. The reduced pulmonary blood flow is reflected in the chest X-ray as pulmonary oligaemia, with a lack of vascular markings in the lung fields. The heart is rarely enlarged.

Example:

Fallot's tetralogy

Ventricular septal defect

This is the commonest congenital lesion. The characteristic murmur is a pan systolic murmur maximal at the lower left sternal edge in the third, fourth and fifth left intercostal spaces. If the shunt is large, there may also be a thrill, cardiomegaly with a displaced apex beat and prominence of the left chest wall in infants, and a *loud* pulmonary second sound. Peripheral pulses are full and bounding and may be 'collapsing' in character. A chest X-ray shows plethoric lung fields, an enlarged heart and prominent pulmonary vessels. The larger the shunt, the earlier will symptoms appear and infants with a large VSD are especially susceptible to intercurrent respiratory infections and heart failure, though after one year of age there tends to be some improvement. Small VSDs are often symptomless and it is now clear that many of these close spontaneously in early childhood.

Atrial septal defect

There are two types of defect:

1. *Ostium secundum* is a simple defect due to failure of the fossa ovalis to close. It is the commonest form of congenital heart disease seen in adults.
2. *Ostium primum* — this defect is situated low down on the atrial septum, just above the atrioventricular valves and may be part of a more complex lesion with abnormal mitral valves, or VSD or a common atrioventricular canal defect.

The characteristic murmur is a soft ejection systolic murmur in the second and third intercostal spaces near the left sternal edges and radiates to the back. There is a fixed widely split second heart sound. A mid-diastolic murmur may sometimes be heard in the tricuspid area, and an apical pansystolic murmur in ostium defects. As with a VSD, the chest X-ray will show some enlargement of the heart and pulmonary conus, and plethoric lung fields. If available, an ECG may be helpful in distinguishing between a secundum defect in which right axis deviation is found and a primum defect in which left axis deviation occurs.

Patent ductus arteriosus

Failure of the ductus to close after birth results in a L → R shunt. Signs will depend on the size of the ductus which in extreme cases may be as large as the pulmonary artery. The characteristic murmur is a continuous 'machinery' murmur in the pulmonary area and under the left clavicle, radiating to the back. A thrill and collapsing pulses may be palpable and a loud pulmonary second sound heard. An apical mid-diastolic murmur is occasionally heard. The chest X-ray is similar to that seen in a VSD.

Obstructive lesions

These are usually due to narrowing of a valve (stenosis) or outflow tract, with reduced blood flow through the valve. They produce back pressure and hypertrophy of the ventricle below the obstruction. Obstructive lesions may also be present in large blood vessels — e.g. aorta and main pulmonary arteries.

Examples:

pulmonary stenosis
aortic stenosis
coarctation of the aorta

Pulmonary stenosis

This is a relatively common lesion. The characteristic murmur is a harsh ejection systolic murmur maximal in second and third left intercostal spaces and radiating to the back. A thrill may be palpable, and an ejection click and widely split second sound heard, though in moderate to severe stenosis the second sound is often soft. A chest X-ray shows relatively oligaemic lung fields. The pulmonary conus may be prominent but the heart is not enlarged. Mild degress of pulmonary stenosis are often symptomless in childhood. In severe stenosis, right ventricular hypertrophy increases and as it does so back pressure in the right atrium also increases and may open up the foramen ovale with the development of a R → L atrial shunt and cyanosis.

Aortic stenosis

The characteristic murmur is a harsh ejection

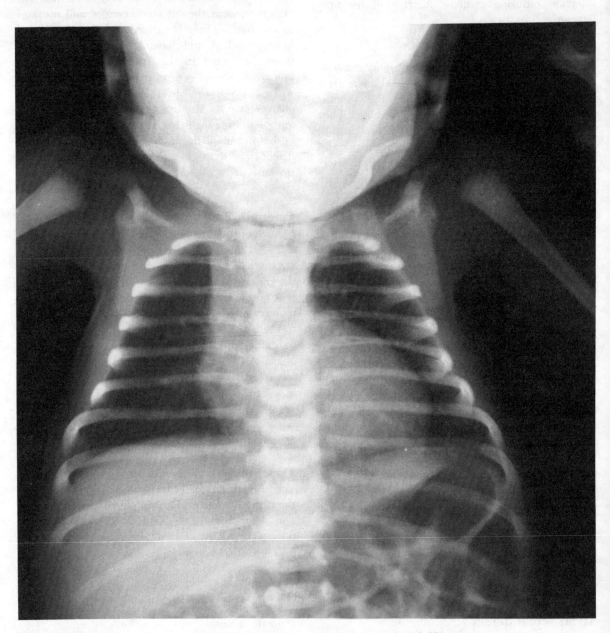

Figure 11.1 Fallot's tetralogy — typical 'boot shaped' heart and oligaemic lungfields

systolic murmur maximal in the aortic area radiating into the neck. There is often an associated thrill and an ejection click. If aortic incompetence is also present, an early diastolic murmur may be heard. Mild degrees of aortic stenosis are often symptomless, but in moderate or severe stenosis exercise tolerance may be limited, and sudden death is an unpredictable hazard. Physical exercise and activity should be restricted.

Coarctation of the aorta
The classical sign is an absent or delayed femoral pulse of poor volume. For comparison, femoral and right radial or brachial pulses should be felt simultaneously. A systolic or continuous murmur may be heard over both the front and back of the chest. The blood pressure in the leg is lower than in the arm. In mild long-standing cases, left ventricular hypertrophy and hypertension eventually develop and pulsation is visible in the anastamotic circulation ciculation around the scapulae and ribs. Severe coarctation quickly produces cardiac failure in infancy.

Abnormal arrangements of vessels

These result in blood entering or leaving the heart from the wrong chambers, and may cause cyanosis.

Total or partial anomalous venous drainage

One or more or all of the pulmonary veins drain into somewhere other than the left atrium — most commonly into the right atrium, or liver or diaphragm.

Transposition of the great arteries
The aorta arises from the right ventricle and the pulmonary artery from the left ventricle, thus there are two independent circulations — a situation incompatible with survival. Affected infants die within a few days of birth unless there is a shunt allowing some mixing of blood between the two circulations.

Truncus arteriosus
The pulmonary arteries, aorta and coronary arteries all arise from a common trunk from the base of the heart. There is always an associated large VSD. Affected infants are cyanosed.

Complex lesions

These are combinations of one or more of any of the above. The best known and commonest is Fallot's tetralogy (Figure 11.1). Many, such as tricuspid stenosis, absence of the right ventricle and hypoplastic left heart syndrome are incompatible with life for any length of time and death occurs soon after birth.

Fallot's tetralogy
The four lesions are:

1. pulmonary stenosis
2. right ventricular hypertrophy — due to obstruction at the pulmonary valve
3. ventricular septal defect
4. aorta overriding the right ventricle

Progressive cyanosis is present from early infancy although it may not be very severe at first and (except in very severe cases) is not present in the neonatal period. The major symptoms are cyanosis, development of finger and toe clubbing and failure to thrive with stunting of growth. Drop attacks, in which the child becomes severely cyanosed and unconscious, are related to the degree of pulmonary stenosis and follow exercise, excitement and emotional outbursts. Affected children often 'squat' when sitting, and this position may relieve the 'drop' attacks, thought to be due to muscle spasm around the pulmonary valve. Recently it has been found that β-blockers e.g. propranolol 0.5−1.0 mg/kg/day divided into three or four doses will relieve symptoms.

There is usually an ejection systolic murmur of varying intensity and a single second sound. A thrill may be palpable. The chest X-ray shows oligaemic lung fields with reduced pulmonary vascular markings and the heart which is seldom enlarged has a characteristic 'boot shape'.

Congestive heart failure

Heart failure is the commonest medical emergency in the paediatric age group. It is defined as the inability of the heart to maintain a cardiac output that is adequate for the body's requirements.

Cardiac output is determined by four basic factors: (1) pre-load or the ventricular end-diastolic pressure; (2) contractile state of the myocardium;

(3) afterload or the forces opposing the ventricular ejection; and (4) heart rate.

The clinical features of heart failure are either the result of changed haemodynamics secondary to mechanical defects or of the compensatory mechanisms. Irrespective of the cause, the cardiac chambers dilate resulting in cardiac enlargement. Pulmonary congestion and an increase in interstitial fluid decrease lung compliance resulting in increased workload, rapid shallow respiration and and increased oxygen requirements. Increased cardiac workload increases cardiac oxygen requirements in the face of decreased oxygen availability. This causes further cardiac dysfunction.

Cardiac enlargement and decreasing cardiac output (and falling blood pressure) lead to stimulation of stretch receptors and baroreceptors respectively, resulting in sympathetic overactivity. This causes circulatory redistribution with decreased supply to limbs, splanchnic area and the kidneys. Fatigue, decreased appetite, oliguria and growth retardation in chronic cases are all related to these circulatory changes. Tachycardia, peripheral vasoconstriction and increased sweating also result from sympathetic overactivity. Raised systemic venous pressure results in engorged neck veins, hepatomegaly and oedema.

Cardiac failure in infants

Raised jugular venous pressure and peripheral oedema, cardinal signs of congestive heart failure in adults and older children, are not useful signs in small infants. Feeding difficulty, failure to thrive, tachypnoea, tachycardia, rales, hepatomegaly and cardiomegaly are helpful in diagnosis. Other features include: excessive sweating, peripheral vasoconstriction and pallor, and gallop rhythm.

Cardiac failure may result from impaired myocardial function (toxic and viral myocarditis, rheumatic carditis, hypoxic damage, hypothyroidism, beri beri, cardiomyopathy), rhythm disturbances or an excessive haemodynamic load (valvular diseases, congenital defects, hypertension, anaemia, thyrotoxicosis) or both.

Treatment

The objectives of treatment are to increase cardiac output, and thereby improve peripheral perfusion and to decrease systemic and pulmonary venous congestion. The following are the principles of treatment:

Rest

The child is nursed in a semi-upright position. Oxygen administration reduces respiratory workload and improves cardiac function. Mild sedation in a restless child helps.

Diet

Congestive heart failure is accompanied by salt retention. Therefore, dietary sodium intake should be restricted. An infant with severe heart failure should preferably be on restricted i.v. fluids, 70 ml/kg/day are given, and not fed orally. If oral feeds are continued, a modified milk with low solute content should be used.

Correction of metabolic abnormalities

Underlying hypoglycaemia, hypocalcaemia, electrolyte disturbances and acidosis should be corrected.

Digitalis

These glycosides have a direct positive inotropic effect on the ventricular myocardium, thus increasing ventricular contractility. There is also a slowing effect on the conducting system.

Several digitalis alkaloids are available; digoxin is the most commonly used preparation. Since these alkaloids are potentially toxic with a narrow safety margin, one should become familiar with one or two commonly available preparations. Sensitivity to digoxin varies with age, therefore, the dosage schedule varies. Since it is a cumulative drug, the dosage has to be reduced for maintenance, after the digitalizing dose has been given. Dosage schedules are given in Table 11.1.

If facilities for monitoring drug levels are available, digoxin levels should be monitored to prevent toxicity; toxic levels for various age groups are given in Table 11.2

Serum digoxin levels correlate poorly with clinical response. Heart rate monitoring and ECG monitoring are more useful. In the ECG, PR interval increases, QT interval increases, there is ST depression and there may be T wave inversion. A prolongation of the PR interval by 0.02 s over pretreatment duration indicates adequate dosage.

Clinical evidence of digoxin toxicity includes:

• anorexia, nausea, vomiting, dizziness, headache

Table 11.1 *Recommended digoxin dosage*

Age group	Total digitalizing dose (TDD)	Maintenance dose
Newborn	30 µg/kg	4–5 µg/kg/day in two doses
Infant	35 µg/kg	5–10 µg/kg/day in two doses
Preschool	40 µg/kg	5–10 µg/kg/day in two doses
Older child	1.0–2.0 mg	0.125–0.250 mg once daily

Notes on TDD:

1. The above doses are for the i.m. route. The i.v. route is not normally recommended. Oral dosage is approximately 20 per cent more.
2. TDD is divided into ½, ¼ and ¼. Second dose is given 8 hours after first and the third 12–16 hours after the second. In older children TDD is given over 48 hours.

Digoxin preparations

Digoxin elixir paediatric is dispensed in bottles containing 50 µg per ml (0.05 mg/ml) and with a dropper marked with 0.2 ml graduations. Each 0.2 ml graduation contains 10 µg.
Digoxin tablets are in strength of 62.5 µg, 125 µg and 250 µg.
Digoxin for injection is in two strengths: 100 µg per ml in 1 ml ampoules; 500 µg in 2 ml ampoules (i.e., 250 µg in 1 ml).

Table 11.2 *Serum digitalis levels (ng/ml)*

	Non-toxic	Borderline toxic	Toxic
Infants and children up to 2 years	<2.0	2.0–5.0	>5.0
Children over 2 years	<1.0	1.0–2.0	>2.0

- bradycardia for age (infant <100/min; child <60–80/min)
- arrhythmia. Any arrhythmia developing during digoxin therapy may be presumed to be due to toxicity

If toxicity occurs, the drug should be stopped immediately, potassium chloride infusion in 5 per cent dextrose (0.5 mmol/kg/day) should be started under ECG monitoring and if bradycardia is marked, a single dose of atropine 0.02 mg i.m. should be given.

Diuretics

Information on commonly used diuretics is given in Table 11.3. Frusemide and spironolactone in early management and hydrochlorothiazide and spironolactone for long-term management are the most commonly used diuretics. Accurate daily weight records and urinary output are good indicators of a diuretic effect. Periodic electrolyte monitoring is necessary to avoid electrolyte depletion. Potassium supplements should be given to patients receiving long-term diuretic therapy with frusemide or hydrochlorothiazide alone.

Afterload reduction

Generally the above measures are adequate. Selected patients may require the use of vasodilators in order to produce arteriolar dilation to facilitate ventricular emptying. Hydralazine is commonly used for this purpose. The dose is 0.5 mg/kg/day orally, divided 8-hourly, the dose may be increased to 7 mg/kg/day (maximum 200 mg daily). When used intravenously the dose is 0.1–0.5 mg/kg/dose (maximum 2 mg/kg/dose).

Inotropic drugs

Isoprenaline and dopamine may be required in emergency conditions when the patient has hypotension.

Intractible heart failure

Although medical management is expected to improve cardiac function, treatment of the underlying cause, including surgical correction of congenital defects is necessary. The following additional factors aggravate heart failure: anaemia, infection, rheumatic activity, subacute bacterial endocarditis, electrolyte disturbance (especially hypokalaemia). Measures to treat these are necessary for effective management.

Acute rheumatic fever

Rheumatic fever is an inflammatory disease involving several organ systems following β-haemolytic streptococcal pharyngitis. Whereas most of the clinical manifestations are self-limiting, involve-

Table 11.3 *Dosage schedule of diuretics*

Drug	Site of action	Dosage		Comments
		Oral	i.v.	
Ethacrynic acid	Ascending limb of loop of Henle	3 mg/kg/day as single dose	0.5−1.0 mg/kg/dose every 12 to 24 h	Not recommended for neonates and infants
Frusemide	Ascending limb of loop of Henle	1−2 mg/kg/dose every 12 h (max 6 mg/kg/day)	1 mg/kg/dose every 8 to 12 h (max 6 mg/kg/day)	Potassium supplements necessary with prolonged use
Hydrochlorothiazide	Distal tubule	2−3 mg/kg/day every 12 h	−	Has a relatively longer duration of action − a single daily dose, early in the morning is recommended for long-term use
Spironolactone	Collecting tubule	2−3.5 mg/kg/day once or twice daily	−	
Triamterene	Collecting tubule	3−4 mg/kg/day every 12 h	−	Relatively potassium sparing

ment of the heart causes significant morbidity (and possible mortality) in the acute phase and frequently leads to persistant valvular damage and chronic disability.

Historical

Individual manifestations of the disease were first described in the seventeenth and eighteenth centuries. Thereafter, Cheadle in 1889 gave a description of the disease as we know it today. The role of streptococcal pharyngitis in its aetiopathogenisis was established in 1931 and the therapeutic role of penicillin was recognized in 1949.

Incidence

Rheumatic fever was a major public health problem in Europe and the United States in the late nineteenth and early twentieth century. Thereafter, the incidence gradually fell and at the present time it is a mere 0.64 per 100 000 in the United States.

No hard data on its prevalence in developing countries were available until the latter half of this century. The figures from these countries are reminiscent of the magnitude of the problem in the West at the turn of the century. An incidence of 16 to 20 per 1000 in Kuwait, 19 per 1000 in Libya, 16 per 1000 in Morocco, 15 per 1000 in Algeria, 10 per 1000 in Egypt and a very high incidence from Iran

of 22 per 1000 of the child population has been reported in recent years. Urban slums, overcrowding, cold damp climate and poor nutrition predispose to the disease. The incidence has a seasonal variation being more common in late winter months. It most commonly affects children in the age group 5−15 years. In the tropics approximately 5 per cent of children have the initial attack below 5 years of age.

Aetiopathogenesis

The disease represents a non-suppurative complication of group A β-haemolytic streptococcal throat infection; rheumatic fever is not known to follow skin infection. Current evidence indicates an immune cross-reaction between streptococcal antibodies and body tissues.

The incidence of rheumatic fever following streptococcal pharyngitis varies from 0.3 to 3.0 per cent; the incidence being higher following severe pharyngitis and during epidemics.

There is evidence to suggest that host factors are significant in its pathogenesis and a genetic predisposition may exist.

Pathology

Initially various organs show an exudative inflammatory reaction with connective tissue oedema and lymphocyte and plasma cell infiltration. This phase is self-limiting and lasts for 2 to 3 weeks. This is followed by a proliferative phase which is characterized by perivascular aggregation of multinuclear cells around fibrinous material. The proliferative phase predominantly involves the myocardium and endocardium and the lesions develop along the valve edges; these lesions may go on to scarring and valvular damage. Scarring increases with each recurrence of the disease.

Pathological changes in the central nervous system do not resemble lesions in other organs or tissues. Widespread degenerative changes in blood vessels are more extensive than the clinical involvement of the central nervous system would suggest.

Clinical features

Symptoms start approximately 10 days after the acute throat infection subsides. Clinical presentation varies with the site of pathology and severity of the disease. General features include high intermittent fever, fatigue, vague pains, weight loss, anaemia and abdominal pain.

The specific clinical manifestations are divided into major and minor depending upon their diagnostic usefulness. Major manifestations include polyarthritis, carditis, chorea, subcutaneous nodules and erythema marginatum. Minor manifestations include fever, arthralgia, previous history of rheumatic fever or presence of rheumatic heart disease and the presence of acute phase reactants (ESR, C-reactive protein).

Polyarthritis is one of the earlier manifestations. It is characteristically described as migratory and fleeting; migratory implies that it shifts from joint to joint and fleeting because it is transitory — lasting usually 2 to 3 days in a joint but never more than a week. Large joints of extremities including knees, ankles, elbows and wrists are involved. Uncommonly the hip joints and the small joints may be involved but are not a regular feature of the disease. Swelling, redness and raised temperature over the joint are usually present, but pain is the most outstanding feature and is out of proportion to the objective signs of arthritis. Arthritis resolves without any residual damage to the joint.

The term arthralgia implies a milder degree of pain experienced by the patient without objective evidence of arthritis.

Carditis (Table 11.4) occurs in 50 to 60 per cent

Table 11.4 *Clinical signs of carditis*

1. Cardiac murmurs: long pansystolic murmur at apex, early diastolic murmur at the base and a mid-diastolic murmur (Carey–Coomb's).
2. Pericardial friction rub and/or pericardial effusion.
3. Presence of congestive cardiac failure.
4. Cardiomegaly on radiology.

Note: Sleep tachycardia and a 'soft' first sound at apex are suggestive but not indicative of carditis.

of cases. It may accompany arthritis but is generally a later manifestation. Pathologically it is a pancarditis because it involves the pericardium, myocardium and the endocardium. Pericarditis is often not detected clinically, but when present it indicates a severe carditis. More commonly carditis presents with the appearance of cardiac murmurs, cardiomegaly and as heart failure. A sleep tachycardia out of proportion to the degree of fever may be suggestive but is not diagnostic. The changing character of a cardiac murmur on repeated auscultation during the course of the disease is strong evidence of carditis.

Carditis may last from 6 weeks to 6 months and may be fatal either due to progressive deterioration of cardiac function or due to complicating infective endocarditis.

Chorea is a late manifestation and may be preceded by polyarthritis and carditis. It is distinctly more common in girls and has been reported in 10 to 15 per cent of cases in the Western literature. It has a lower incidence in tropical countries and in the Middle East the incidence is less than 5 per cent. It may constitute the only manifestation of activity, but carditis and arthritis can co-exist.

Emotional lability, involuntary grimacing, deteriorating handwriting and school performance and clumsiness are some of the earlier features. Characteristic choreiform movements can be highlighted objectively by signs such as the 'milk-maid' grip, Adar's darting tongue and 'dinner fork' deformity of outstretched hands. Hypotonia may be a dominant feature in some cases (chorea mollis), or the movements may be limited to or more severe in one half of the body (hemichorea). Chorea may last from a few weeks to several months but recovers completely.

Subcutaneous nodules are small (a few mm to 1 cm), firm and painless, presenting symmetrically over bony prominences. These appear several weeks after the onset of rheumatic activity, are seen in about 5 per cent of the cases and usually accompany severe carditis. The skin over the nodules moves freely and they are better felt than seen.

Erythema marginatum is recorded in less than 5 per cent of cases. It is pink, non-pruritic rash with well-demarcated margins (Figure 11.2). The rash appears in fair-skinned subjects and is transient. It occurs only in patients with carditis.

Laboratory manifestations

Throat culture is generally negative by the time the clinical features of rheumatic fever develop. However, evidence of streptococcal infection is reflected by demonstration of antibodies such as antistreptolysin O (ASO), anti-DNase B and anti-DPNase. Of these ASO titre is the most important. After uncomplicated streptococcal throat infections ASO titres rarely exceed 200 Todd units (TU). In acute rheumatic fever the values generally exceed 500 TU but values over 300TU are considered significant; the titres begin to decline 2 months after infection. Significantly high ASO titres are recorded in 80 per cent of cases with rheumatic fever. The height of the ASO titre bears no relation to the severity and course of the disease. Acute phase reactants such as C-reactive protein (CRP) are helpful in both diagnosis and assessment of the course of the disease. The ESR is high in all cases.

The electrocardiogram (ECG) may show a prolonged PR-interval; values over 0.18 s indicate an abnormal PR-interval. Ideally the PR-interval should be related to the heart rate and if it exceeds the maximum PR-interval for the recorded heart rate it should be considered abnormal. A prolonged PR-interval does not indicate carditis. Other ECG changes include flattening or inversion of T-wave due to myocarditis and ST-segment changes due to pericarditis. Chest radiology may show cardiomegaly in cases with carditis.

Diagnosis

All the manifestations are unlikely to be seen in a single patient. Modified Jones' criteria (Table 11.5) have, therefore, been used to make a diagnosis of the disease. Using these criteria, a diagnosis of acute rheumatic fever may be made if:

• two major criteria are present, or

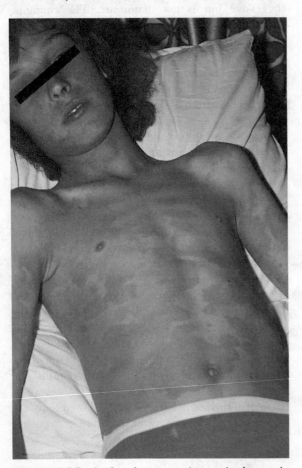

Figure 11.2 Rash of erythema marginatum in rheumatic fever

Table 11.5 *Modified Jones' criteria for diagnosis of acute rheumatic fever*

Major manifestations:	Minor manifestations:
Polyarthritis	*Clinical:*
Carditis	Fever
Chorea	Arthralgia
Subcutaneous nodules	Previous rheumatic fever or
Erythema marginatum	rheumatic heart disease
	Laboratory:
	Raised ESR or C-reactive protein
	Leucocytosis
	Prolonged PR interval in ECG

Plus: Supportive evidence of preceding streptococcal infection; increased ASO or other streptococcal antibodies; positive throat culture for group A β-haemolytic streptococci; recent scarlet fever.

- one major and two minor criteria with supporting evidence of a preceding streptococcal infection are present.

Using these criteria there is a possibility of both false positive and false negative diagnosis.

Diagnosis of rheumatic chorea and of low grade carditis can be made in the absence of Jones' criteria.

Differential diagnosis

The differential diagnosis depends upon presentation and a number of conditions have to be differentiated. Several diseases may present with polyarthritis or a combination of polyarthritis and cardiac disease.

1. Juvenile rheumatoid arthritis may present with polyarthritis, skin rash and a raised ESR. Pericarditis may be present. However, the arthritis is never migratory and persists for a longer period with the possibility of residual limitation of movement. The rash is transient, salmon-pink, macular and is present over the trunk.
2. Systemic lupus erythematosus may also present with joint symptoms. Characteristic extra-articular manifestations as well as laboratory evidence of antinuclear antibodies are helpful in differentiation.
3. Polyarthritis is also a feature of infectious diseases, e.g., rubella and parvovirus infection and of other disorders such as serum sickness and Henoch–Schönlein purpura.
4. Infective endocarditis may present with cardiac manifestations and arthralgia. There is often a hectic temperature and several extra-cardiac manifestations such as a soft spleen, petechiae, splinter haemorrhages, Osler's nodes, Janeway's spots and haematuria which help in diagnosis. Blood cultures should be taken and endocarditis vegetations looked for on real-time echocardiography.
5. *Yersinia enterocolitica* infection (mainly seen in the Scandinavian countries) causes arthritis which may be associated with cardiac manifestations. Cardiac involvement is in the form of myocarditis and pericarditis, valvular involvement being uncommon.
6. Lyme disease is caused by a spirochaete and transmitted by a tick. The clinical spectrum includes arthritis, carditis, central nervous system involvement and a skin rash which spreads from the site of the tick bite.
7. Gonococcal arthritis may present as a polyarthritis closely resembling rheumatic fever and whenever suspected appropriate cultures should be taken to make a diagnosis.
8. Patients presenting dominantly with cardiac disease have to be differentiated from viral and toxic myocarditis and viral pericarditis. Viral and toxic cardiac disease does not involve the valves, but cardiac murmurs may be present.

Rheumatic chorea is perhaps the only pure chorea and usually causes no diagnostic problems. Occasionally complex tics may be mistaken for chorea. A fidgety child may also present like early chorea.

Management

Rest is mandatory and patients should be admitted to hospital. All cases, irrespective of throat culture results, must receive a 10-day course of penicillin to eradicate any persisting streptococcal infection. For specific therapy salicylates and corticosteroids are used. There is, however, no difference in the final outcome with relation to chronic valvular disease whether salicylates or corticosteroids are used. For all cases of arthritis and mild carditis salicylates are recommended. Aspirin in doses of 100 mg/kg/day divided in three or four doses for the first 2 weeks followed by 75 mg/kg/day for the next 4 to 8 weeks is given, the total duration depending on clinical response and fall in the ESR. Ideally the dose of aspirin should be adjusted to maintain serum salicylate levels of 25 mg/dl (values above 30 mg/dl are in the toxic range). Some patients may require aspirin in the range of 125 to 150 mg/kg for optimum blood levels but such high doses should only be given under constant monitoring.

Indications for corticosteroids include:

- patients with moderate to severe carditis,
- patients with hypersensitivity to salicylates,
- patients who are very toxic, and
- patients not showing satisfactory response to aspirin.

Prednisone (or prednisolone) in a dose of 2 mg/kg/day (maximum 60 mg) is given for 2 weeks. Aspirin 75 mg/kg/day is added in the third week (except in patients sensitive to salicylates) and prednisone is tapered over the following 2 weeks. Patients with carditis generally receive treatment for from 8 to 12 weeks; some patients may require treatment for up to 6 months. Patients with congestive heart failure do not respond well to digoxin because the myocardium itself is diseased. Heart failure has to be managed mainly with diuretics. In some cases with intractable heart failure surgery may have to be undertaken in the presence of rheumatic activity.

Chorea, unless accompanied by arthritis or carditis (which is not uncommon) requires no anti-inflammatory treatment. If the involuntary movements are severe, the patient has to be protected from trauma and he may have to be assisted in feeding. Sedation with phenobarbitone 3 to 4 mg/kg/day or chlorpromazine 1.0 to 2.0 mg/kg/day is effective.

Secondary prevention (chemoprophylaxis)

One of the main problems with rheumatic fever is that each successive streptococcal throat infection exposes the patient to the risk of recurring rheumatic fever and potential further cardiac damage. It is, therefore, mandatory to take measures to prevent streptococcal infection. Chemoprophylaxis (Table 11.6) is started immediately after the 10-day course of oral penicillin is completed.

Primary prevention

It has been observed that rheumatic fever can be completely prevented if group A β-haemolytic

Table 11.6 *Prophylactic therapy for prevention of rheumatic fever recurrence*

Drug	Dosage	Remarks
Benzathine penicillin	1.2 million units i.m. every 3 weeks	Not recommended for patients allergic to penicillin
Phenoxymethyl penicillin	125 mg twice daily	Compliance of oral medication is poor
Sulphadiazine	1 g/day with body weight >30 kg 0.5 g/day with body weight <30 kg	For patients allergic to penicillin

streptococcal throat infection is effectively treated early in its course (first 9 days). Streptococcal screening for all throat infections followed by a 10-day course of penicillin V (or erythromycin in penicillin-sensitive subjects) is ideal. When streptococcal screening facilities are not available, penicillin therapy should be undertaken on the basis of clinical suspicion.

Pericarditis

Pericarditis is common in the tropics, and is usually secondary to other diseases:

- tuberculous pericarditis — which may be either a constrictive pericarditis or with effusion
- purulent (pyogenic) pericarditis — especially staphylococcal or pneumococcal, following which constrictive pericarditis may quickly develop necessitating pericardiotomy — it is always secondary to infection elsewhere
- rheumatic fever
- EMF
- viral — e.g. Coxsackie or influenzal
- 'idiopathic'

Symptoms

Some degree of praecordial pain is almost invariably present, together with dyspnoea and cough. Other symptoms, fever, malaise etc., depend on the underlying cause (Figure 11.3). The heart is enlarged and heart sounds may be muffled and soft. The classical superficial scratchy pericardial friction rub (heard both in systolic and diastole) may not always be detected.

Diagnosis

This is based on clinical findings and confirmed by pericardial aspiration in most cases.
ECG findings include:
- elevation of S−T segment especially leads I and II and chest leads (except VI);
- flattening or inversion of T waves;
- low voltage QRS complexes

Treatment

Treatment is that of the underlying cause. Purulent pericarditis always requires surgical drainage and appropriate antibiotics.

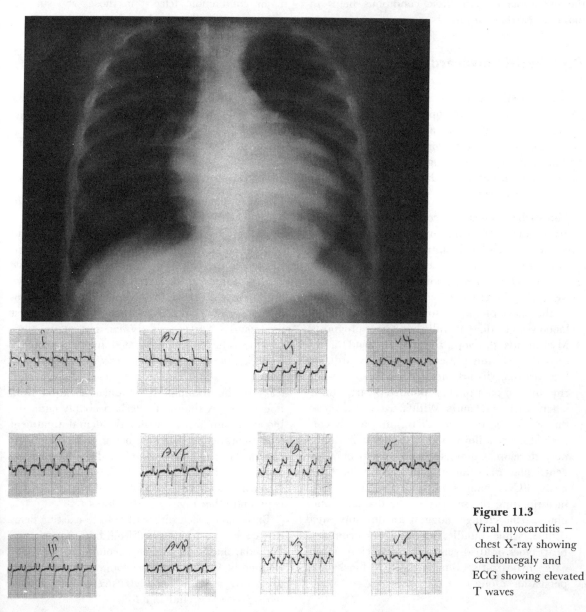

Figure 11.3
Viral myocarditis – chest X-ray showing cardiomegaly and ECG showing elevated T waves

Cardiac tamponade

Cardiac tamponade may result from constrictive pericarditis or a large effusion. Both compress the heart reducing diastolic filling of the ventricles. In chronic constrictive pericarditis, there is gradually increasing enlargement of the liver, ascites and peripheral oedema, dyspnoea being relatively mild until cardiac output is severely reduced. In addition, the neck veins are distended, the pulse is of poor volume and a paradoxical pulse is typically felt. The heart size, clinically and on X-ray, is smaller than might be expected but X-ray findings are not diagnostic. Chronic constrictive disease requires pericardiectomy as well as treatment of the underlying cause.

In acute tamponade the neck veins are grossly distended, there is cyanosis, tachycardia and a weak and paradoxical pulse with low blood pressure. Urgent decompression of the heart by aspiration is essential, followed by thoractomy and appropriate surgery. Digitalis may be required to treat cardiac failure but diuretics should be given cautiously as the hypervolaemia in these conditions helps to maintain cardiac output.

Diphtheritic myocarditis

It is estimated that the heart is affected in 10 to 25 per cent of cases of diphtheria, although the original illness may not always be recognized. Cardiac involvement results from toxic damage to the myocardium and conducting tissues by circulating exotoxins and not from direct infection. Three effects may be seen.

1. The earliest signs are conduction defects and disturbances of heart rhythm with partial or complete heart block, and bundle branch block, causing bradycardia or tachycardia.
2. Another early event, about the end of the first week, may be circulatory failure and shock due to the effect of the exotoxin on the peripheral blood vessels; this generally has a poor prognosis.
3. Myocarditis develops towards the end of the second week and presents with tachycardia or bradycardia, disturbances of rhythm, a gallop rhythm and poor quality 'muffled' heart sounds. There are no murmurs. With increasing myocardial weakness, the heart dilates and finally congestive heart failure, with varying arrhythmias may develop. Complete heart block, or atrio-ventricular dissociation indicate a poor prognosis. ECG changes (if available) are helpful in estimating the severity of the disease; minor non-specific changes suggest an uncomplicated course, while bundle branch block, complete heart block or atrio-ventricular dissociation indicate myocarditis. Bundle branch block may persist for a long time after recovery.

Treatment

Anti-diphtheria serum should be given immediately in appropriate doses (after a test dose) together with penicillin or erythromycin.

Bed rest is essential even in mild cases. Cardiac failure and arrythmias are treated in the usual way but care should be taken in giving digoxin which may itself be toxic. Small doses of a short acting cardiac glycoside may be indicated. Corticosteroids are of no value in established myocarditis.

The highest mortality is in those who develop major conduction defects; in those who survive recovery is usually complete.

Dose of anti-diphtheria serum varies with age and weight of child from 20 000 units to maximum of 100 000 units by intramuscular injection, divided if necessary into more than one site.

A test dose for hypersensitivity should *always* be given, 0.05 ml subantaneously and the patient watched for 30 minutes.

Infective endocarditis

Infective (bacterial) endocarditis may develop in patients with congenital or acquired heart disease, when organisms in the blood stream settle and implant on an abnormal myocardium or damaged thickened valves. It may also follow corrective cardiac surgery, the insertion of grafts or valve replacements, and in hydrocephalic children from infected ventriculo-atrial shunts. The commonest organism is *Streptococcus viridans*, but many other organisms have been implicated, including staphylococci, enterococci, *Escherichia coli*, *Haemophilus influenzae* and the organism of Q fever. *Staphylococcus albus* is the commonest organism isolated from infected V−A shunts. Bacteria probably enter the blood stream from the mouth, dental treatment and poor dental hygiene being the commonest causes. The importance of infected skin lesions as a portal of entry is not known. Bacteraemia and endocarditis are known to follow cystoscopy, endoscopy and other invasive procedures.

Bacterial endocarditis without pre-existing heart disease has been described from both Nigeria and Uganda, and seems to be encountered relatively frequently. Organisms most commonly responsible are *Staph. aureus*, β-haemolytic streptococci, *Streptococcus pneumoniae*, and *E. coli*.

Pathology

Infecting organisms settle on the damaged parts and the fibrinous inflammatory exudate produces vegetations on which a further growth of organisms results in progressive damage to the endothelium and valve. The vegetations are very friable and small emboli break off entering the circulation, and if infected produce mycotic aneurysms in peripheral vessels. Chronic vegetations become more organized and less friable.

Clinical features

Initially, the symptoms are vague with irregular fever of obscure or unknown origin, malaise, anorexia and weight loss. As the illness progresses the child is clearly unwell, with constant fever, lethargy, breathlessness and progressive anaemia. Night sweating and rigors are common. Although a recent history of dental treatment, tonsillectomy or skin infection is helpful, it is by no means always forthcoming. Even when the child is known to have congenital or rheumatic heart disease, the recognition of infective endocarditis may be slow.

On examination, there is generally a cardiac murmur whose quality may have changed recently. Splenomagaly develops sooner or later, it is modest, and the spleen is soft. In the full blown picture other signs include:

1. Petechiae in the skin, due to micro-emboli
2. Osler's nodes — tender red nodules on the pulp of fingers and toes, thenar and hypothenar eminences
3. Splinter haemorrhages — linear reddish brown streaks under the finger and toe nails
4. Finger clubbing is common
5. Microscopic haematuria
6. Release of emboli into (a) the systemic circulation, lodging in any organ, but especially the spleen, kidneys, lungs and brain, producing a sudden hemiplegia, convulsions, blindness, meningitis, microscopic or macroscopic haematuria, and infarcts; (b) the pulmonary circulation, producing pulmonary emboli, haemoptysis or pleurisy if lesions are on the right of the heart

Diagnosis

Although the causes of fever are almost legion, the diagnosis should be suspected in any child known to have heart disease who presents with persistent fever, splenomegaly and any of the above features. Diagnosis is confirmed by blood culture. When suspected, frequent cultures — anaerobic and aerobic — should be taken, 6, 8 or 10 over at least 48 hours or several days if necessary. No antibiotics should be given until sufficient cultures have been taken. Sub-cultures may be necessary to isolate the organism. Sensitivity tests are essential and where possible the m.i.c. of the antibiotic estimated against the organism in the presence of the patient's serum.

Treatment

Strict bed rest is essential to prevent cardiac failure.

Appropriate antibiotics are given for at least 6 weeks with an absolute minimum of 2 weeks intravenously. High doses at frequent intervals are necessary to achieve bactericidal concentrations in the blood. Ideally, blood levels of antibiotics should be monitored, just before and 1 hour after injections to measure 'peak and trough' levels. Unfortunately this is seldom possible in the tropics, but if the organism has been cultured, it may be possible to estimate the bactericidal effect of the blood on the organism at the above times.

Suggested treatment regimes

Streptococcus viridans. (α haemolytic streptoccus)
Benzyl penicillin 2 megaunits (1.2 g) × four hourly intravenously for 4 weeks at least, (through an indwelling cannula if possible).

Probenecid 50 mg/kg/day ÷ 12 hourly doses orally to inhibit renal excretion of penicillin.

The addition of gentamicin 6 mg/kg/day ÷ eight hourly doses provides a synergistic effect and can be reduced after 2 or 3 weeks to a lower dose of 2 mg/kg/day ÷ 12 hourly doses.

Staphylococcus
If penicillin sensitive: benzyl penicillin 20 megaunits (6.0 g) daily or 4 megaunits (2.4 g) 4-hourly intravenously for 3–4 weeks minimum, longer if possible.

If penicillin resistant: use flucloxacillin 200–300 mg/kg/day ÷ four or six doses intravenously for 3–4 weeks (plus oral probenecid), continuing for a further 4–6 weeks as necessary.

Enterococci
Benzyl penicillin as above for *Streptococcus viridans*, intravenously plus gentamicin 6 mg/kg/day ÷ three doses. A more effective combination may be ampicillin 400 mg/kg/day (or amoxycillin) and gentamicin since some enterococci are more sensitive to ampicillin than to penicillin.

Unidentified organisms
Benzyl penicillin 5 to 20 megaunits (3–12 g) per day in divided doses for 6 weeks in a continuous intravenous drip; plus gentamicin 6 mg/kg/day ÷

eight hourly doses and flucloxacillin 200–300 mg/ kg/day ÷ six hourly doses, both intravenously for 6 weeks, and oral probenecid. Ampicillin 400 mg/kg/ day in divided doses intravenously may be substituted for benzyl penicillin if clinically appropriate.

Prognosis

Strept. viridans – 80 per cent recover with full treatment.

Staphylococci – including *Staph. albus* – and *Candida* have a 40 per cent mortality rate.

The prognosis is worse if:

- congestive heart failure develops
- the aortic valve is involved
- child is under 3 years of age, because of high rate of staphylococcal infection

Remember that sterile emboli may continue to be thrown off for some weeks after vegetations become sterile.

Prophylaxis of endocarditis

Dental procedures
Either
1. Single oral dose of amoxycillin:
    - 1.5 g up to 10 years old
    - 3.0 g aged 11 years and over
    ½–1 hour before operative procedures.
or
2. Benethamine penicillin (Triplopen™) (dose according to age) by intramuscular injection ½ hour before procedure.
3. If hypersensitive to penicillin or if penicillin has been given within the previous 2 weeks use erythromycin:
    - 0.5 g up to 10 years of age
    - 1.0 g 11 years and over
    ½–1 hour before the procedure.

Endoscopic procedures
Ampicillin 25 mg/kg
    - intramuscular 30 minutes before
    - intravenously immediately before
plus gentamicin 2 mg/kg intravenously or intramuscularly and repeat at 8 and 16 hours afterwards.

Endomyocardial fibrosis

Endomyocardial fibrosis, (EMF), is the commonest of several cardiomyopathies of unknown cause found in the tropics and subtropics. Although it is widespread throughout tropical Africa, especially in the wetter rainforest areas, cases have also been reported from the Indian subcontinent, Thailand and South America, as well as in Europeans who have lived for long periods in endemic areas. It is essentially a disease of children, in whom symptoms may appear as early as 2 years of age, and young adults. In endemic areas in Africa it is almost as common as rheumatic heart disease.

Pathology

The characteristic feature of EMF is a dense endocardial plaque of fibrous tissue situated usually in the apex of either the right ventricle or left ventricle, or quite often in both ventricles. This spreads to involve the inflow tracts, papillary muscles and chordae tendinae, and so the atrioventricular valves become increasingly incompetent. At this point, the atria become involved, the extent depending on the severity of the ventricular lesions. The right atrium may become enormously dilated and hypertrophied with prominent trabeculation, with right atrial pressure almost identical to that in the right ventricle. The pulmonary and aortic valves remain normal although in right sided EMF the pulmonary conus may be dilated and infundibulum hypertrophied. It seems likely that the earliest lesion at the apex is endocardial damage and a fibrin deposit, followed by thrombus formation and ultimately fibrous scarring. Antemortem thrombus penetrating into the myocardium (from which emboli may develop) is sometimes found over recent scars. In contrast to the endocardium, the pericardium remains thin, in spite of the large pericardial effusion (Figure 11.4) – quite different from tuberculosis in which it becomes grossly thickened.

Aetiology

The cause of EMF remains unknown. Evidence suggests that environmental factors may be important, possibly acting as triggering events and that further damage results from stimulation of immunological mechanisms. Antibodies to heart muscles are high. In Uganda changes of both EMF and

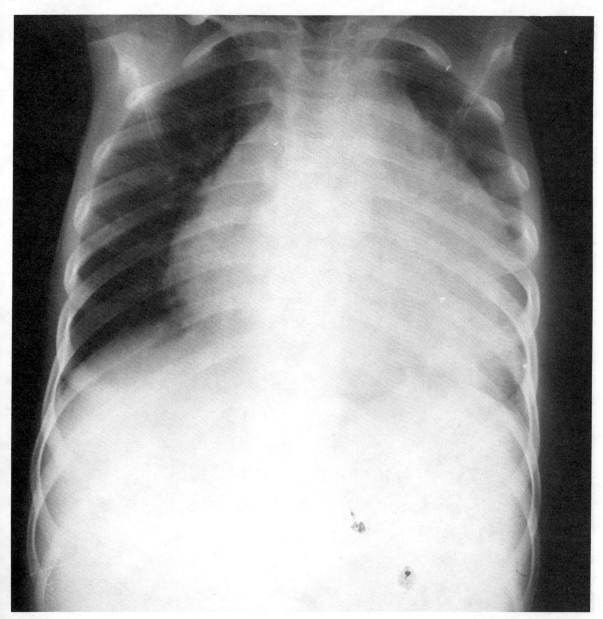

Figure 11.4a

rheumatic heart disease have been found in the same patient at autopsy, the two conditions occurring more frequently than might be expected by chance. The epidemiology of the two diseases is similar in age, sex, familial incidence and tendency to recurrence and progression.

The similarity of the geographical distribution of both *Loa loa* and EMF in Nigeria and India has suggested an aetiological relationship. Free microfilariae have occasionally been seen in the myocardium and pericardial effusion in some cases, and filarial antibodies demonstrated in Europeans who have developed the disease in the tropics.

Clinical features

In young children the onset may be abrupt, but in older children is classically insidious, with increased oedema, dyspnoea on exertion, chest pain and abdominal pain due to an enlarged, congested and firm liver. There may be a long vague history of preceeding anorexia, malaise and episodes of fever.

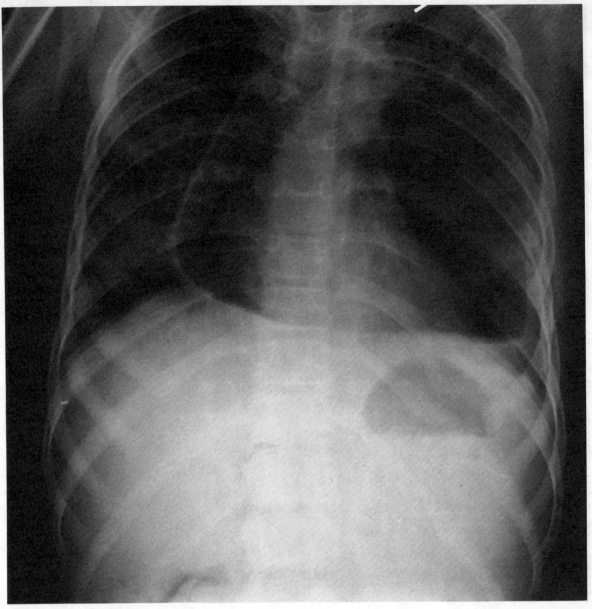

Figure 11.4b Pericardial effusion in EMF (a) before and (b) after tapping and air insufflation. Note the thin pericardium

The physical findings depend to some extent which ventricle is predominantly involved. (Table 11.7). On examination the eyes are often prominent with periorbital oedema. Cyanosis and clubbing may be present, liver and spleen enlarged and abdomen distended with ascites. A large pericardial effusion is invariably present in right-sided EMF. The chest wall may be covered with scars as a result of traditional treatment and pulsation noted in the third and fourth left intercostal spaces due to infundibular hypertrophy in right ventricular EMF. The apex beat may be difficult to localize. A pulsus paradoxus can sometimes be demonstrated, most easily in the femoral pulses. The lung fields are generally clear, although in left ventricular failure crepitations or a pleural effusion may be present.

Table 11.7 *Signs found in right and left ventricular endomyocardial fibrosis*

Signs suggestive of predominantly right ventricular EMF

1. raised jugular venous pressure with prominent pulsation
2. tricuspid incompetence − early or pansystolic murmur louder on inspiration
3. an infundibular impulse
4. pulsus paradoxus
5. gallop rhythm with prominent third heart sound at left sternal edge
6. gross hepatic enlargement with ascites

Signs suggestive of predominantly left ventricular EMF

1. minimal apical displacement
2. mild or moderate mitral incompetence − murmur heard best over the apex
3. pulmonary hypertension − loud P_2, right ventricular hypertrophy, split second HS, and Graham Steel murmur of pulmonary incompetence (in which case P_2 will be diminished in intensity)
4. fine crepitations in lung fields or pleural effusion

Signs suggestive of biventricular EMF
A combination of some or all of the above features.

Chest X-ray

In right-sided EMF the right atrium may be grossly dilated, the heart moderately enlarged, the pulmonary conus prominent and a pericardial effusion present which may be massive. This can be distinguished from a dilated heart due to congestive failure by (1) the globular shape of the heart, (2) the lung fields are not congested as they are in heart failure.

In left-sided EMF the pulmonary arteries may be prominent and the left atrium enlarged − best demonstrated by a barium swallow in the left lateral or oblique position. The left ventricle is usually normal in size.

Differential diagnosis

This includes rheumatic heart disease, neprhotic syndrome in young children with generalized oedema, constrictive pericarditis, tuberculous peritonitis and pericarditis, other cardiomyopathies, myocarditis, cirrhosis and kwashiorkor. Resem-

blance to thyrotoxicosis due to proptosis is very superficial and easily excluded clinically.

The pericardial fluid can be tapped as a diagnostic procedure to exclude a pyogenic or tuberculous effusion. The fluid in EMF has a high protein and lymphocyte count. If a small volume of air is injected into the pericardial sac after tapping, a chest X-ray taken in the erect position will reveal the classical picture. (See Figure 11.4a and b)

Progress and management

Unfortunately the disease is only recognized once irreversible fibrosis has developed and is at an advanced stage, with the patient in a state of resistent cardiac failure. Survival depends on the extent and severity of the lesion, and haemodynamic changes, and varies from a few weeks to several years, with some evidence of relapses and remissions.

The major complications are (1) cardiac tamponade resulting from a large pericardial effusion; this must then be aspirated; (2) pulmonary emboli and, less often, systemic emboli.

Treatment is that of cardiac failure, using digoxin and diuretics − frusemide, thiazides, or spironolactone, together with a good diet, low in salt and high in protein. Paracentesis of pleural effusions and ascites should be avoided if possible because the loss of protein can be ill-afforded. Death is usually from myocardial failure or an intercurrent respiratory infection.

Hypertension

Although hypertension is uncommon in children, blood pressure should always be measured as part of the routine examination of every child in both outpatient clinics and in hospital. A selection of cuffs of different sizes is available for children of all ages; the size selected should be the widest that can be wrapped comfortably round the upper arm. Use of too small a cuff will result in erroneously high readings, especially in obese children. It is the author's practice to tell the child that he is putting a bandage on the arm, it will be blown up and make the arm feel 'tight' and 'funny' but will not hurt. The child is asked to keep the arm still. It is often surprisingly difficult to obtain the blood pressure even in co-operative children and it is useful to obtain the systolic pressure by palpation first before auscultation.

Aetiology

The various causes can be classified into two main groups: acute transient hypertension due to intercurrent illness and chronic persistent hypertension.

Acute transient hypertension due to intercurrent illness

The commonest causes are:

- *acute glomerular nephritis*
- *acute renal failure*

Less commonly hypertension may complicate:

- *CNS disease* − brain damage from any cause, e.g. encephalitis, trauma and head injury, Guillain− Barré syndrome
- excessive *corticosteroid therapy*
- *burns, dehydration or relapses of the nephrotic syndrome*

In each of these there is an acute depletion of circulatory fluids, followed by an excessive secretion of angiotensin II by the kidneys and rise in blood pressure. Treatment is by infusing normal saline.

Chronic persistent hypertension

- *Chronic renal disease* is the commonest cause, secondary to dysplastic kidneys, scarred kidneys, chronic pyelonephritis and vesico-ureteric reflux, glomerulo-nephritis, neurogenic bladder, renal vascular abnormalities etc.
- *Co-arctation of the aorta.* This can be readily diagnosed clinically by finding absent or delayed femoral pulses. These should be palpated simultaneously with the right brachial or radial pulse − normally synchronous and of equal volume.
- *Neuroblastoma* due to excessive catecholamine secretions.
- *Corticosteroids* either from excessive therapy (usually clinically obvious) or unrecognized cases of congenital adrenal hyperplasia.
- *Wilms' tumour* − occasionally.

Investigations

Investigations are directed towards the obvious causes, and include i.v.u., cystogram and retrograde pyelography and abdominal ultrasound.

Cardiac emergencies

Cardio-respiratory arrest

A 'cardiac arrest' may be the sequel to many paediatric emergencies. Most 'cardiac arrests' are preceded by respiratory difficulties such as hypoxia and respiratory arrest. In addition, electrolyte abnormalities, anaemia and hypoglycaemia may complicate the picture.

There should be a well-established procedure for summoning staff. Resuscitation equipment and drugs should be kept on a trolley specifically for this purpose (see Table 11.8). This should be readily accessible in emergency rooms and the childrens' ward. Equipment should be checked daily and should not be 'raided' to provide drugs or equipment for routine use.

Table 11.8 *Suggested list of drugs and equipment*

Drug	Number of ampoules
Adrenaline 1:1 000	2
1:10 000	1
Atropine 0.4 mg in 1 ml	2
Calcium gluconate 10 per cent solution 10 ml	1 (or calcium chloride 10 per cent solution 10 ml)
Potassium chloride 1 g in 10 ml	1
Diazepam 10 mg in 2 ml	2
Paraldehyde 5 ml	2
Hydrocortisone 100 mg	2
Dexamethasone 5 mg in 1 ml	1
Frusemide 20 mg in 2 ml	1
Paediatric digoxin 0.1 mg in 1 ml	1
Aminophylline 250 mg in 10 ml	1
Hydralazine 20 mg	1
Methyldopa 250 mg in 5 ml	1
Isoprenaline 2 mg in 2 ml	1
Phenytoin 250 mg in 5 ml	1
Lignocaine 2 per cent (100 mg in 5 ml)	1
Chlorpheniramine 10 mg in 1 ml	1
Normal saline 5 ml	2
Water for injection 2 ml	2
Ampoule file	2
Sodium bicarbonate 8.4 per cent solution	50 ml
Dextrose 25 or 50 per cent for injection (i.v.)	50 ml
Mannitol 20 per cent solution	500 ml
Dextran or other plasma expander	500 ml

- i.v. giving set − adult   1
                   − paediatric with burette   1
- Sterile syringes: 1 ml, 2 ml, 5 ml and
                         10 ml   2 of each
                         20 ml   1
- Disposable needles for injection
                    21 g−4 cm   5
                    23 g−2.5 cm   5
                    18 g   3
- i.v. cannulae and catheters and
  butterfly needles, assorted sizes 21, 22,
  23, 24 and 25   5 of each
  3-taps and Ý connectors − sterile
- Cardiac board
- ECG paediatric pads and gel, and paper if ECG machine is available.
- Ambu (or other hand resuscitator) bag and face masks of varying sizes with appropriate connectors to corrugated tubing and endotracheal tubes.
- Guedal airways sizes 000, 00, 0 and 1.
- Connecting tubing for oxygen cylinders.
- Paediatric laryngoscope and batteries, with curved and straight blades sizes, 0, 1 and 2, with spare bulbs and batteries.
- Endotracheal tubes* with introducers − two of each size:

Age	Size in mm
0−6 months	3.0−3.5
6−12 months	3.5−4.0
12−18 months	4.0−4.5
4−6 years	5.5−6.5
Over 6 years	6.5−7.0

- Disposable mucus extractors.
- Foot and electric operated sucker.
- Suction catheters 5FG, 6FG, 10FG and 12FG − 5 of each
- Arm board and splints for i.v. drips.
- Alcohol and cotton wool swabs.
- Guaze squares (sterile) 10 cm × 10 cm
- Tourniquet
- Cut down tray (sterile) List of contents:
  Tape, spatulas, artery forceps (2), scissors, razor blades, scalpel, KY jelly, open wove gauze bandages, lignocaine 2 per cent for local anaethesia, and suture materials of varying sizes.
- Oxygen cylinder. Turn off when not in use. Key to be firmly attached by string so that it can't be lost.

---

* Portex Ltd. make an infant resuscitation set containing an endotracheal tube with sidearm and 5FG suction catheter for mucus extraction.

The A−B−C−D of resuscitation

Begin resuscitation on the spot as this is an emergency, by establishing an airway and re-establishing the circulation. Summon help.

A = Airway
clear the airway of vomit and mucus

B = Breathing
- begin mouth to mouth respiration using gauze between your lips and the baby's, *N B*. use your cheeks only for a bellows, and not your lungs
- insert an oral airway
- use a bag and mask attached to the oxygen supply if available.

C = Circulation and closed cardiac massage
1. Place the baby on his back on a firm surface, thus helping effective compression of the heart.
2. In infants place your hands around the chest. encircling it; rhythmically compress both thumbs over the mid-sternum at the rate of 100 times per minute.
3. In older children, place the heel of your hand on the sternum and depress the sternum at the rate of 80 per minute. Your assistant will monitor the heart rate by feeling the femoral pulses. However, if you are on your own, stop every 30 seconds and give four mouth to mouth respirations. Then return to cardiac massage.

D = Drugs
An intravenous drip should be set up as soon as assistance is available. Use the largest accessible vein. In infants this is generally the scalp vein. In desperate situations drugs can be given directly into the heart. However, this may cause haemorrhage into the pericardium, or even cardiac arrest.

Correction of acidosis
An 8.4 per cent solution sodium bicarbonate given intravenously at a dose of 1 ml/kg body weight. This is only beneficial if ventilation has been established.

Bradycardia
Atropine given intramuscularly at a dose of 0.01 mg/kg body weight.

Adrenaline 1:10 000 solution at a dose of 0.1 ml/kg body weight given subcutaneously.

Asystole
- adrenaline 1:10 000 solution as above.
- calcium gluconate 10 per cent solution 0.1 ml/kg, or calcium chloride 10 per cent solution 0.1 ml/kg
- leakage of calcium gluconate or chloride produces severe necrosis in muscle tissue, so great care must be taken when giving intravenous injections
- do not give directly into the heart

Ventricular tachycardia or fibrillation
Lignocaine 2 per cent (= 20 mg/ml). Dose 1 mg/kg body weight.

These conditions can only be detected if the facilities of an ECG are available.

E = ECG
Not all hospitals will have access to ECG facilities. 'Arrest' may be due to either asystole or ventricular fibrillation. In most children it is safe to assume that severe bradycardia or asystole has occurred.

F = Follow-up
A dose of 2 ml/kg body weight of 25 or 50 per cent dextrose should be given intravenously to correct hypoglycaemia that will have developed. After a period of severe hypoxia (lack of oxygen) some degree of cerebral oedema will develop as the child recovers. It is therefore important to avoid excessive fluid intake for 2 to 3 days.

How long to continue resuscitation?

If there is no response of any sort after 10–15 minutes of strenuous resuscitation and the pupils are fixed and dilated, with no response to light, then survival is unlikely and resuscitation should be abandoned.

Equipment for the resuscitation trolley

The following list is not intended to be a comprehensive one. Personal experience or preference together with local circumstances will decide what needs to be added and what can be omitted.

- The trolley should be kept in an area that is easily accessible.
- A named person should be responsible for checking the equipment daily to make sure that everything is in working order and present.
- The emergency trolley should be reserved for emergencies and not 'raided' to provide drugs not immediately on hand in the ward.
- All drugs and equipment should be replaced immediately after use.

12

Abdominal Disorders

The abdomen is the site of many problems in childhood in every country in the world. These problems are both physical and psychological, but in developing countries the health worker is wise to place psychological causes of symptoms very low on his list of suspected diagnosis. The swollen belly of a child in a developing country is a very common sight.

The acute abdomen

This condition is a surgical emergency and is generally the result of:

1. inflammation (as in acute appendicitis)
2. acute obstruction (as in twisted bowel or intussusception)
3. perforation of the gut (as in the second and third week of typhoid fever)
4. infarction (as in sickle cell crisis)

Conditions (1) and (3) are more likely to occur in children over the age of 4 years and condition (2) more likely to occur in children under 1 year but may occur at any age.

When examining the abdomen of a child at any age, it is preferable to ensure that he is lying on a firm surface and to kneel if possible so that you are at the level of the child's abdomen. For very small children it may be preferable to examine them on the mother's lap as this prevents crying which automatically stiffens the abdominal wall.

Observation is the most important part of the abdominal examination.

Direct observation of the abdominal wall may reveal the presence of peristaltic movement of the child's gut. This is suspicious of intestinal obstruction, but may also be normally present in a marasmic baby's abdominal wall with no obstruction.

After careful observation, gentle palpation should follow, but the child's face should be observed and not his abdomen. This is very important because this is where pain is first registered.

These aids to examination will be helpful if the child has an acute abdomen or a swollen abdomen. The main conditions causing an acute abdomen are as follows:

Inflammation

This commonly occurs in acute appendicitis or peritonitis. In the first condition the abdomen may be soft or firm on gentle palpation but the child will develop severe acute pain if the hand is suddenly released. This is known as 'rebound' reflex and is a very important sign. A kinder way to produce rebound is to gently percuss the abdomen. In peritonitis the abdomen is rigid and it is difficult to palpate without causing severe pain. Peritonitis occasionally occurs on its own but generally follows acute inflammation of the appendix. In both cases on auscultation no bowel sounds can be heard. The abdomen is quiet. A good aid to the diagnosis of acute appendicitis is the fact that a child never sleeps when suffering from acute appendicitis. He may vomit and the vomit relieves the pain temporarily. In acute peritonitis the child looks ill and is toxic. Fever may be low grade.

In acute appendicitis rectal examination may demonstrate tenderness in the pelvis.

The treatment in both cases is surgical, preceded by gastric suction and i.v. therapy.

In acute obstruction outside the new born period the child's abdomen may be swollen. There may also be visible peristalsis. Both these signs can be detected on inspection alone. The child looks anxious and vomiting is early. Diarrhoea is rare but initially there may be one massive bowel action.

Intussusception

This occurs at any age but is commonest under the

age of 6 months. The baby has bouts of 'colic' and may be shocked during the attack. He appears reasonably well between the attacks at first. If the condition is suspected early, a rectal examination may reveal the 'apex' of the intussusception and there will be blood on the examining finger. A 'sausage shaped' swelling may be palpated in the epigastrium or the right iliac fossa. Later, if a diagnosis is not made, blood and mucus may be passed per rectum and this should lead to the diagnosis although many cases are referred to the gastro-enteritis ward.

The differential diagnosis from bacillary dysentery may be difficult. Figure 12.1 shows X-ray findings after barium enema.

Volvulus

The main symptoms are severe colicky abdominal pain followed by vomiting. The abdomen may be

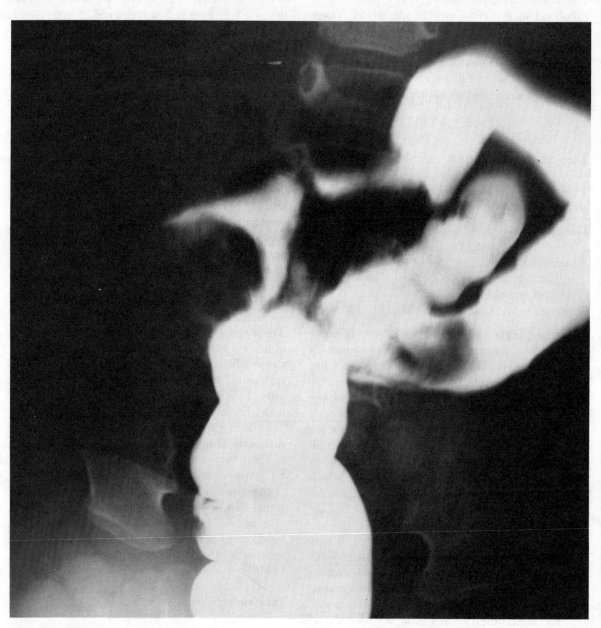

Figure 12.1 Barium enema showing intussusception

146

swollen and there may be 'rebound' present. Bowel sounds are numerous and are high pitched. The treatment in all cases is surgical but gastric suction and intravenous therapy should be started by the medical attendant if possible before the surgeon arrives.

Perforation of the gut

This is not common in children and the signs are the same as in acute peritonitis but the child is generally more shocked. It may be found in the comparatively rare condition of Hirschsprung's disease, but more commonly is seen as a complication of typhoid fever. The treatment is surgical, preceded by gastric suction and intravenous therapy.

Intestinal helminths

Ascariasis may cause intestinal obstruction due to the accumulation of a very large number of worms.

Sickle cell crisis

Severe acute abdominal pain with some 'rebound' reflex may occur during a crises in sickle cell anaemia. The pain may be due to the infarcted liver or bowel. Treatment is generally conservative.

The swollen abdomen

The swollen abdomen is a very common sight in many children in developing countries and may be the result of a combination of the conditions mentioned below.

Muscle wasting and poor muscle tone

This is generally due to malnutrition including conditions such as rickets. Cretinism and mongolism will also give this picture.

On examination there may also be an umbilical hernia. There is a marked absence of abdominal fat and the peripheral veins are visible but not dilated. Peristalsis may be visible.

On palpation there may be a loss of skin elasticity. No enlarged organs will be palpated in the abdomen and on auscultation the bowel sounds are present and normal.

Gas

This is a cause of a swollen abdomen in many children who have chronic diarrhoea as well as in cases of malnutrition. It may be a sign of obstructed bowel or enlarged colon (megacolon). The condition may occur in malnutrition. It should be suspected when diarrhoea is present and numerous bowel sounds are heard. The absence of bowel sounds would make the examiner suspect obstruction.

Hepatosplenomegaly

This is a common cause of swollen abdomen. In some diseases both organs may be below the umbilicus. Both organs are superficial in the abdomen and there is no bowel above them. Palpation should start very low in the abdomen with the hand lying flat and slowly moved until the leading edge of the hand, the fore finger, meets the leading edge of the liver or spleen. The finger tips should not be used to feel the liver. The spleen curves round from the left flank, and when it is large enough to cause a swollen abdomen a notch can be felt in its lower border.

There are very many medical causes of large liver and spleen and this condition should be thoroughly investigated. Apart from blood disorders such as leukaemia and thalassaemia, malaria is the most likely cause in a malarious area. In the Mediterranean and parts of North Africa it may be kala-azar (visceral leishmaniasis).

Ascites

Ascites is the medical term for free fluid in the abdomen. It is generally caused by liver disease but may be caused by abdominal tuberculosis. It is often present with a large liver.

On examination the abdomen is swollen, tight and shiny with large veins radiating from the umbilicus. On palpation it is difficult to feel any organ in the abdomen, and it sometimes feels like a balloon full of water. If a colleague places his hand along the centre line of the abdomen, and you place a hand on either flank a fluid thrill can be felt in one flank if the other is flicked with the finger and thumb. Smaller amounts of fluid cannot be detected by this method, but only large amounts of fluid cause a swollen abdomen.

Tumours

Tumours in the abdomen most commonly arise from the kidney (hypernephromas or Wilms' tumours, polycystic kidneys and hydronephrosis), adrenal medulla (neuroblastoma) and mesenteric lymph glanmds (lymphomas including Burkitt's lymphoma and tuberculosis). Ultrasound may be very helpful but if not available diagnosis can only be made by laparotomy. If malignancy is suspected frequent palpation of the abdomen should be discouraged as this may move tumour cells into the general circulation. An intravenous pyelogram may help in the diagnosis of a suspected kidney tumour.

The bladder

In small babies and teenage girls, a full bladder may cause a swelling in the abdomen rising from the pelvis. The cause is often as a result of an acute urinary tract infection. Children on treatment with the drug imipramine hydrochloride for enuresis may also develop retention of urine with similar results. The bladder presents as a swelling in the lower abdomen but may extend up to the umbilicus. On palpation it is a firm swelling which may also be tender. When percussed it is dull. The diagnosis is usually confirmed by passing a catheter.

Blood in the stool

This is a fairly common condition and it is sometimes difficult to discover the cause. The bleeding may be heavy or light and occur in any age group. In adults bleeding in the upper intestinal tract becomes altered during passage through the gut and appears black in the stool. This is not necessarily so in children. Intestinal bleeding may produce unaltered blood in the stool.

The easiest way to classify this problem is by age groups.

Infancy

1. *Late onset haemorrhagic disease* of the newborn.
2. *Anal fissure*. A tear in the anal mucosa following a bout of constipation causes pain on defaecation but also blood in the stool. Treatment: The fissure will heal if there is no constipation and the baby may need extra fluids. An anaesthetic cream applied locally may help to relieve spasm.
3. *Cow's milk allergy*. This may cause quite heavy bleeding with resultant anaemia. The baby often suffers from colicky abdominal pains which cease when the cow's milk is discontinued. In rare cases the baby may suffer from acute anaphylactic shock.
4. *Intussusception*. See above (page 145).
5. *Bacterial enteritis* or any inflammatory bowel disease including amoebiasis, infection with *Campylobacter*, *Salmonella* and *Shigella* are common causes of bloody diarrhoea. It may sometimes be difficult to distinguish from intussusception.
6. *Haemangioma* and *polyps* of the bowel. These, particularly polyps, are a relatively common cause of rectal bleeding and polyps may occur at any age during childhood.
   Treatment: polyps should be removed surgically.

Older children

1. *Inserted foreign bodies*. These may also be inserted into the bladder resulting in haematuria, or in the vagina resulting in a bloody discharge.
   Treatment: surgical removal may be required.
2. *Peptic ulcer*. This condition is commoner in childhood than originally thought and fresh blood may occur in the faeces.
3. *Oesophageal varices*. Rare in children but associated with hepatic cirrhosis and portal hypertension. Diagnosis is by barium swallow.
   Treatment: surgery.
4. *Meckel's diverticulum* of the bowel should always be considered.
   Treatment: surgery.
5. *Systemic blood diseases*, such as leukaemia. There is generally evidence of other bleeding.
   Treatment: acute leukaemia treatment.

Often it may not be easy to find a cause for the bleeding.

Liver disease

Common causes of liver disease

Outside the neonatal period and infancy liver disease in childhood in general presents as jaundice and is commonly due to infection. Other causes of liver disease are relatively rare.

1. Viral hepatitis (See page 54)
2. Amoebic hepatitis (See amoebiasis page 236)
3. Jaundice in sickle cell disease. Two types of jaundice occur in sickle cell disease:
- haemolytic jaundice
- jaundice due to hepatocellular damage

Haemolytic jaundice
This is mild and common. It is similar to other haemolytic jaundices, and is due to a raised serum indirect bilirubin as a result of increased breakdown in the sickled r.b.c.s.

Jaundice due to hepatocellular damage
The aetiology (cause) of this jaundice is not certain, but is probably due to hepatocellular damage caused by multiple infarcts of liver tissue as a result of blockage of liver blood vessels by clumps of sickled r.b.c.s.

The condition resembles viral hepatitis and the jaundice may be deep. The condition occurs during a sickling crisis (see sickle cell disease page 164).

The liver is enlarged and tender and the child feels ill. The jaundice may take several weeks to clear. The treatment for the jaundice is as for viral hepatitis.

Rarer causes of liver disease

Veno-occlusive disease
This is a disease first described in malnourished West Indian children between the ages of 1 and 6 years. It has more recently been reported in malnourished children in India, South Africa and South America. It has a high mortality but the cause has not yet been found. It would appear, however, that local food poisons may play a part.

Clinical features

1. *Acute disease* — after a period of fever and malaise lasting about a week, there is a rapid enlargement of the liver with ascites. Jaundice may occur, but it is rare. Veno-occlusive disease often follows on from an acute infectious disease. The condition may clear up spontaneously, or pass on to the sub-acute phase.
2. *Sub-acute disease* — there is generally marked hepatosplenomegaly which may be detected on routine examination. Acute flare-ups may occur,

but, as in the acute phase, jaundice is rare. The disease may resolve, or pass on to the chronic phase.
3. *Chronic disease* — this is the stage of cirrhosis of the liver and may occur several years after the initial attack. Cases have been reported, however, 3 months after the initial acute stage. Death may occur as a result of acute liver failure or from haemmorhage of oesophageal varices.

Treatment
There is little in the way of specific treatment apart from a high energy diet, salt restriction and diuretics for the ascites.

Prognosis
There is a 50 per cent recovery rate in the acute disease, but this rapidly decreases in the sub-acute and chronic disease. Jaundice is a poor prognostic sign.

Indian childhood cirrhosis
This is a disease that affects Indian children between the ages of 1 and 3 years. Male infants are more commonly affected and it is commoner in Hindus than Muslims. There is a familial incidence and siblings are often affected. It is said to be a disease of the middle classes and malnourished children are seldom affected. The actual cause is still to be found but toxic factors are implicated. The most important of these is copper in cooking pots.

Clinical features
The onset of the disease is gradual with loss of appetite, constipation or diarrhoea and abdominal distension due to hepatomegaly. Some cases have an acute onset and a fulminent course. The stools are pale and jaundice becomes deep. There is much muscle wasting. Later the spleen and liver enlarge to 3 to 4 cm and portal hypertension develops. At this stage there is also massive oedema of the legs. This is generally a sign of approaching death.

Treatment
There is no specific treatment for the disease and so it has to be supportive as in the other liver diseases.

Cystic fibrosis
This is a disease that is inherited as an autosomal

recessive gene and has a high incidence in the Caucasian race. The incidence in Europe is as high as 1:2000, with a carrier rate of 1:25. Other branches of the Caucasian race include peoples in the Middle East and the Indian sub-continent.

In the United States of America the incidence of the disease in black Americans is 1:17 000, and in Caucasians in that country the incidence is the same as in Europe.

It is rare in Chinese and Japanese races.

Pathology

Cystic fibrosis is a disease affecting the secretions of the exocrine glands throughout the body with a susceptibility to infection of the lower respiratory tract. Death generally results from chronic infection of the lower respiratory tract.

Pancreas

In 80 per cent of cases the pancreas is involved. There is a failure to produce water and bicarbonate in the gland although the enzymes are produced normally. As a result, the secretions become thick and the ducts are blocked. The enzymes cannot therefore be excreted.

As a result of this foods requiring the enzymes for digestion before absorption cannot be absorbed. This includes fats and carbohydrates, and results in the malabsorption syndrome. As there is no defect in absorption of the small intestine (unlike in coeliac disease and milk protein allergy) other foods, particularly iron, can be absorbed normally.

Respiratory system

At birth the lungs are normal but have an increased susceptibility to infection. In early childhood these infections are chiefly in the upper respiratory tract. The infection spreads to the lower tract and there is a hypertrophy of the goblet cells of the respiratory epithelium with increased secretion of viscid mucus and decrease in ciliary action. This results in bronchiole obstruction and development of bronchiectasis and airway obstruction.

Intestine

Ten per cent of all cases present with meconium ileus at birth. This obstruction is caused by inspissated meconium as a result of a lack of water secretion and proteolytic enzymes from the pancreas.

Liver and bile ducts

There is an accumulation of mucus in the bile ducts, resulting in obstruction, dilatation and proliferation. This eventually results in biliary cirrhosis. Hepatocellular damage is rare, but portal hypertension will follow.

Sweat glands

Sodium and chloride values are in normal concentrations at the base of the gland. Under normal heat conditions these ions pass up the sweat ducts to the skin and the concentrations on the skin remain within normal limits.

Under excessive heat stimulation there is a defect in the absorption in the sweat duct and abnormally high concentrations occur on the skin surface. Values of 60 mmol/l or more are abnormal; this is of diagnostic value. In very hot climates there could be a dangerous loss of salt.

Diabetes mellitus

The incidence increases with age but the diabetes is mild and controllable.

Reproductive system

Nearly 100 per cent of all males with fibrocystic disease are sterile due to bilateral absence of epididymous vas deferens and seminal vesicles. Impotency is not present.

In females, fertility is reduced to 20 per cent of the normal population due to increased viscosity of cervical mucus.

Diagnosis

Between the age of 1 year and adolescence the sweat test is invaluable and levels over 60 mmol/l of sodium are diagnostic. Mothers can sometimes make the diagnosis by saying that the child tastes salty when kissed.

In the malabsorption syndrome jejunal biopsy is normal, as are the levels of red cell folate and iron. Aspiration of jejunal juices show absence or low level of pancreatic enzymes.

In the neonatal period the Boehringer-Mannheim strip test is positive in the meconium of 80 per cent of cases.

Clinical picture

About 10 per cent of all cases present with intestinal

obstruction in the neonatal period. This is diagnosed by X-ray. The main clinical problem is concerned with the respiratory tract, which presents late in the first year of life as recurrent upper respiratory tract infections that do not respond easily to treatment and the malabsorption syndrome, which presents a little later, up to 2 years of age, and may even present as a rectal prolapse which is very common in fibrocystic disease. Steatorrhoea is more marked than in coeliac disease but anaemia is absent.

Disease of the respiratory tract leads to widespread bronchiectasis. Death from fibrocystic disease results from respiratory tract involvement. Respiratory function becomes increasingly diminished, pulmonary hypertension develops and death results from chronic respiratory failure, often aggravated by chronic *Psuedomonas* and *Staphylococcus* infections. Diabetes mellitus is a late complication of the disease. In hot climates salt loss is a very great problem which must not be overlooked.

Treatment

There is no specific treatment. Surgery is necessary for meconium ileus. Pancreatic deficiency requires pancreatic enzymes replacement therapy and a high protein diet should be given to help overcome the low growth rate.

The respiratory tract is the main problem. Prophylactic antibiotics help but it is not possible to keep the lower respiratory tract sterile. Exacerbations of infections should be treated with the appropriate antibiotic.

Exercise, particularly swimming and trampoline work, is very important for children with fibrocystic lung disease. More important still is postural drainage, which may have to be carried out three times per day, and regular physiotherapy.

Screening in the neonatal period

This depends on the presence of protein of more than 20 mg/g dry weight of meconium. The test is a paper strip test called the Boehringer-Mannheim strip test. The test paper turns blue when positive.

Prognosis

This really depends on several factors, depending on lung damage. Early diagnosis is very important

and in countries where the condition is rare, it should always be kept in mind.

Chronic diarrhoea

After an acute bout of gastro-enteritis, many children and infants may have persistent diarrhoea. Others will have persistent diarrhoea and loss of weight with no history of an acute episode. The first group of children suffer from the 'post-diarrhoeal syndrome' and the second group from the primary malabsorption syndrome.

Post-diarrhoeal syndrome

After a bout of acute and severe diarrhoea, the superficial epithelium (the 'brush border') of the small intestine is temporarily 'wiped off' (Figure 12.2). This epithelium contains the enzyme lactase which helps break down lactose, the sugar in the milk, to facilitate its absorption from the bowel. If lactose is not absorbed it enters the large bowel and draws fluid from the colon by osmosis, resulting in a watery diarrhoea. Some breakdown of lactose in the large bowel by bacteria may also occur resulting in the production of organic acids which cause irritation to the perineum and buttocks. Provided no more lactose is given by mouth, the 'brush border' will heal and regenerate within 3 to 4 weeks and the baby can again digest lactose.

Treatment
Replace milk containing lactose with milk preparations containing no lactose, such as

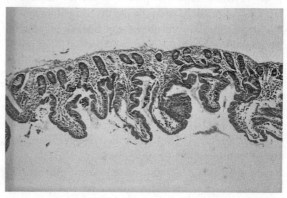

Figure 12.2 A section of jejunum under high-power microscope, with damaged villi, absent brush epithelium and increase in round cell infiltration of the crypts in a case of gluten enteropathy

'galactamine' or soya milk. Yoghurt is also acceptable. Should none of these be available, lactose in milk can be broken down to the absorbable monosaccharide by making the milk sour with the addition of vinegar or lemon juice. After 3 weeks milk should be gradually re-introduced. Should diarrhoea persist, re-introduction of milk should be delayed a further week.

Primary malabsorption syndrome

The major part of the absorption of protein, carbohydrate, fat, iron and folic acid takes part in the small intestine (jejunum chiefly but also ileum). This is a very large absorption area but all of it is needed. Damage and destruction of this area causes considerable defect in the absorption of all foods, resulting in severe malnutrition. Two particular foods, the gliadin factor of gluten (which is present in the cereals wheat, rye, barley and oats) and cow's milk protein (casein) cause damage to the mucosa of the gut by allergy in certain susceptible children. Antibody/antigen complexes severely damage the jejunal mucosa. This results in a loss of epithelial cells and flattening of the great absorptive area. Whereas cow's milk allergy is comparatively rare and may present with symptoms outside the gastrointestinal tract, such as eczema and even asthma, gluten enteropathy, or coeliac disease as it is usually called, is relatively common in those areas where wheat, rye, barley or oats are the staple part of the diet (Figure 12.3). In susceptible infants, symptoms occur within 3 to 6 months after the cereal is introduced into the diet, generally after the weaning period. Cow's milk allergy may present with similar symptoms as coeliac disease in the gastrointestinal tract, but as already mentioned, it is rare. Similar symptoms can also be produced by infestation with the parasite *Giardia*. This parasite lives on the jejunal mucosa damaging it, but also produces malabsorption by literally covering the mucosa.

Clinical picture
This is similar in presentation irrespective of the three different pathologies mentioned above, i.e. cow's milk allergy, coeliac disease and giardiasis.

Young children

- diarrhoea with bulky, offensive stools
- loss of appetite and vomiting

- abdominal distension
- irritability and apathy
- muscle wasting

Older children
Because of the absence of diarrhoea in many cases the diagnosis may be missed and the child presents later with growth retardation and delayed puberty.

Infestation with *Giardia* is relatively common and may occur in the presence of coeliac disease. If coeliac disease is not present symptoms of malabsorption may occur fairly suddenly in a previously healthy child. Symptoms of cow's milk allergy tend to be acute. Vomiting predominates eczema and skin rashes may also occur, as well as asthma.

Complications of coeliac disease
- growth retardation
- rickets
- anaemia (iron and folic acid deficiency)
- cancer (lymphoma) in untreated adults

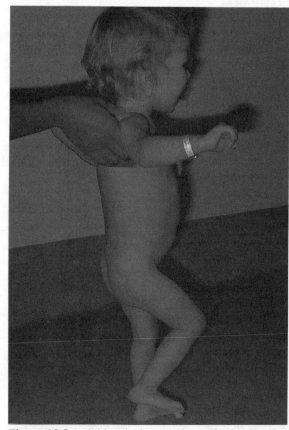

Figure 12.3 A child with gluten enteropathy (coeliac disease), note the distended abdomen and wasted buttocks.

Diagnosis

This is not easy without the aid of laboratory facilities. Jejunal biopsy is the only satisfactory way of confirming the diagnosis. At the same time as the biopsy jejunal juices can be aspirated to examine for the presence of active *Giardia*. The stools will contain fat globules and the presence of giardial cysts can be detected if infestation is present.

Cystic fibrosis commonly presents as a malabsorption syndrome. It differs from other forms of malabsorption as follows:

1. Under the age of puberty the sweat test is abnormal.
2. The jejunal mucosa is normal (malabsorption being due to absence of pancreatic enzymes in the jejunum.)
3. Serum iron and red cell folate have normal levels.
4. Respiratory problems usually predominate.

General screening tests for malabsorption include:

1. The 1 hour D-xylose screening test. Xylose powder (5 g) is given orally after overnight fasting. Serum xylose levels are estimated after 1 hour. If less than 20 per cent has been absorbed there is a suspicion of malabsorption, but this is not specific for coeliac disease.
2. Serum iron and red cell folate estimations. These are low in malabsorption.
3. Gliadin and cow's milk antibodies are specific for the conditions and may be estimated in specialist laboratories.

Management

In most rural clinics none of these tests can be carried out. Giardial cysts are often difficult to find in the stools. However, giardiasis is common and a 5-day course of metronidazole (7.5 mg/kg three times per day) should be given to start with. Within a few days dramatic improvement in the patient's condition will be noted if giardiasis is the sole cause.

If coeliac disease is suspected the child should be placed on a gluten-free diet. Rice is a good staple substitute.

Improvement is slow and early signs are a return of appetite, smile and loss of apathy. The child should be kept in hospital for 3–4 weeks and daily weighing should be recorded. This is the only true indication of improvement. Oral iron and folic acid should also be given.

Whereas gluten enteropathy may take some months or even years to develop, cow's milk allergy develops quickly and goes as quickly on the withdrawal of cow's milk.

Children with suspected coeliac disease should be monitored by jejunal biopsy before and after a gluten challenge after 2 years on a gluten-free diet. As this is not possible for most health workers, 3-monthly weight and symptom checks in the first year of treatment should be carried out. When the condition appears stable and the patient and parents have accepted the situation, yearly checks may be all that is necessary. A child with coeliac disease must remain on his diet for the rest of his ife. This helps to reduce the possibility of developing a lymphoma in adult life.

Non-compliance (dietary failure) is common and full understanding of the disease by the parents is essential for their co-operation. A dietician if available would be very helpful, as would leaflets in the local vernacular.

The vomiting child

Infants and young children vomit much more readily than adults. It is one of the commonest presenting symptoms seen in outpatient clinics. It is a feature of many illnesses and not necessarily indicative of 'gastro-enteritis'. Some of the commoner causes are considered here.

Possetting and regurgitation, feeding problems

'Possetting'. The regurgitation of small mouthfuls of milk is harmless and relatively common in infants soon after birth. More serious vomiting, occurring intermittently from the end of one feed to the beginning of the next, may be due to the free reflux or regurgitation of stomach contents up the oesophagus. This is caused by the relative incompetence of the sphincter at the lower end of the oesophagus. Control improves steadily throughout the first year of life, and is seldom a problem by the age of one year. Occasionally a hiatus hernia is present. In this case the vomiting may be quite forceful, suggesting pyloric stenosis. The vomitus may contain stale curds or mucus, and even streaks of blood if peptic ulceration or inflammation present at the lower end of the oesophagus. It is, however, never bile-stained. Occasionally the vomiting is severe enough to prevent the baby from gaining weight, but this is not common. Vomiting in babies is increased by excessive or rough handling after feeds. Forced feeding and giving the wrong weaning feeds (particularly highly spiced feeds) will very often produce vomiting.

When presented with a case of vomiting in this age group it is therefore very important to obtain a good feeding history. Management of excessive reflux consists of thickening the feeds and keeping the baby in an upright position in between feeds. Many African babies are carried on their mother's backs and 'reflux' vomiting is seldom a problem.

Congenital hypertrophic pyloric stenosis

This is commonly seen between the age of 3 to 12 weeks, and is seldom seen after the age of 3 months. It presents with increasingly severe vomiting which becomes projectile immediately after feeds. It is never bile-stained. Visible peristalsis may be seen over the stomach after a feed and a 'tumour' may be felt to the right of the rectus muscle in the epigastrium during a feed.

It is best felt by deep gentle palpation about 2 cm to the right and 2 cm above the umbilicus. Treatment is surgical. An untreated baby will die of marasmus and dehydration.

Infections

Vomiting is a common non-specific symptom and may occur as a presenting sign in almost any infection. In infectious hepatitis nausea and abdominal pain may also be present.

In upper respiratory tract infections the copious mucous secretions are usually swallowed and then vomited back, as they are extremely irritant to the stomach. Sometimes this vomiting can be quite severe. Coughing may also induce vomiting. Again a careful history is important and may show the relationship between vomiting and coughing.

Whooping cough and virus infections involving the respiratory tract such as measles are examples.

Intestinal obstruction

The classical signs are vomiting, progressive abdominal distension and constipation.

Intussusception

Infants present with episodes of screaming and abdominal pain, drawing up their knees and pass-

ing blood-stained stools often with mucus. It is sometimes very difficult to distinguish the condition from bacillary dysentery.

Strangulated hernia

This is not rare in children, and hernial orifices should always be closely examined.

Peritonitis

This condition should be considered when there is a distended silent abdomen.

Malabsorption

Any of the causes of malabsorption may be associated with vomiting. This is particularly so after a bout of gastro-enteritis.

Poisoning

Vomiting is usually acute in onset although lead poisoning may produce chronic vomiting. Almost any poison will produce vomiting, it is a natural defence, but a careful look-out must be kept for vegetable poisons ('bush teas'), or local medicines. Parents should never be sent home with iron tablets or aspirin as these are becoming a common cause of poisoning and may present with vomiting.

Intracranial causes

1. Tumours — vomiting is an early sign of raised intercranial pressure. It typically occurs in the early morning.
2. Cerebral abscess — for the same reasons as above.
3. Tuberculous meningitis — this may also be an early sign and is associated with progressive drowsiness.

These three conditions are, of course, relatively rare.

Psychological causes

These causes occur commonly in older children, generally in a fairly affluent environment. Vomiting is generally related to stress and unhappiness, particularly at school. Abdominal pain is usually associated with the vomiting and may be a form of school phobia.

13

Musculo-skeletal Disorders

Juvenile rheumatoid arthritis

This is a disease of the connective tissues involving most of the connective tissue of the body including joints, heart, blood vessels, lungs, lymph glands, skin and subcutaneous tissue. It is believed to be a manifestation of an auto-immune disease.

Clinical diagnostic criteria (Ansell and Bywater, 1959)

- The disease must commence before the age of 16.
- Inflammatory involvement of four or more joints for at least 3 months.
- Biopsy of synovial membrane must show histological changes of rheumatoid arthritis if only one joint is involved.
- Other causes of arthritis must be excluded.

The disease may start from early infancy up to the age of 16. Early onset juvenile rheumatoid arthritis (EOJRA) more commonly presents with extra articular manifestations. Late onset juvenile rheumatoid arthritis (LOJRA) commonly presents with predominantly articular manifestations and may present with one large joint only (large joint or mono-articular rheumatoid arthritis).

EOJRA tends to occur in children under the age of 5 years. LOJRA tends to occur in older children but there is a wide overlap. Mono-articular disease occurs in the younger age group. Polyarthritis occurs in the older age group.

Clinical picture

Early onset juvenile rheumatoid arthritis (EOJRA)

Articular involvement is mild and the disease generally presents with a high swinging fever which lasts several weeks with lymphadenopathy and spleno-

megaly. The child is toxic and may die during this phase.

Mono-articular involvement presents later when the systemic disease has settled. The hip and the knee are the most common joints to be involved.

Late onset juvenile rheumatoid arthritis (LOJRA)

Mono-articular disease.
The joints that may be involved are the large joints. The knee, hip, ankle, elbow or wrist (Figure 13.1)

Polyarthritis
This resembles the rheumatoid arthritis of adults. The earliest joints involved are often the cervical spine or the temperomandibular joint. Commonest joints to be involved are the interphalangeal joints, followed by the wrist, elbow, knee and ankle. Involvement is symmetrical. The joints are swollen and tender but the onset may be insidious. The

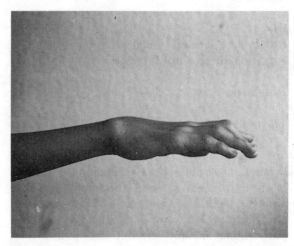

Figure 13.1 The wrist of a child with LOJRA showing fusiform swelling of the interphalangeal joints and wrist

joint pains are not as severe as in rheumatic fever.

The acute phase may last several weeks. Untreated the joints become contracted due to muscle wasting and ligament fibrosis. The disease is a long one and will result in growth retardation.

Rash
The rash is commoner in EOJRA and may resemble the 'butterfly' rash of systemic lupus erythematosus. It is pink and presents in small macules which may coalesce.

It occurs on any part of the body and on the abdomen may present as erythema marginatum. It may last for several weeks. It may be the only manifestation of EOJRA in the early part of the disease.

Nodules
These resemble those found in acute rheumatic fever but are a rare manifestation.

Fever
This is very common in EOJRA and may last for several weeks or months. It is high and swinging. It is one of the differential diagnoses of a pyrexia of unknown origin.

Carditis
This occurs but is rare.

Lungs
The 'rheumatic lung' (an interstitial fibrosis) that occurs in adult rheumatoid arthritis is very rare in children.

Eyes
Iridocyclitis, generally unilateral, is not uncommon but tends to occur in EOJRA.

Diagnosis

The criteria of Ansell and Bywater are helpful.

EOJRA presents often as a pyrexia of unknown origin in early childhood and must always be kept in mind. It resembles the rarer condition of systemic lupus erythematosus. Acute rheumatic fever may also be a diagnostic problem in LOJRA, but generally the diagnosis is obvious. Henoch-Schönlein purpura may initially resemble large joint disease (mono-articular rheumatoid arthritis) but the rash is diagnostic.

Laboratory
Rheumatoid factor related to raised levels of IgM antibody may be present late in the disease but only about 20 per cent of children have detectable IgM antibodies. Raised levels of IgG antibodies may also be present. They are detected using the Rose-Waaler or latex foams fixation tests.

Some children may have raised IgG levels and not raised IgM. These tests are not very useful in diagnosis.

The ESR is always very high (above 100 fall in the first hour) during the acute phase of the illness and this is helpful.

Leucocytosis is common. Normochromic normocytic anaemia occurs in LOJRA.

Course of the disease

Early onset disease may present as a systemic illness lasting several months and passing into mono- or polyarthritis, which can lead to permanent disability. Fulminant disease may terminate in death.

LOJRA may progress slowly to chronic rheumatoid arthritis with joint deformities. The disease may exacerbate from time to time, leaving greater deformity. Some children may develop the severe deformities of adult rheumatoid arthritis (the 'burnt out' case). Amyloid disease may occur in these cases. LOJRA may regress spontaneously and not recur.

Treatment

Drug therapy
During the acute phase of LOJRA aspirin (100 mg/kg/day) is the most useful drug and is anti-inflammatory. In some very specific cases and under strict medical supervision gold therapy may be of help. Chloroquine is not recommended for use in children. Recent experience with the newer non-steroid anti-inflammatory drugs is promising. In severe EOJRA a course of steroids (prednisolone 5 mg/kg/day) may be life-saving in children with severe systemic upset. They should never be used in any other case.

General
In LOJRA early splinting of the joints in the position of maximum use is essential. After one week night splints alone may be sufficient. The

splints should be in the form of plaster of Paris back splints that are kept in place by bandage. Bed rest is important in the early stages.

In the chronic form with permanent deformity, surgical treatment may be necessary to attempt to fix the joint in the most useful position.

Osteitis and septic arthritis

The common organisms causing these infections in healthy children are *Staphylococcus pyogenes*, group A and group B *Streptococcus*, *Haemophilus influenzae* and *Streptococcus pneumoniae*. Septic arthritis is more likely to occur under the age of 3 years and in this condition, as well as all cases of osteitis in the neonatal period, Gram-negative organisms as well as group B haemolytic *Streptococcus* are more important casual agents. In sickle cell disease, *Salmonella osteitis* is the recognized complication.

The differential diagnosis between osteitis and septic arthritis may be difficult clinically and septic arthritis may occur with osteitis in a long bone.

Pathology

Often there is a history of minor trauma around the metaphysis of a long bone. The area is invaded by the pathogen and abscess formation occurs. When virulence is low this may remain localized in the metaphysis and form a chronic abscess (Brodie's abscess). More commonly, there is spread through the cortex to the periosteum and a subperiosteal abscess may form. If the condition is chronic and untreated, the raised periosteum produces new bone (involucrum). The underlying cortex becomes devitalized, dies and pieces of dead bone may work through the skin, accompanied by discharging pus.

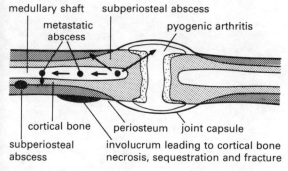

medullary shaft   subperiosteal abscess
    metastatic   pyogenic arthritis
    abscess

cortical bone   periosteum   joint capsule
subperiosteal   involucrum leading to cortical bone
abscess   necrosis, sequestration and fracture

Figure 13.2 The sequence of events following a bacterial infection of the long bone

The primary focus may also spread into the shaft of the long bone, where multiple abscess formation may occur throughout the shaft (Figure 13.2). Septicaemia, meningitis and multiple pathological features may occur. Any bone in the body may be affected.

If the primary focus is in a long bone near a joint capsule, it may spread into the joint capsule, resulting in a septic arthritis. Septic arthritis may also result from a primary septic focus in the joint capsule itself.

Clinical

The onset is generally sudden, often following minor trauma or a septic spot in the skin. There may be severe tenderness at the site of the infection and occasionally some adjacent joint effusion (not a septic arthritis). Untreated, there is overlying local tenderness, swelling and erythema. Fever is high and there is severe constitutional upset. The child may not be able to move the limb (if this is the site of infection) because of pain.

Early diagnosis and early use of antibiotics will prevent the lesion developing. If the diagnosis and treatment are late, it may be necessary to drill the bone to release the pus.

However, the acute phase may resolve quickly under antibiotic therapy but if the antibiotics are then discontinued, an insidious chronic osteitis may develop.

Diagnosis

Clinical diagnosis will give a high level of suspicion.

1. A full blood count will show a leucocytosis of 20 000 per mm^3 polymorphs or more.
2. Blood culture will be positive in 50 per cent of cases.
3. Bone X-ray shows no changes for 10 days.
4. Technetium bone scan shows evidence of osteitis in 3 to 4 days.
5. Serological tests for the responsible pathogen may be helpful.
6. Trauma, leukaemia, acute rheumatic fever and scurvy should be excluded.

Treatment

Early diagnosis and treatment are essential. The

organisms should be isolated from the blood culture. This may not be possible, so the following combination of antibiotics may be used empirically:

1. bacterocidal antibiotic penicillinase-resistants, such as methicillin or cloxacillin, should be given parenterally 200 mg/kg/day, together with:
2. kanamycin (200 mg/kg/day or ampicillin (200 mg/kg/day) to cover non-staphylococcal organisms.

Intravenous therapy should be given for 24 hours, followed by intramuscular therapy for 7 days. It is then reasonable to change to oral therapy for at least 4 weeks.

Clindamycin, cephalosporin and carbenicillin may also be used. If the organism isolated is a non-penicillinase *Staphylococcus*, then benzylpenicillin may be used.

For subacute and chronic osteitis long-term antibiotics, with surgical bone drilling and sequestron removal, are necessary.

In pyogenic arthritis, the same anti-microbial therapy should be carried out and the joint may have to be aspirated. In infants and toddlers with osteitis and pyogenic arthritis, chloramphenicol or ampicillin are the drugs of choice.

In both conditions joints may have to be immobilized for a short period and of course when surgical drilling and sequestration occurs, the limb has to be plastered.

Myositis and pyomyositis

Viral myositis

This often accompanies most viral infections but is most severe in those due to Coxsackie B virus. Treatment is symptomatic.

Pyomyositis

Haematomas (severe bruises) may become infected and result in local cellulitis. The cellulitis may spread into the muscle of the arms and legs (particularly the thighs) resulting in a pyomyositis. Tropical myositis is relatively common in Central Africa. These conditions are generally accompanied by high fever and inability to walk. The pathogenic organism is generally the *Staphylococcus*.

Treatment
Systemic penicillin and probably surgical incision to release the pus.

Further reading

Ansell, B.M. and Bywater, E.G.C. (1959). Prognosis in Still's disease. *Bulletin on Rheumatic Disease*, **9**, 189.

14

Blood Disorders and Childhood Malignancies

Unicellular organisms fulfil their metabolic needs by simple diffusion from the surroundings. With the development of multicellular and multi-organ life, a transport system for delivery of oxygen and nutrients to the various tissues became essential. The transport system evolved in the form of blood and the vasculature to contain it. Blood, besides performing the functions of gas transport and nutrient absorption and transport, is also responsible for host defence against infection, haemostasis and maintenance of a stable milieu.

The three formed elements of blood are assigned three different haematological functions: red cells are primarily responsible for gaseous exchange; white cells perform the phagocytic function and set up an immune response, and the platelets partake in haemostasis. Each of these elements, singly or in combination, are liable to several disorders.

Anaemia

Anaemia is defined as a deficit in the circulating haemoglobin (Hb) mass and is said to be present when red cell volume or Hb concentration in an individual is below the normal range for age and sex (Table 14.1). A large number of causes may be responsible for anaemia. A working aetiological classification is given in Table 14.2

Physiological anaemia of infancy

From a polycythaemic state in fetal life, a precipitous fall in Hb occurs in the neonate to reach a nadir around 3 months of age, in the fullterm infant the average is around 10 g/dl, the value being lower in the preterm baby (7 to 9 g/dl). Several factors contribute:

- improved oxygenation leads to a marked decrease in erythropoiesis
- a fall in erythropoietin occurs
- rapid destruction of fetal red cells
- expansion in plasma volume due to rapid increase in body size
- relatively non-responsive bone marrow

There are no clinical effects and since it represents a phase in normal development no treatment is required.

Anaemia may be aggravated in the preterm baby by folate and vitamin E deficiency. Such deficiencies must be corrected. Some babies may need a transfusion of packed cells.

Megaloblastic anaemia of infancy

Megaloblastic anaemia may be caused by folate or vitamin B_{12} deficiency. In infancy folate deficiency is by far the commoner of the two. Normal folate

Table 14.1 *Normal Hb and Hct (PCV) values (mean)*

| | Birth | 3 months | 6 months–6 years | 7–12 years | 12–15 years | |
					M	F
Haemoglobin (g/dl)	16.5	10.0	12.5	13.0	14.0	13.5
Haematocrit (PCV) (%)	55	35	37	40	43	41

Table 14.2 *Aetiological classification of anaemia*

1. Inadequate production of red cells:
   (a) Normal red cell precursors:
      – Anaemia of infection
      – Anaemia of chronic renal failure
   (b) Decreased precursors:
      – Congenital pure red cell aplasia (Diamond–Blackfan syndrome)
      – Aplastic anaemia
      – Bone marrow replacement (leukaemias, other malignancies, osteopetrosis)
   (c) Deficiency of specific factors:
      Iron, folate, B_{12}
2. Excessive red cell destruction (haemolytic anaemias):
   (a) Acute haemolytic anaemia
      – Glucose-6-phosphate dehydrogenase deficiency (favism)
      – Immune haemolytic anaemias
      – Non-immune haemolytic anaemias (malaria)
   (b) Chronic haemolytic anaemias:
      – Spherocytosis
      – Haemoglobinopathies
      – Thalassaemia
      – Hypersplenism
3. Acute or chronic blood loss

requirement is $50-70\,\mu g$/day. Besides deficient intake several other factors may lead to a deficiency state. Requirements are increased in infancy due to rapid growth. The presence of infection or chronic haemolytic anaemia also leads to increased requirements. Absorption may be defective in states of intestinal malabsorption.

Peak incidence is in the 4 to 7 months age group. Besides anaemia, the other features include irritability, failure to gain weight, chronic diarrhoea, and, in severe deficiency, thrombocytopenia.

A macrocytic picture in the peripheral blood smear with neutropenia, thrombocytopenia and large hypersegmented neutrophils should suggest folate deficiency. The bone marrow shows megaloblastic erythropoiesis with giant megakaryocytes and hypersegmented neutrophils.

Diagnosis is confirmed by decreased serum folate (normal $5-20\,$ng/ml) and red cell folate (normal $150-600\,$ng/ml). Serum iron and B_{12} may be increased. Treatment is oral replacement with folic acid $2-5\,$mg daily.

Iron deficiency anaemia

A newborn infant has $0.5\,$g body iron derived from the mother. Iron intake has to be adequate not only to provide for the rapidly expanding blood volume during periods of rapid growth but must also build up iron stores to an adult value of approximately $5\,$g. To achieve this target 1 to $1.5\,$mg iron must be absorbed daily. Under physiological circumstances only 10 per cent of dietary iron is absorbed. Thus an optimum intake should be $10-15\,$mg daily. A deficiency state may exist in a variety of conditions (Table 14.3). However, deficient dietary intake, hookworm infestation, infections and malabsorption states remain the leading medical causes of iron deficiency in the developing countries.

Generally the storage iron transferred from the mother is expected to be adequate for the infant's needs during the first 4 to 6 months and in the Western countries iron deficiency anaemia is rare before 9 months of age. The situation is different in the developing countries where economic deprivation and multiple pregnancies with inadequate antenatal care deplete maternal iron stores, with the result that babies are born with inadequate body iron. In such a setting iron deficiency in early infancy is common. Since most of the iron in the

Table 14.3 *Aetiological factors in iron deficiency*

1. Inadequate intake/stores:
   – Deficient intake
   – Maternal iron deficiency
   – Prematurity
2. Malabsorption syndromes
3. Increased demands:
   – Periods of rapid growth
   – Pregnancy
4. Chronic blood loss:
   – Hookworm infestation
   – Peptic ulcer
   – Meckel's diverticulum
   – Intestinal polyps
   – Excessive use of cow's milk and cow's milk allergy
5. Impaired utilization:
   – Chronic infection
   – Malignancies
   – Collagen diseases
   – Pyridoxine deficiency

fetus is transferred near term, preterm babies are much more likely to become iron deficient.

Clinical manifestations

Different degrees of iron deficiency exist:

1. *Latent iron deficiency*: iron stores are deficient but serum iron and Hb levels remain within the normal range.
2. *Subclinical deficiency*: both storage iron and serum iron are decreased but Hb level is still normal.
3. *Overt iron deficiency*: it presents as microcytic hypochromic anaemia.

There is no classical presentation of iron deficiency anaemia in children. Atrophic glossitis, dysphagia, koilonychia so commonly described as characteristic signs of iron deficiency in adults, are seldom observed in children. Most of the symptoms and signs are due to anaemia itself. Subclinical iron deficiency, though asymptomatic, does give rise to subtle manifestations. Irritability, poor physical performance and minor effects on neurological and intellectual function, including poor school performance, have been ascribed to iron deficiency. More severe deficiency produces clinical symptoms such as pallor, tiredness and fatigue, breathlessness, and in extreme cases, cardiac failure. Anaemia also increases the morbidity and mortality from all infections.

Laboratory data

The blood picture is that of microcytic hypochromic anaemia and as such has to be differentiated from other causes of microcytic anaemia, such as chronic lead poisoning and thalassaemia minor. Besides other characteristic features of these disorders, free erythrocyte protoporphyrin levels are helpful in differentiating them. The value is normal in thalassaemia minor, slightly elevated in iron deficiency and markedly elevated in chronic lead intoxication (normal $60-120\,\mu g/dl$).

Serum iron is reduced and total iron-building capacity elevated (normal $250-500\,\mu g/dl$). Serum ferritin levels (normal $35\,ng/ml$) provide the best indicator of storage iron, which may also be assessed from iron staining of bone marrow aspirates.

Treatment

In states of iron deficiency gastrointestinal iron absorption is markedly increased and oral iron administration is the preferred route. Ferrous sulphate is cheap, effective and well tolerated by children. It provides 20 per cent of elemental iron. An oral dose of $3-6\,mg/kg/day$ of elemental iron is the recommended dose. A reticulocyte response in 4 to 7 days indicates a good response.

Iron should be administered in divided doses in between meals (uptakes in food and iron-binding proteins in milk decrease absorption). However, if nausea and vomiting occur, the dose may be given soon after a meal. Vitamin C increases iron absorption.

Iron therapy should be continued for 2 to 3 months after Hb values return to normal; this is essential to build up iron stores.

There are very few indications for parenteral iron which is given by a deep intramuscular injection in the form of iron-dextran complex.

Often deficiencies are combined, and so for optimum response, these deficiencies, especially folate, should be treated simultaneously.

Haemolytic anaemias

The normal lifespan of a red cell is 100 to 120 days. When the lifespan is shortened, the red cell production in the marrow can increase up to six to eight times (compensated haemolytic state). Anaemia develops when the erythrocyte lifespan is markedly reduced to less than 15 to 20 days. Anaemias due to a shortened red cell lifespan are termed 'haemolytic anaemias' (Table 14.4).

In this section only hereditary red cell defects are discussed.

Hereditary spherocytosis

This is inherited through a Mendelian dominant gene. The basic defect is in the red cell membrane which results in a passive influx of sodium into the cell. At the same time glucose consumption is increased and there is a rapid decline in ATP and 2, 3-diphosphoglycerate on glucose deprivation. The resultant cells become spherical, relatively non-deformable and get trapped in the oxygen- and glucose-poor environment in the spleen and are lysed.

Clinical manifestations

The first manifestation may be hyperbilirubinaemia

Table 14.4 Classification of haemolytic anaemias

1. Extracorpuscular causes:
   a. Acquired defects with antibodies (Coombs' positive)
      - Erythroblastosis fetalis
      - Transfusion reactions
      - Acquired haemolytic disorders:
         - Autoimmune idiopathic haemolytic anaemia (AIHA)
         - Drug induced
         - Systemic diseases – SLE, lymphoma, lymphocytic leukaemia
   b. Non-immune (Coombs' negative)
      - Chemical toxins – snake venom
      - Physical agents – radiation, burns
      - Infectious agents – malaria
      - Microangiopathic – DIC
      - Hypersplenism
2. Intracorpuscular causes:
   a. Hereditary red cell defects:
      - Hereditary spherocytosis
      - Hereditary ovalocytosis
      - Thalassaemia
      - Enzyme deficiencies: G-6-PD, pyruvate kinase (PK)
      - Haemoglobinopathies
   b. Acquired defects:
      - Paroxysmal nocturnal haemoglobinuria (PNH)
      - Nutritional deficiences
3. Interaction of intracorpuscular and extracorpuscular abnormalities:
   - Favism
   - Lead poisoning
   - Pernicious anaemia

in the neonatal period. Later, anaemia of varying degree, mild jaundice and splenomegaly develop. Gallstones may develop as early as 4 to 5 years of age and 50 per cent of unsplenectomized subjects develop gallstones by adolescence.

Haemolytic crises

Patients may become profoundly anaemic due to rapid haemolysis without apparent reason.

Aplastic crises

Infection and/or folate deficiency may result in bone marrow erythroid hypoplasia and reticulocytopenia. A rapid fall in haemoglobin and haematocrit occurs. Recently, infection with parvovirus has been shown to be a cause of acute aplastic crises.

Laboratory findings

Classically there is anaemia, marked reticulocytosis, increased indirect bilirubin and bone marrow erythroid hyperplasia.

Red cell osmotic fragility

In normal subjects, red cell haemolysis begins in a saline concentration of 0.55 per cent; in spherocytosis it may begin at 0.7 per cent. Both normal subjects and patients with hereditary spherocytosis have a tendency to osmotic lysis after incubation of red cells at 37°C for 24 h, but the effect is more marked in the latter when haemolysis may occur at a saline concentration of 0.8 per cent.

Autohaemolysis

Red cells are incubated in normal saline at 37°C for 48 hours. There is haemolysis of 10 to 50 per cent of cells in spherocytosis compared to less than 4 per cent of normal red cells.

Differential diagnosis

Hereditary spherocytosis has to be differentiated from other congenital haemolytic anaemias which also present with anaemia and splenomegaly.

Autoimmune idiopathic haemolytic anaemia may show a large number of spherocytes in the peripheral blood. The history is short in this disorder, splenomegaly is not gross and direct Coombs' test is positive.

Management

Prompt control of infection is important since it may precipitate an aplastic crisis. Folic acid supplements should be given because the requirements are increased

Splenectomy improves the clinical status of the patient. It should preferably be postponed until the age of 5 years or over because of the risk of overwhelming pneumococcal infection in small children. Splenectomized patients should receive prophylactic penicillin therapy throughout childhood, and possibly for life.

Glucose-6-phosphate-dehydrogenase deficiency

This affects over a million people around the world. American blacks, Italians, Greeks, South-east Asians, Africans and Middle Eastern ethnic groups are affected. The defect is transmitted as a sex-linked trait. Female heterozygotes have widely varying enzyme levels.

There are more than one hundred structural variants of the enzyme glucose-6-phosphate-dehydrogenase (G-6-PD). The three most important are A+, B+ and G-6-PD Canton which is found in the Chinese population.

American blacks have A⁻ type of deficiency and the enzyme activity in such subjects is 5 to 15 per cent. The Mediterranean type of deficiency (B⁻) has an activity below 1 per cent, consequently these patients have a more profound haemolytic disease. The enzyme activity in G-6-PD Canton deficiency is approximately 5 per cent.

The enzyme G-6-PD is essential for the hexose monophosphate pathway and in its absence free oxygen radicals damage the red cell membrane and lead to Hb denaturation.

Clinical manifestations

Deficiencies of G-6-PD B⁻ type and G-6-PD Canton may be associated with severe neonatal hyper-bilirubinaemia with a high risk of kernicterus. Deficient patients may develop a chronic haemo-lytic state.

The most common presentation of the deficiency is with acute haemolysis which is triggered by a drug, infection, or more commonly ingestion of fava beans. Anaemia develops rapidly with haemo-globinuria and jaundice. Acute haemolysis causes a rapid and precipitous fall in haemoglobin severe enough to cause cardiac failure, and renal function may be impaired because of profound haemoglobinuria.

Laboratory findings

Peripheral blood shows fragmented red cells, reticu-locytosis and Heinz bodies (on supravital staining). Plasma haemoglobin is high and haptoglobin low or absent. There is gross haemoglobinuria. Renal function may be compromised.

The bone marrow shows erythroid hyperplasia. Red cell G-6-PD assay done during a non-haemolytic phase shows marked decrease in enzyme levels. The enzyme level may be near-normal after an acute haemolytic episode since reticulocytes and young red blood corpuscles have a higher concentration of the enzyme.

Management

- Hyperbilirubinaemia in the neonate may require exchange transfusion.
- Manage acute haemolysis with intravenous fluids, blood transfusions and alkalinization of urine (ideal pH 7.0).
- Monitor renal function during acute haemolytic episodes.
- Avoid fava beans and drugs (see Table 14.5)

Table 14.5 *Compounds associated with haemolysis in individuals with G-6-PD deficiency*

1. Analgesics and antipyretics
   Aminopyrine
   Antipyrine
   Acetanilid
   Aspirin
   Phenacetin

2. Antimalarials
   Pamaquin
   Primaquine
   Mepacrine
   Quinine

3. Nitrofurans
   Nitrofurantoin
   Furazolidone

4. Sulpha drugs
   Sulphasoxazole
   Co-trimoxazole

5. Sulphones
   Dapsone
   DDS (diaminodiphenyl sulphone)

6. Miscellaneous
   Chloramphenicol
   Dimercaprol
   Fava beans
   Isoniazid
   Methylene blue
   Naphthalene (moth balls)
   Para-amino salicylic acid (PAS)
   Phenylhydrazine
   Probenecid
   Quinidine
   Vitamin K analogues.

Note: Haemolysis has been observed in G-6-PD deficient patients in association with viral or bacterial infection, diabetic ketoacidosis, acute or chronic hepatitis, nephritis.

known to cause haemolysis to prevent acute haemolytic complication.

Pyruvate kinase deficiency (PK)

This is the second commonest red cell enzyme deficiency and is transmitted as an autosomal recessive trait. In the absence of the enzyme, the mature red cell is unable to produce its energy requirements.

Clinical manifestations
The heterozygotes generally have no overt clinical disease. Neonates may present with hyperbilirubinaemia.

Pallor, splenomegaly and jaundice are present in the homozygous state. Patients may develop gallstones. Aplastic and haemolytic crises may develop in association with infection. Certain American ethnic groups are known to have a relatively severe disease.

Laboratory findings
Peripheral blood shows microcytosis, polychromasia, reticulocytosis and burr cells. Autohaemolysis is markedly increased and is not corrected by glucose, but is corrected by ATP. Unincubated osmotic fragility is normal.

Spectrophotometric assay of PK in red cells demonstrates the enzyme deficiency.

Management
- exchange transfusion may be required in neonates
- folate supplementation and transfusions for anaemia
- prompt management of infection
- splenectomy may help severe cases; it should not be undertaken before 5 to 6 years of age

Haemoglobinopathies

Haemoglobinopathies are structural haemoglobin variants resulting from the substitution of a single (occasionally two) amino acids in one of the globin chains. These variants are genetically determined. More than 200 structural variants of the molecule have been found; most of these do not cause clinical disease. The ones which lead to clinical disorders may express as:

1. shortened red cell lifespan
2. easy denaturation of haemoglobin (unstable haemoglobin)
3. altered oxygen affinity (haemoglobin Rainier, Malmo)
4. altered haemoglobin solubility (HbS)
5. methaemoglobinaemia (HbM)

Haemoglobin nomenclature

Each Hb has been assigned a letter of the alphabet based on its electrophoretic mobility. If a newly discovered Hb resembles structurally an already identified Hb, it is designated further according to geographic location, e.g., HbJ Capetown.

Structure of normal haemoglobins
HbA: 2 alpha and 2 beta chains.
HbA2: 2 alpha and 2 delta chains.
HbF: 2 alpha and 2 gamma chains.

Important abnormal haemoglobins
Since the haemoglobinopathies are transmitted by an autosomal recessive gene, they exist in a heterozygous state or trait and homozygous state expressed clinically as the disease. Clinically important haemoglobinopathies are HbS, HbC, HbD, HbE, HbM.

Geographic distribution
(Figure 14.1)
HbS: Tropical Africa, Saudi Arabia, Greece, Italy, Turkey, India, West Indies, USA (blacks)
HbC: West Africa
HbD: India
HbE: South East Asia

Sickling disorders

Sickling most commonly occurs in a homozygous state of HbS (HbSS, sickle cell anaemia), the double heterozygous state (HbSC, HbS β-thalassaemia) and certain variants of HbC.

Sickle cell haemoglobinopathy

The substitution of glutamic acid, which is a hydrophilic amino acid, for valine at position 6 leads to an altered configuration of haemoglobin on deoxygenation. Rigid microfilaments are formed which

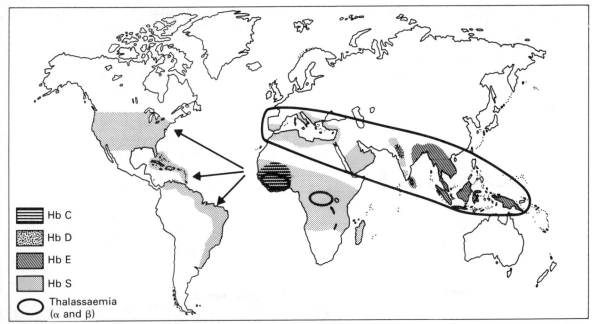

Figure 14.1 Geographical distribution of haemoglobinopathies

lead to sickle cell formation. Mild changes are reversible. HbA and HbF have a protective effect against sickling.

Sickle cell trait

This has a fairly benign course. Individual cells have a mixture of both HbA and HbS. HbS varies from 35 to 45 per cent and significant sickling does not occur. These cells are protected from infection with *Plasmodium falciparum*. Severe hypoxia, such as at very high altitudes, may produce vaso-occlusion. Spontaneous haematuria may occur. The disorder does not affect longevity.

Sickle cell disease

Symptoms usually begin in the second half of the first year. This coincides with a decrease in HbF from the cell and simultaneous rise in HbS. The following clinical states may develop:

1. *Vaso-occlusive crises*: There is intravascular sickling *in vivo* secondary to deoxygenation and slowing of the circulation in small blood vessels. Vaso-occlusion leads to infarcts in various organ systems – abdominal organs, lungs, CNS, bones, etc. Factors leading to vaso-occlusive crises are given in Figure 14.2.

2. *Hand–foot syndrome* (sickle cell dactylitis): Small infarcts in bones of the hands and feet cause bone destruction and periosteal reaction. Clinically these are painful swellings of the hands and feet. Bone changes can be seen radiologically.

3. *Sequestration crises*: These occur in the younger age group. Blood pools acutely in the liver and spleen. The spleen becomes massively enlarged. There is a rapid fall in Hb, abdominal pain, jaundice and circulatory collapse. It is a frequent cause of death in infancy.

4. *Aplastic crises*: Marrow erythropoiesis suddenly stops and severe anaemia with circulatory failure follows. It may be related to an acute infection, bacterial or viral, or folate deficiency.

5. *Hyperhaemolytic crises*. It occurs uncommonly in sickle cell disease.

Patients develop progressive liver cell dysfunction and gallstone formation. Diffuse glomerular and tubular fibrosis results in renal impairment. Initially the spleen is considerably enlarged, but following repeated infarcts, it becomes fibrotic and small (autosplenectomy). This produces a situation similar to that in splenectomized subjects, and patients become susceptible to severe pneumococcal infections including septicaemia and meningitis. *Salmonella osteomyelitis* may also complicate the disease.

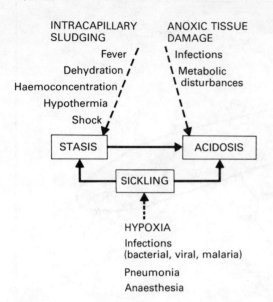

INTRACAPILLARY SLUDGING

ANOXIC TISSUE DAMAGE

Fever

Dehydration

Haemoconcentration

Hypothermia

Shock

Infections

Metabolic disturbances

STASIS

ACIDOSIS

SICKLING

HYPOXIA

Infections
(bacterial, viral, malaria)

Pneumonia

Anaesthesia

Figure 14.2 Factors leading to sickling and vaso-occlusive crises

Growth retardation, delayed puberty and chronic leg ulcers are other manifestations.

Differential diagnosis
Because of the probability of infarcts in any of the organs, the disease can mimic various acute illnesses and emergencies. An abdominal crisis may mimic an acute surgical emergency. A CNS infarct may resemble a cerebral 'stroke' or subarachnoid haemorrhage; bone infarcts have to be differentiated from acute osteomyelitis; a patient presenting with anaemia and bone pains may mimic acute leukaemia or acute rheumatic fever.

Laboratory findings
The peripheral blood shows changes of a haemolytic state. Sickling can be demonstrated in vitro. Definite diagnosis is made from Hb electrophoresis.

Management
There is no specific treatment. Management consists mainly in the prevention of complications. Any condition predisposing to dehydration should be avoided. Folic acid supplements are given daily for life.

Transfusions are generally not required because anaemia is usually well compensated and not profound. Anaemia is preferably corrected with whole blood rather than packed red cells because the latter may increase blood viscosity.

Sickle cell disease in Arabia
Sickle cell disease is common in many of the oasis areas of the Arabian Peninsula where the incidence may be as high as 1 in 250. However, there is an associated high level of HbF in these patients. This is because of increased synthesis of HbF.

In view of the high HbF level, these patients run a mild clinical course and early deaths are rare. Moderate anaemia develops by 1 year of age and the Hb level rises to 9.5 g/dl by 3 years of age. Vaso-occlusive crises are the commonest reason for seeking medical help. These patients also have an increased risk of pneumococcal infections.

Thalassaemia

The thalassaemias are a group of inherited disorders in which there is a reduction in the rate of production of one or more globin chains of haemoglobin, producing an imbalance of globin chain synthesis and resulting in anaemia.

Genetic control of globulin synthesis
- There are 2 α chain genes on chromosome 16.
- Non α chains, γ, δ, β are on chromosome 11.
- Production of α and non α chains is more or less synchronous. Deletion of a gene results in the absence of production of the corresponding globin chain. Partial deletion of the gene results in globin chain production at a reduced rate.

Gene:	α	γ	δ	β
Corresponding globin chain:	α	γ	δ	β
Haemoglobin:	$\alpha_2\beta_2$	$\alpha_2\gamma_2$	$\alpha_2\delta_2$	
	HbA	HbF	HbA$_2$	
Cord blood level	15–40%	50–85%	1.8%	
3 months	90–95%	5%	2%	
6 months	95%	2%	2%	
Adult level	97%	1%	1.5–3.5%	

Pathophysiology of thalassaemias
- There is a reduced rate of synthesis of one globin chain.
- This results in an excess of partner chains pro-

duced at a normal rate and ineffective erythropoiesis.

- Red cell survival is shortened.
- Anaemia and haemodilution are the final results.

β *thalassaemia*

This is a common condition throughout the Mediterranean, Middle East and South East Asia and wherever descendents of these people are found (see Figure 14.1).

Very few α chains are produced, although β chain synthesis is unaffected, hence there is very little or no HbA, and some increase in HbA_2 occurs. γ chains continue to be produced, so HbF production continues and is the principal form of Hb. Although HbF constitutes 70–80 per cent of the total haemoglobin, the total amount in each red cell is low. Many of the chains are released into red cell precursors but are precipitated in the immature red cells as Heinz bodies and are destroyed in the marrow causing 'ineffective erythropoeisis'. The molecular structure of β globin genes is now known revealing a complex genetic background to β thalassaemia. Some 40 different mutations or alterations in the structure of the gene have been identified that can produce the clinical features of β thalassaemia. Some mutations result in a total absence of β chain production, others in the production of β chains at a slower or very slow rate. Many patients apparently homozygous for β thalassaemia have been found to be compound heterozygotes for two different molecular types. β Thalassaemia also interacts with β chain structural haemoglobin variants. The most important ones are HbS-thalassaemia, a condition as severe as sickle cell anaemia, and HbE-thalassaemia.

β Thalassaemia is inherited as an autosomal recessive condition, although perhaps more accurately it should be termed 'intermediate inheritance' because the heterozygous carrier of the gene is not absolutely normal.

For practical purposes, thalassaemia clinically falls into three groups:

- severe transfusion dependent homozygous β thalassaemia
- milder intermediate β thalassaemia requiring only occasional or no transfusion
- symptomless heterozygotes

Clinical features of homozygous β thalassaemia

Anaemia is usually apparent by 6 months of age, sometimes earlier, though occasionally not until 2 years of age. Infants fail to thrive and have non-specific signs of ill health such as lethargy, fever and poor feeding. Chronic anaemia results in stunting of growth and delayed puberty. Untreated, severe anaemia causes cardiac failure. It may be complicated by folate deficiency. The characteristic bone changes due to marrow hyperplasia include bossing of the skull, overgrowth of the maxillary bones (the 'leonine' or thalassaemia face) and long slender limbs (Figure 14.3). There is an increased susceptibility to infection, especially streptococcal. Gross splenomegaly may cause hypersplenism. Death in the late teens is due to iron overload and complication of multiple transfusions.

Haematological findings

There is a severe anaemia, with Hb between 2 and

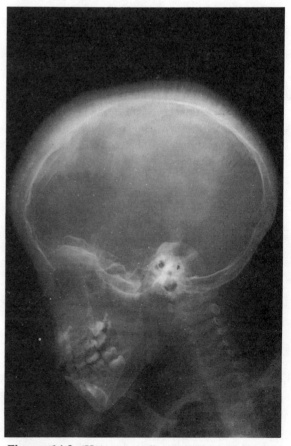

Figure 14.3 'Hair on end' appearance of skull in thalassaemia

5 g/dl. The peripheral blood contains hypochromic, microcytic red cells, with anisocytosis, poikilocytosis, target cells, teardrop cells and fragments. Normoblasts stained with methyl-violet show granular cytoplasmic inclusion bodies (Heinz bodies), aggregates of α-chains.

Hb electrophoresis shows HbF (from 10 to 90 per cent), normal or increased levels of HbA_2 and low or absent HbA.

Management
Erythropoiesis is ineffective to maintain an adequate level of Hb without transfusion, and there is a progressive fall in Hb with fatigue, breathlessness and cardiac failure. Blood transfusions have to be given regularly. The aim should be to maintain a Hb around 10 g/dl. At this level, regular transfusions should:

- improve the quality of life
- reduce the frequency of transfusions
- enable normal growth and pubertal development to occur
- reduce marrow activity and iron absorption

Folic acid supplements, 5 mg daily, are required for life to meet the increased demands of the hyperplastic marrow. Vitamin C and E deficiencies may also develop. Splenectomy may be necessary if hypersplenism develops, shortening red cell life and increasing the frequency of blood transfusions.

Iron overload develops as a consequence of multiple transfusions; each unit of blood contains 200 mg iron which is ultimately stored throughout body tissues (see below). To some extent iron excretion can be increased by giving the iron-chelating agent desferrioxamine, as intramuscular injections 0.5−1.0 g on alternate days. Continuous subcutaneous injections are however more effective in removing iron and more acceptable to most children. Ascorbic acid, given orally, increases mobilization and excretion of iron when combined with desferrioxamine.

Prognosis
Death usually occurs by the late teens due to haemosiderosis and iron overload. Bone marrow transplantation in early infancy or at the latest by 2 to 3 years of age from a histocompatible sibling is still very experimental and not possible on a large scale; it is a complex procedure and carries considerable risks. Chorionic villous biopsy in early pregnancy with DNA and gene analysis to detect homozygotes offers the possibility of therapeutic termination of pregnancy if this is acceptable in the community. It must be done between 8 and 12 weeks.

Complications of transfusion
1. Iron deposits in many organs result in haemosiderosis and eventually organ failure, and the development of further complications, thus in:
   - the liver − cirrhosis
   - the myocardium − heart failure
   - the pancreas − diabetes
   - the pituitary − panendocrine failure with hypothyroidism, hypoadrenalism and delayed puberty
   - the skin − pigmentation
2. Development of antibodies to blood groups, and possibly leucocytes.
3. Transmission of infections such as hepatitis B, cytomegalovirus, Epstein−Barr virus, and human immunodeficiency virus. Immunity may also be altered.

Thalassaemia intermedia and heterozygous β thalassaemia

These are usually symptom-free, although symptomatic anaemias may occur during periods of stress, e.g., infection or pregnancy, when increased folate demands may result in a secondary megaloblastic anaemia.

The anaemia is usually mild, with Hb between 9 and 11 g/dl. The mean cell haemoglobin (MCH) and mean cell volume (MCV) are low. HbA_2 is elevated (3.4−6.5 per cent) in most cases. The main differential diagnosis is from iron deficiency anaemia.

The α thalassaemias

Severe α thalassaemia is common in South-east Asia, parts of the Middle East, Greece and Cyprus. Milder forms are common in West Africa. In South East Asia α thalassaemia is frequently associated with HbE to produce HbE-thalassaemia.

Many different disorders resulting from inherited defects of α chain production have been discovered, but all result in two clinical disorders from excessive production of γ and β chains:

$\gamma 4 = \text{HbBart's}$
$\beta 4 = \text{HbH}$

Hb Bart's is useless as an oxygen carrier; the fetus becomes severely anaemic and is still-born with hydrops fetalis (homozygous α thalassaemia).

HbH disease produces a moderately severe haemolytic anaemia, Hb between 7 and 10 g/dl and survival to adult life. Splenomegaly and occasional episodes of haemolytic anaemia occur. The blood film shows microcytic red cells. HbH is susceptible to oxidation by oxidant drugs such as sulphonamides.

In Saudi Arabia 52 per cent of Shi'ite newborn infants have been found to have Hb Bart's in the cord blood, ranging from 0.5 per cent to 16 per cent of the total haemoglobin. These elevated levels of Hb Bart's, a low mean red cell haemoglobin (MCH) and abnormal red cell morphology are due to the presence of α-thalassaemia. Hydrops fetalis due to Hb Bart's and HbH diseases are rare.

Bleeding disorders in children

Any loss of vascular integrity leads to bleeding. Whenever this happens three mechanisms come into action to control it. First there is vascular spasm and aggregation of platelets which forms the haemostatic plug. Simultaneously the coagulation cascade starts which lays down a fibrin meshwork to strengthen the plug. Since the process of clot formation is self-perpetuating, it needs to be checked in order to prevent progressive intra-vascular clotting. The cessation of coagulation is brought about by the limiting reactions. Disorders of any of the three mechanisms of coagulation factors may lead to an abnormal bleeding tendency. Vascular and platelet disorders tend to cause spontaneous haemorrhages into the skin in the form of petechiae or bruises; known generally as purpura. Coagulopathies, on the other hand, more commonly lead to prolonged bleeding after trauma and to haemorrhage into the tissues and organs; these are discussed under the coagulation disorders. A simplified classification of bleeding disorders is given in Table 14.6.

Purpuras

Thrombocytopenia

Irrespective of the cause, thrombocytopenia results

Table 14.6 *Bleeding disorders*

1. Purpuras:
   a. Platelet disorders:
      i. Thrombocytopenia:
         ● Normal precursors:
            Idiopathic thrombocytopenic purpura (ITP)
            Disseminated intravascular coagulopathy (DIC)
            Drug induced (quinidine)
            Wiskott−Aldrich syndrome
            SLE and auto-immune disorders
            Cyanotic congenital heart disease
            Giant haemangiomata
         ● Reduced precursors:
            Marrow replacement (malignancies, metabolic disorders)
            Marrow depression (aplastic anaemia and thrombocytopenia)
            Folate and B_{12} deficiency
      ii. Platelets in normal numbers:
          Thrombasthenias
          Drug induced abnormalities (aspirin etc.)
   b. Vascular:
      Henoch−Schönlein purpura
      Scurvy
2. Coagulation disorders:
   Haemophilia A (classical factor VIII deficiency)
   Haemophilia B (Christmas disease, factor IX deficiency)
   Haemophilia C (Von Willebrand's disease)
   Deficiency of specific coagulation factors
   Congenital afibrinogenemia
   Acquired deficiency of vitamin K dependent factors
   Consumption coagulopathy (DIC)

in bleeding into the skin in the form of purpuric spots and larger ecchymoses, epistaxis which may be severe, haemorrhagic bullae into the mucous membrane of mouth, conjunctival haemorrhages and bleeding into the gastrointestinal and genitourinary systems. Spontaneous bleeding seldom occurs with platelet counts above 20 000/μl. Serious bleeding develops spontaneously when the count falls below 10 000/μl. Deep haematomas and bleeding into the peritoneal and pleural cavities may occur. The most serious type of bleeding is in the CNS, where it may be fatal. Bleeding into the eye may lead to permanent blindness.

Severe bleeding in thrombocytopenia is a more serious hazard in acute forms of platelet deficiency;

patients with chronic, moderate thrombocytopenia have a lower risk of spontaneous bleeding.

Idiopathic thrombocytopenic purpura (ITP)

This is a disorder of unknown aetiology in which thrombocytopenia occurs in the presence of normal (or increased) megakaryocytes in the bone marrow. It is often preceeded by a virus infection. There is considerable evidence that platelet destruction is the result of an immunological reaction. IgG type platelet antibodies have been demonstrated in the serum of patients, but are not consistantly present in all the patients. Additional support for an auto-immune mechanism comes from the demonstration of autoantibodies on the red cells by the direct antiglobulin test, a positive LE cell test and from the therapeutic response to corticosteroids and immunosuppressive drugs.

The disease occurs at all ages but children are affected much more commonly than adults, and unlike adults, both sexes are equally affected.

Clinical manifestations

The majority of cases have a mild illness with bleeding after trauma, or spontaneous bleeding into the skin, mucous membranes and from the nose. Occasionally bleeding from these sites may lead to considerable blood loss. Profound thrombocytopenia with counts below 10 000/µl carries a considerable risk of serious bleeding into the CNS.

Apart from the presence of purpura, and possibly anaemia, physical examination is generally unremarkable; enlargement of liver and spleen is rare.

The course is benign in the majority of cases and over 90 per cent of cases recover spontaneously. When marked thrombocytopenia persists for more than a year ITP is considered to be chronic.

Laboratory findings

The peripheral blood picture is unremarkable except for the presence of thrombocytopenia and mild eosinophilia in 25 per cent of cases.

Bone marrow morphology is normal with normal or increased megakaryocytes. When blood loss is significant, erythroid hyperplasia may occur. Bleeding time is prolonged and prothrombin time is normal; clot retraction is poor.

Management

Blood losses, if significant, are replaced, otherwise

management is conservative. If thrombocytopenia is profound, there is danger of serious bleeding. Such cases benefit from a short course of low-dose prednisolone; recommended doses vary from 0.5 to 2 mg/kg/day. The duration of treatment should seldom exceed 3 weeks.

In chronic ITP prolonged steroid therapy appears to be of benefit. Azathioprine, an immunosuppressive agent, may be used in cases not responding to steroids. Splenectomy may raise platelet counts to a level where serious bleeding is not a hazard. The benefits however, should be carefully weighed against the risk of overwhelming sepsis in splenectomized patients undergoing splenectomy.

Wiskott–Aldrich syndrome

This sex-linked recessive disease affects male children and presents within the first year of life. The main features are recurrent infections and failure to thrive, eczema and thrombocytopenia. The increased risk of infection is due to defective macrophage function and deficient antibody response to infection. Thrombocytopenia is due to defective platelets and their peripheral destruction. Death results from overwhelming infection or later from lymphoreticular malignancy.

Laboratory findings

Thrombocytopenia is present from birth and the platelets are small. Serum IgM is low and IgA is elevated. Cell-mediated immunity is defective. Bone marrow is normal.

Management

The only treatment which appears to improve the clinical picture is bone marrow transplantation.

Henoch–Schönlein purpura (anaphylactoid purpura)

This is a common disorder of school age children and adolescents and is characterized by purpura, abdominal symptoms and joint pains. The exact aetiology is not known but it has characteristics of an allergic reaction. It often follows a mild viral infection and tends to be seasonal in incidence. The basic pathological lesion is a widespread vasculitis.

Clinical manifestations

Skin lesions consisting of purpura and bruising are characteristically distributed over the legs, buttocks and extensor surfaces of forearms. Sometimes the lesions may be present on the upper arms over the deltoid area but are rarely seen on the face and the trunk.

Abdominal pain and bleeding into the gut are due to vasculitis and oedema of the bowel wall. Malaena is more common than haematemesis. Intussusception may complicate abdominal involvement.

Pain and swelling of joints, especially knees and ankles, is transient and disappears within a few days without sequelae.

Renal involvement may occur. Microscopic haematuria and mild proteinuria are symptomless and common. A few cases develop frank gross haematuria and acute glomerular nephritis. Renal involvement may occur late in the course of the disease.

In the majority of cases the clinical course is mild and complete recovery takes place in 3 to 4 weeks. However, microscopic haematuria may persist for several months.

Although rare, patients developing frank nephritis are at risk of developing nephrotic syndrome or chronic renal failure.

Differential diagnosis
Many conditions both medical and surgical need to be distinguished depending upon the presentation. Purpura has to be differentiated from thrombocytopenic purpura. Abdominal pain and bleeding have to be distinguished from surgical causes. Joint manifestations may be severe enough to mimic rheumatoid arthritis.

Laboratory findings
The peripheral blood picture may be of anaemia of blood loss. The urine may show haematuria proteinuria and casts. Erythrocyte sedimentation rate is high and serum IgA may be elevated.

Management
The majority of children do not require any treatment except for symptomatic relief of pain. Severe bleeding requires blood replacement. In severe or recurrent cases a short course of prednisolone 1 to 2 mg/kg/day may be helpful. It however does not affect the incidence of renal complications.

South-east Asian acute haemorrhagic fever
This is one of several types of haemorrhagic fever.

Dengue virus has been recovered from the patients and is considered to be the cause. The virus is transmitted by the mosquito *Aedes aegypti*.

Though the virus is ubiquitous, epidemics of the disease are only seen in South-east Asia. The disease results from a secondary infection when high levels of circulating antibody to the virus are present.

The onset is acute with fever, chills, headache and severe body aches. Nausea, vomiting, abdominal pain and respiratory symptoms may be present. Hepatomegaly is a constant feature. Purpura, epistaxis, melaena and other haemorrhagic manifestations are due to thrombocytopenia and disseminated intravascular coagulation. Shock develops in almost one-third of cases. It carries a high mortality.

Laboratory investigations show thrombocytopenia, decreased C3 complement and evidence of DIC. Chest X-ray may show an interstitial pneumonia and pleural effusion.

Treatment is mainly symptomatic.

Coagulation disorders

Haemophilia A: factor VIII deficiency
Haemophilia is the commonest of the hereditary deficiencies of clotting factors. It was recognized in China and the Middle East 3000 years ago. It is transmitted as a sex linked recessive condition and affects males. Females are symptomless carriers of the abnormal gene and can be detected by measuring levels of inactive immunoreactive factor VIII. The basic defect is due to an abnormal gene that produces a functionally inactive variant of factor VIII.

The incidence in the general population appears to be in the range of 4 to 8 per 100 000, though regional variations occur.

Clinical manifestations
The deficiency presents from birth and early features are prolonged bleeding from injury sites. Infants have profuse bleeding after circumcision. Bruises in the skin, haemarthroses and painful soft tissue swellings due to bleeds in the muscles are common as the child grows. Excessive bleeding after dental extraction or tonsillectomy, epistaxis, haematuria, etc. are other manifestations of the bleeding tendency. The severity of bleeding depends on the amount of functional factor VIII

concentration in the circulation. Values up to 50 per cent of normal are not associated with significant bleeding; values between 25 and 50 per cent will lead to excessive blood loss after major trauma and levels below 25 per cent will result in excessive bleeding even after minor trauma. Repeated bleeding into the joints results in chronic deformities and disability.

Laboratory findings
Screening tests are useful in deciding whether there is a defect in the clotting mechanism. The partial thromboplastin time tests the integrity of the early stages of coagulation (intrinsic pathway) and is prolonged in haemophilia. The prothrombin time which tests the later stages (extrinsic pathway) is normal as are platelet count and bleeding time. The clotting time is not a good test because it is normal until factor VIII levels fall to $1-2$ per cent. The definitive test is an assay of factor VIII.

Management
In the event of bleeding, however minor it may be, replacement therapy with fresh frozen plasma, cryoprecipitate or factor VIII concentrate is mandatory.

Fresh frozen plasma (contains 0.7 units/ml)* is suitable only for minor bleeds; a dose of 15 ml/kg raises factor VIII level to 20 per cent. This should be followed with 10 ml/kg every 12 hours since the half life of factor VIII is 12 hours (half life is decreased in the presence of fever, infection or presence of circulatory factor VIII inhibitors). Cryoprecipitate contains between 75 to 150 units* of factor VIII per bag. Factor VIII concentrate (Haemofil) has 250 units/10 ml and when given to a 10 kg child will raise factor VIII level from zero to about 50 per cent. The requirements of factor VIII relate to the type or risk of bleeding. The following guidelines may be useful:

Condition	Factor VIII level required
Haemarthrosis, haematuria	10 to 20 per cent
Surface wound bleeding	20 to 40 per cent
Surgery	60 per cent
Intracranial haemorrhage	100 per cent

* One unit is defined as the factor VIII activity in 1 ml of average fresh plasma (assumed to have 100 per cent factor VIII activity).

Stored blood is not a satisfactory source of factor VIII since it virtually disappears from fresh blood within 24 hours of withdrawal from the donor. Children with haemophilia should never be given intramuscular injections or aspirin. They need good dental care because of risk of excessive bleeding. They should not be trained for vocations which may expose them to trauma. Since they require repeated i.v. infusions, they have increased risk of AIDS and hepatitis B infection, therefore their liver function should be monitored from time to time. Haemarthroses, particularly in the lower limbs may lead to crippling unless proper physiotherapy is given.

ε-Aminocaproic acid (EACA) given in dose of 200 mg/kg, and later in dose of 100 mg/kg every 6 hours for 3 to 5 days helps to control local bleeding from the mouth, teeth and nose in mild cases, but should never be used to control haematuria.

Haemophilia B (Christmas disease); factor IX deficiency
Factor IX deficiency is also transmitted as a sex linked recessive trait. Clinically the disease is indistinguishable from haemophilia. The incidence is almost one-sixth that of classical haemophilia.

Factor IX is stable and sufficient quantities are present even in blood stored up to 3 weeks. There is some loss of activity in fresh frozen plasma but it can be used. Factor IX concentrates are available commercially. The initial replacement is done with 1 unit/kg. The half life is 22 hours.

Haemophilia C (Von Willebrand's disease)
This is an uncommon inherited bleeding disorder transmitted as an autosomal dominant trait. The main abnormalities are defective platelets which have decreased adhesiveness, and defective factor VIII molecule. Clinically skin bruising, mucous membrane bleeding and epistaxis are common. Excessive bleeding may follow dental extraction and trauma. In females menorrhagia may be a problem. The severity of bleeding is variable and it may vary even in the same individual at different times. The main laboratory findings are a prolonged bleeding time, prolonged partial thrombo plastin time and abnormal platelet adhesiveness; platelet aggregation *in vitro* is normal. Factor VIII cryoprecipitates are used for serious bleeding as in haemophilia. ε-aminocaproic acid is useful in epistaxis.

Childhood malignancies

In the developed countries cancer is the commonest cause of death, second only to accidents, in the paediatric age group beyond infancy. This is not true of the developing world which is still dominated by infection, diarrhoeal disease and malnutrition. Nevertheless malignant disease does cause significant morbidity and mortality amongst ethnic groups, though there are differences in incidence of various tumour types in different geographic regions. Thus Burkitt's lymphoma is common in African blacks; liver cancer is common in the Far East and central America and retinoblastoma has a high incidence in India.

The annual incidence of malignancies in the 1 to 15 year ago group is 110 per 10^6. One-third of these are accounted for by leukaemias, one-third by brain tumours and the rest are other solid tumours. In the paediatric age group different malignancies tend to cluster in different age periods. Acute lymphoblastic leukaemia. Wilms' tumour, retinoblastoma, hepatoblastoma and neuroblastoma occur in infancy and early childhood; non-Hodgkin's lymphoma and Ewing's sarcoma are common in school years and Hodgkin's lymphoma osteogenic sarcoma, acute myeloid leukaemia and rhabdomyosarcoma are more common in older children.

With improved management the prognosis of various malignancies in childhood years has improved vastly, and with the exception of acute myeloid leukaemia and neuroblastoma a 5-year survival rate of over 50 per cent can be expected in good centres. A considerably better prognosis can be expected with regard to Hodgkin's lymphoma, retinoblastoma and Wilms' tumour. Factors that have contributed to the improved prognosis include early diagnosis, proper staging and a multi-disciplinary approach and teamwork involving the paediatrician, paediatric surgeon and the radiologist.

Risk factors

In adults 60 to 90 per cent of malignancy is related to environmental factors. The same is not true of childhood cancer and in them host factors are more important.

Immunodeficiency states are associated with an increased risk of malignancy particularly with regard to lymphomata.

Defective DNA repair as in ataxia telangiectasia and xeroderma pigmentosum increase the risk of lymphoma and skin cancer respectively.

Congenital anomalies such as aniridia and hemihypertrophy have an increased associated risk of Wilms' tumour and hepatoma. Down's syndrome patients have a higher incidence of leukaemia. Deletion of the long arm of chromosome 13 is associated with an increased incidence of retinoblastoma.

Presentation

Early diagnosis needs a high index of suspicion. Cancer in childhood may present with lumps, lymphadenopathy, unexplained fever, weight loss, anaemia, bleeding or may be detected on routine check-ups in an otherwise asymptomatic patient. Intracranial tumours generally present with visual disturbance, ataxia or symptoms of raised intracranial tension.

Diagnosis

An accurate diagnosis, both clinical and histological, is essential to plan proper therapy and to assess prognosis. A skeletal survey, bone marrow aspiration, ultrasound scan, computerized tomography, radionucleotide scanning, α-fetoprotein (hepatoblastoma, malignant germ cell tumour) and urinary VMA (neuroblastoma) are some of the important diagnostic aids.

Staging

Several solid tumours have specific staging systems. In general the staging is as follows:

Stage I: Tumour localized to the tissue of origin and totally resectable.
Stage II: Localized, with spread to local nodes and not totally resectable.
Stage III: Regional spread.
Stage IV: Distant metastases.

The following abbreviations are used in the sections on childhood malignancies:

Actino-D   Actinomycin D
ADM   Adriamycin (doxorubicin)
ALL   Acute lymphoblastic leukaemia

AML	Acute myeloblastic leukaemia
ASP	Asparaginase
Ara-C	Cytosine arabinoside
BMT	Bone marrow transplant/transplantation
CML	Chronic myeloid leukaemia
CNS	Central nervous system
CSF	Cerebro spinal fluid
Cyclo	Cyclophosphamide
CT	Computerized axial tomography
EBV	Epstein—Barr virus
FAB	French/American/British Co-operative Group
HD	Hodgkin's Disease
HMA	Homovanillic acid
IT	Intrathecal
HLA	Human lymphocyte antigen
6MP	6 Mercaptopurine
MTX	Methotrexate
NHL	Non-Hodgkin's lymphoma
Pred.	Prednisolone
6TG	6 Thioguanine
VBL	Vinblastine
VCR	Vincristine
VMA	Vanillylmandelic acid

The leukaemias

Leukaemias are malignancies characterized by circulation of large numbers of leukocytes in the peripheral blood. An accompanying infiltration of various organs with immature and mature leukocytes is an important pathological component. Leukaemias may occur at any age from birth to old age but the peak incidence is from 2 to 4 years with an overall incidence in childhood years of 4 to 5 per 100 000 children. Males and females are equally affected.

In children the majority of leukaemias are acute in type. About 85 per cent are acute lymphoblastic (ALL) and 13 per cent are of the acute myelogenous type (AML); chronic granulocytic leukaemia and other related disorders account for only 1–2 per cent of cases. Chronic lymphocytic leukaemia is not seen in children.

Definitions

The following terms are important with regard to haematological malignancies:

- *Aleukaemic leukaemia*: refers to acute leukaemia in which the peripheral blood is free of immature forms and the white cell count is normal. Diagnosis depends upon bone marrow examination.
- *Subleukaemic leukaemia*: immature white cells are present in the peripheral circulation but the total white cell count is normal.
- *Hyperleukocytosis*: the leukocyte count in the per-

ipheral circulation is very high and band forms of granulocytes are present.
- *Leukaemoid reaction*: the white cell count in the peripheral circulation is very high and immature forms are present. The bone marrow is normal.

Classification

Leukaemias are classified according to cell morphology and natural history of the disease. The various morphological types are further subclassified.

Acute lymphoblastic leukaemia is divided into the following sub-groups:

1. Common ALL: 70 per cent cases. Equally common in boys and girls. White cell count is usually not very high. Generally good prognosis.
2. T-cell type: 15 per cent of all cases. Usually presents with a mediastinal mass. More common in older boys. Prognosis is poor.
3. B-cell type: 1.5 per cent cases. It has a very poor prognosis.
4. 'Null' cell type: 10 per cent. It has no immunological surface markers. It is commoner in adults and has a poor prognosis.

ALL is also sub-classified into six types L1 to L6 according to the French/American/British co-operative group classification (FAB classification). Acute myeloblastic leukaemia (AML) is subclassified also into six types as per the FAB classification:

FAB classification	Morphologic type
M1	Myeloblastic, no maturation
M2	Myeloblastic, with maturation
M3	Hypergranular, premyelocytic
M4	Myelomonocytic
M5	Monocytic
M6	Erythroleukaemia

Chronic myeloid leukaemia (CML) is classified into the juvenile and adult forms:

	Juvenile form	Adult form
1. Philadelphia chromosome	Negative	Positive
2. Thrombocytopenia	Common	None
3. Response to therapy	Unresponsive	Relatively good
4. Median survival	One year	Three years

Aetiology

A combination of genetic and environmental factors seems important. Viruses have been implicated and human T-cell lymphoma virus was isolated in 1982; Epstein–Barr virus has been related to Burkitt's lymphoma. The following have been associated with an increased incidence of leukaemia:

- maternal irradiation during pregnancy,
- chromosomal anomalies as in Down's syndrome, Klinefelter's syndrome,
- Fanconi's anaemia, and
- immunological disorders such as hypogamma-globulinaemia, Wiscott–Aldrich syndrome, ataxia telangiectasia.

Clinical presentation

Acute leukaemias, irrespective of the morphological type have a common clinical picture. The various symptoms and signs are the result of:

- replacement of normal marrow by the blast cells with with failure of erythropoiesis
- extramedullary infiltration of blast cells

Early features are non-specific and are in the form of anorexia, fatigue, irregular fever etc. Pallor, infection, bleeding (bruising, purpura, petechiae, epistaxis, bleeding gums, haematuria), joint and bone pains, lymph node enlargement or hepato-megaly may be presenting features. Bone pains and sternal tenderness are important clinical features. Certain uncommon presentations are:

- mediastinal mass
- raised intracranial tension (due to infiltration/ bleeding)
- Mikulicz syndrome (enlargement of salivary glands and lachrymal glands)
- bony masses (chloroma in AML)

Differential diagnosis

This varies with the clinical presentation:

- bleeding: ITP and other bleeding diatheses, scurvy
- bone pains: rheumatic fever, rheumatoid arthritis, sickle cell disease
- lymphadenopathy: infectious mononucleosis, other lymphoreticular malignancies

- pancytopenia: aplastic anaemia
- bone marrow infiltration: disseminated neuro-blastoma, rhabdomyosarcoma

Bad prognostic signs (ALL)

- age below 2 years or above 10 years
- black races
- marked organomegaly
- mediastinal mass (T-cell type)
- B-cell type, 'null' cell type, L3 (FAB)
- CNS disease on presentation
- profound leukocytosis, thrombocytopenia

Good prognostic signs (ALL)

- female sex
- FAB L1 type
- leukocyte count $<20 \times 10^9/l$

Management

Includes general measures and specific chemotherapy.

General measures (prior to chemotherapy):

- treat anaemia, infection and metabolic abnormalities
- provide granulocyte support for profound granulocytopenia
- platelets, only if the child is bleeding – ABO and HLA matching if possible
- Prophylactic antibiotics if febrile and neutropenic – neutrophils $< 1 \times 10^9/l$
- allopurinol to avoid uric acid nephropathy
- DIC which often complicates AML (M3) may be managed with fibrinogen replacement, platelets and anticoagulation

Note: HLA-matched relatives should be avoided as donors for blood products if bone marrow transplantation (BMT) is possible and planned at a later date.

Specific therapy:

- remission induction with combination chemotherapy – if two to three cycles fail to induce remission, an alternative combination may be tried
- consolidation: a more intensive course with the same drugs to achieve a 'maximum kill'

- CNS prophylaxis is recommended for ALL and monoblastic (M5) leukaemia
- maintenance therapy is recommended only for ALL for a period of 2–3 years

Therapy for ALL:

1. Induction: vincristine (VCR), prednisolone (pred), daunorubicin and/or L-asparaginase (ASP) (both are used for high risk cases).
2. Consolidation: good risk cases need less extensive medication.
3. CNS prophylaxis: a combination of intrathecal methotrexate (IT-MTX) and cranial irradiation or high dose IV-MTX and IT-MTX is used.
4. Maintenance: combination of cyclophosphamide (cyclo), MTX and 6-mercaptopurine (6-MP) with periodic reinduction with VCR, pred and ADM is used.
5. Relapses: during the course of maintenance or afterwards when all treatment is stopped, a patient may develop a bone marrow relapse. This can be treated with the same drugs or with more aggressive therapy. A second remission can be achieved but long-term survival after a relapse is unlikely. If an HLA-matched sibling or relative is available, bone marrow transplantation (BMT) may be considered.
6. One of the important sites of relapse may be one of the 'sanctuaries'. In the natural history of ALL the two most important sanctuaries are the CNS and testes in boys. Testicular relapse may occur in almost 15 per cent. Testicular biopsies should be taken when a relapse is suspected. Management is with intensive chemotherapy, irradiation of testes and possibly BMT.
7. Relapse in the CNS may present as headache, cranial nerve palsies or papilloedema. Management is with intensive therapy and intrathecal MTX and cytosine arabinoside (ara-C) and possibly irradiation.

Therapy for AML:

Remission is induced by using a combination of anthracycline antibiotics (daunomycin etc.), ara-C and 6-thioguanine (6-TG). The same drugs in the highest tolerated dosage are used for consolidation. Consolidation with cyclo, total body irradiation (TBI) and BMT from an HLA-matched sibling is recommended in highly specialized centres. Maintenance therapy is not undertaken because it does not alter relapse rates.

In the patients with leukaemia who achieve a long-term survival, the after-effects of medication and more importantly irradiation may be seen in the form of psychomotor and intellectual impairment, hypothalamic or pituitary dysfunction, with growth failure and hypothyroidism, and possible sterility.

Lymphomas

Lymphomas are malignancies arising in lymph nodes or in the lymphoid tissue of other organs. These disorders constitute the second major group of lymphoreticular malignancies and account for 10 per cent of childhood cancer. These are divided into Hodgkin's disease (HD) and non-Hodgkin's lymphoma (NHL).

Aetiology

Viruses

Since the implication of Epstein–Barr (EB) virus in the aetiology of Burkitt's lymphoma, the viral aetiology of malignancies in the lymphoreticular system has gained credibility. Genetically predisposed experimental animals have developed cancer as a result of virus infection and there is epidemiological data which supports a viral aetiology. However, to date, no other human malignancy (except Burkitt) has been associated with a specific virus.

Immunological disturbance

Lymphomas have been shown to be associated with disturbed cell mediated immunity. Antigenic alteration of T lymphocytes has also been demonstrated. Tumour-associated antigen has been detected in Hodgkin's disease. Furthermore, there is a high association of several immunological disorders such as agammaglobulinaemia, ataxia telangiectasia, Wiskott–Aldrich syndrome, Chediak–Higashi syndrome, Hashimoto's disease and autoimmune haemolytic anaemia with lymphomas. Therapeutic immunosuppression (as in patients with renal transplants) also has an increased incidence of lymphomas.

Hodgkin's disease (HD)

This is characterized by progressive, painless enlargement of a group of lymph nodes. It is said to arise in a single node and then spreads to other nodes. The disease is uncommon before 5 years of age, after which the incidence rises with a peak at the 15—34 year age group; a second peak is observed around 50 years. Male:female ratio in 5—10 year age group is 3:1 and in older children is 1.5:1.

Aetiology

Association with collagen disorders, infectious mononucleosis and immune disturbances has been recorded.

Patients receiving the hydantoin group of anticonvulsants develop pseudolymphomas, which regress on drug withdrawal. However, in some cases lesions persist even after drug withdrawal. (Comments on the aetiology of lymphomas also applies to HD.)

Pathology

The characteristic histological change is the presence of Reed—Sternberg cells. Other cell constituents represent lymphoid and reticulum cells similar to other lymphomas.

Histological classification (Rye)

1. lymphocytic predominance
2. nodular sclerosis
3. mixed cellularity
4. lymphocytic depletion

The lymphocytic depletion type has the worse prognosis. Spread is by direct extension as well as to distant organs such as liver and spleen.

Clinical manifestations

Most commonly the cervical glands are involved (60 per cent); supraclavicular and axillary glands may also be involved. Involvement of mediastinal glands may cause compression symptoms (thoracic outlet syndrome).

Initially, apart from local swelling, there are few symptoms. Later Pel-Ebstein type fever, anorexia, nausea and weight loss appear. Pruritus, which is common in adults, is not often seen in children.

Involvement of the lungs leads to fluffy shadows on X-ray which may resemble in appearance that of fungal infection.

Involvement of the liver leads to intrahepatic biliary obstruction. Bone marrow infiltration leads to neutropenia and thrombocytopenia. Gastrointestinal lesions may cause ulceration and bleeding.

Impaired cellular immunity causes an increased risk of infection (varicella, pneumocystis). Immunohaemolytic anaemia and immunothrombocytopenia may occur.

Diagnosis

Any unexplained lymphadenopathy must be investigated histologically. Differentiation has to be made from inflammatory lymphadenopathies such as chronic inflammatory adenitis (tuberculous), cat-scratch disease and infectious mononucleosis. Patients with hydantoin pseudolymphoma have a history of drug intake. Hodgkin's disease has to be differentiated from other malignancies — lymphomas and secondaries into lymph nodes.

Investigations

Include routine haematology, urinalysis, chest X-ray, skeletal survey, i.v.p., lymphangiography, liver function tests. Most clinicians also prefer to do a staging laparotomy and splenectomy. Clinical staging is important for planning management.

Clinical staging (Ann Arbor)

Stage I: Involvement of single lymph node area, or a single extranodal site.

Stage II: Involvement of two or more lymph node areas on same side of the diaphragm or involvement of one extranodal site and one or more groups of glands on the same side of the diaphragm.

Stage III: Involvement of lymph node groups on both sides of the diaphragm, which may include localized extranodal involvement, splenic involvement or both.

Stage IV: Disseminated extranodal disease with or without lymph node lesions e.g. liver or bone marrow.

Note: All stages are subdivided into A or B depending upon absence or presence of fever, night sweats or weight loss of 10 per cent or more during the preceding 6 months.

Therapy

Radiation therapy is the mainstay of treatment in stages, I, II and IIIA. It may be in the form of 'extended field' to include involved nodes and adjacent nodes, or 'total nodal' to include most lymphoid tissue.

Chemotherapy using almost all known chemotherapeutic agents has been tried but the standard regimen includes nitrogen mustard, vincristine, prednisone and procarbazine (MOPP) given as 14 day courses with 14 days rest in between. Other drugs are used in advanced disease.

The risks of immediate and late effects of irradiation and chemotherapy are compounded when both modalities are used together, therefore, the decision to combine the two must be made judiciously. Radiation also is sufficient for stages I and IIA and chemotherapy alone is used for stage IV. Differences of opinion exist about stages IIB, IIIA and IIIB.

Late effects of combined irradiation and chemotherapy include a high incidence of acute leukaemia (4 per cent).

Prognosis
Patients with stages I and II have a relatively good prognosis. Overall 5-year survival is 80 per cent and 50 per cent survive disease-free for 10 years.

Non-Hodgkin lymphoma (NHL)

This represents a group of lymphoid malignancies which are histologically distinct from HD. Reed—Sternberg cells are not seen and the malignant cells are monotypic. NHL is more commoner in children than HD and is more common in boys — male: female ratio is 3:1.

Pathology
Malignancy may arise in the lymphoid tissue of lymph nodes or in extranodal structures such as tonsils, adenoids and Peyer's patches: the malignant tissue replaces the normal architecture.

Histological classification is not as useful as in HD, but the Rappaport classification is used:

1. undifferentiated Burkitt and non-Burkitt
2. lymphocytic, well and poorly differentiated
3. mixed, histiocytic and lymphocytic
4. histiocytic

Each type is further classified into nodular and diffuse. Most of the histological types of adult lymphoma are not seen in children. A more useful classification in children is:

1. Burkitt and non-Burkitt lymphoma
2. immunoblastic form
3. lymphoblastic form

Certain markers such as the response to mitogens, the ability to synthesize immunoglobulins, and T and cell markers are more useful in children than the histology.

Mediastinal lymphomas are more likely to be T-cell type and abdominal ones B-cell. Lymphomas tend to have a haematogenous and lymphatic spread early. About one-third of NHL undergo leukaemic transformation and CNS involvement occurs in approximately 30 per cent of cases. Diffuse bone marrow involvement may occur. It is more common with mediastinal lymphomas. Differentiation from ALL becomes difficult once the bone marrow is infiltrated.

Clinical manifestations
Clinical presentation depends upon the site. Patients may present with regional lymphadenopathy, and mediastinal tumours may cause compression symptoms. Primary disease in the abdomen often presents as intussusception. Low grade fever, anorexia and weight loss are not prominent with localized disease and are late manifestations. Diffuse bone pains may indicate dissemination.

Clinical staging of lymphomas is unsatisfactory.

Diagnosis
This is basically histological. Differentiation has to be made from rhabdomyosarcoma, Ewing's sarcoma, neuroblastoma, Hodgkin's disease and sometimes from non-malignant lymphadenopathy.

Investigations
Include histological diagnosis and radiology as indicated. Routine haematology, bone marrow aspiration, CSF and fluid collections such as ascitic and pleural fluid are examined for malignant cells.

A skeletal survey, radio-isotope scan and computerized tomography are performed as indicated. LDH and uric acid levels are raised in disseminated disease.

Therapy
Surgery has no role except for excision of localized disease. Radiotherapy and chemotherapy are the mainstay of treatment. The various drugs used include vincristine, cyclophosphamide, prednisone, daunorubicin, methotrexate and 6-mercaptopurine

Prognosis

Long-term survival in children is about 50 per cent, and may be as high as 90 per cent in localized disease. Mediastinal and large abdominal tumours have unfavourable prognosis.

Burkitt's lymphoma

This is a non-Hodgkin type of lymphoma which was classically described from tropical central Africa with a distinct clinical and histological picture.* Histologically the description is that of uniform-sized dark-stained cells interspersed with pale-staining macrophages giving a classical 'starry-sky' appearance. There appear to be two clinical types of Burkitt's lymphoma, the original African Burkitt's and the other reported from the West, see Table 14.7.

Solid tumours

Wilms' tumour

This ranks fourth in overall incidence of solid tumours and is one of the commonest intra-abdominal tumours in children. Most cases are below 5 years of age with a peak at 3.5 years. It is equally common in the two sexes. The tumour may be bilateral in 10 per cent of cases. There is a high association with non-malignant renal disorders such as metanephric hamartoma and Wilms' tumourlet, glomerular abnormalities and cortical cystic lesions. Several non-renal anomalies are associated with a high incidence of Wilms' tumour. These include hemihypertrophy, aniridia, deletion of the short arm of chromosome 11 and translocation, and Beckwith's syndrome. Malignancy occurring in children with anomalies is more often bilateral and occurs at a younger age. Almost one-third of unilateral and almost all bilateral tumours are inherited, the transmission being autosomal dominant.

Pathology

The tumour is derived from metanephric blastoma and consists of both ectodermal and mesenchymal elements. It may be solitary or multifocal and may

* Epstein-Barr virus (EBV) has been isolated from all tumours.

Table 14.7 *Burkitt's lymphoma*

	African Burkitt's	Non-African Burkitt's
Age	5–7 years	8–10 years
Sex	M:F 4.7:1	M:F 1.3:1
Clinical presentation	Jaw and orbit most commonly affected. Marked bone destruction. Abdominal involvement in one-third cases.	Soft tissues of face affected. Bone destruction minimal. Abdominal involvement more common.
Neurological involvement	Paraplegia in 18% cases on presentation	More commonly cranial nerve palsies
Marrow involvement and leukaemia	Uncommon	Leukaemic transformation common
Staging	1. Facial tumour 2. Two or more facial tumours 3. Intrathoracic, intra-abdominal, paraspinal or osseous tumours (excluding facial bones) 4. CNS or marrow involvement	As for Hodgkin's
Response to chemotherapy	Good	Not so good

be located in the centre or at the poles. Left-sided tumours are more common. Spread is by local extension and by the haematogenous route early in the disease. Most commonly metastases are seen in the lungs but also occur in bones and liver. Bone marrow and CNS are rarely involved.

Staging (National Wilms' Tumour Study Group)

Stage I – limited to kidney and completely resectable

Stage II – extends beyond kidney but is completely resectable

Stage III – non-haematogenous spread, limited to abdomen

Stage IV – haematogenous metastases

Stage V – bilateral renal involvement

Clinical manifestations

Most patients are first found to have an abdominal mass since the tumour causes few symptoms in the early stages. A small number of patients may present with haematuria or hypertension. Abdominal pain, nausea, vomiting, weight loss and fever may occur but usually are late features.

Diagnosis

An abdominal mass suggestive of renal origin in a small child should arouse suspicion of a Wilm's tumour. The mass, unless very large in size, seldom crosses the midline. It has to be differentiated from other kidney masses, most commonly hydronephrosis and from other malignancies such as a neuroblastoma and lymphoma. Repeated abdominal palpation should be avoided since it may cause the tumour to spread.

Laboratory investigations

These include urine examination, plain X-ray of the abdomen, i.v.p., assessment of renal function, chest X-ray, abdominal ultrasound and CT scan. Liver function and serum uric acid also need to be monitored.

Management

Very early stage I tumours can be removed completely surgically, followed by adjuvent chemotherapy over the next 6 months. Others with unfavourable histology require more aggressive chemotherapy with vincristine and actinomycin D for a period of 6 to 12 months.

Patients in stages II and III receive chemotherapy with vincristine, actinomycin D and adriamycin and the duration may be up to 15 months. Group IV patients have an unfavourable prognosis which justifies the use of a four-drug regimen with addition of cyclophosphamide. The area of irradiation varies with the extent of disease.

Prognosis

This varies with the age of presentation, stage at the time of diagnosis and histological type. Children under 2 years, those with early stage I and histologically more differentiated tumours have a good prognosis and up to 90 per cent are expected to have long-term survival. Children who have a 2-year disease-free survival may be presumed to be cured.

Neuroblastoma

This tumour arises from the immature and undifferentiated neuronal cells of the neural crest ectoderm. It has a reported incidence of 9 per 10^6, but may be higher because spontaneous involution may occur. Most cases occur under the age of 3 years and 25 per cent present before 1 year of age. The incidence is slightly higher in boys and some cases are familial. The tumour may arise at any site along the sympathetic chain from the neck to the pelvis, but the most common site is the adrenal gland. The tumour may be unilateral, bilateral or multicentric in origin. The histological picture varies from the most undifferentiated to mature ganglion cells.

Clinical manifestations

Early disease has few clinical features. Failure to thrive, irritability, anorexia, weight loss and anaemia appear as the disease advances.

An abdominal mass is the most common presenting feature. Not infrequently secondaries are the reason for medical advice and sometimes the primary site is difficult to locate. Masses in extra-abdominal sites may cause pressure symptoms. A mediastinal mass may cause a thoracic outlet syndrome. An intraspinal or retroperitoneal tumour may cause cord compression.

The tumour cells may secrete large quantities of catecholamines and vanillylmandelic acid (VMA) and homovanillic acid (HVA) may be present in the urine.

Clinically these patients have flushing, perspiration, diarrhoea, tachycardia or hypertension.

Metastases are blood-borne and the most common sites are the liver, skull bones and the orbit. Bone marrow involvement may cause bone pains and pancytopenia. Intracranial secondaries cause raised intracranial tension. Seventy per cent of tumours have already metastasized when first diagnosed.

Staging
Stage I − confined to the organ of origin
Stage II − extension beyond the organ of origin but not across the midline
Stage III − extension beyond midline
Stage IV − distant metastases
Stage IVS − stage I or II with remote disease confined to liver, spleen or bone marrow but no other evidence of metastases.

Differential diagnosis
This depends upon presentation. An abdominal mass has to be differentiated from Wilms' tumour and lymphoma. Bone marrow infiltration may mimic acute leukaemia.

Investigations
A plain X-ray of the abdomen may show calcification in the mass. Intrathoracic tumours may appear as a mediastinal mass in the chest X-ray. An intravenous pyelogram may show downward displacement of the kidney by the adrenal tumour. Myelography is done in patients presenting with spinal cord compression.

Bone marrow aspiration is a prerequisite for proper staging. Other investigations include ultrasound, CT scan, radionucleotide skeletal survey, liver and brain scan and urinary VMA and HVA estimation.

Management
In localized disease surgical excision is the treatment of choice. Even for tumours which have already metastasized partial surgical removal is still helpful. The tumour is radiosensitive and irradiation helps to reduce tumour size in large growths. Chemotherapy combines the use of vincristine, cyclophosphamide and adriamycin. Alternatively the 'OPEC' regime using vincristine, cyclophosphamide, cisplatin and VM 26 may be used. Excision and irradiation are recommended for localized disease and chemotherapy for disseminated disease.

Prognosis
Neuroblastoma remains one of the most frustrating of malignancies to treat in childhood. In spite of a multiple therapeutic approach, the recurrence rate and ultimate prognosis remains bad. Overall 3-year survival is approximately 25 per cent. The following are good prognostic signs:

- stages I and IVS
- patient under 1 year of age
- patients with cervical and thoracic tumours
- histologically well-differentiated tumours
- if urinary catecholamine secretion returns to normal after treatment

Retinoblastoma

This is a malignant tumour arising from embryonal retinal cells. It is the commonest intraocular tumour in the paediatric age and most cases present before 3 years of age. Some cases are familial and are inherited as an autosomal dominant. Inherited familial cases are always bilateral. A chromosomal anomaly with deletion of the long arm of chromosome 13 is present in some cases of retinoblastoma. In the familial type the anomaly is present in all the body cells, whereas in the more common non-hereditary type the deletion is found only in the tumour cells.

Clinical manifestations
The earliest presentation is with loss of the red reflex and leukocoria or white pupil (cat's eye reflex). Occasionally very small tumours present with a squint due to visual impairment in the affected eye. Therefore, every small child with a squint should have a complete eye examination including the fundus examination. The tumour may grow anteriorly and present as a fungating mass with proptosis or may extend posteriorly leading to retinal detachment and infiltration into the optic nerve and spread into the CNS.

Management
Early diagnosis is extremely important since treatment in early stages may preserve the eye and vision. Transillumination of the eye, radiography including that of the optic foramen, ultrasound and

CT scan help in assessing the extent of the tumour.

If the tumour is very small radiotherapy, photo-coagulation or cryotherapy may be used to ablate the growth. Bigger tumours require enucleation. Advanced tumours require chemotherapy with vincristine, cyclophosphamide and intrathecal methotrexate, combined with surgery and possibly irradiation.

Prognosis
Early treatment of a unilateral tumour has a 90 per cent chance of survival. With more extensive growths, the survival rate is about 50 per cent.

Rhabdomyosarcoma

This is the most common of soft tissue sarcomas in the paediatric age group and accounts for 4 per cent of all tumours. It is commoner in boys, and in Western countries. White children have a higher incidence than black children. There is a higher occurrence in siblings and adult female relatives have a higher incidence of breast cancer. There are two peaks of incidence, first around 4 years when tumours of the head and neck region are common and the second during adolescence when genitourinary growths are more frequent.

Pathology
The tumour arises from embryonal muscle cells and classified into four histological types.

Clinical manifestations
Presentation is with a mass which has symptoms and signs varying with the anatomical site. The various common sites are:

- head and neck (nasopharynx, ear)
- orbit
- trunk (retroperitoneal)
- limbs
- genitourinary (bladder, prostate, vagina, pelvis, peritesticular)

The tumour is extremely malignant and besides local infiltration there is early dissemination to lung and bones.

Management
Only a small percentage of tumours are resectable because early diagnosis is difficult and secondaries develop early in the disease. Irradiation is effective in causing local regression. Patients also require combination chemotherapy using three or four drugs, including vincristine, cyclophosphamide, adriamycin and actinomycin-D.

Prognosis
This depends upon:

1. Age and sex − children in the age group 1−7 years have a better prognosis, boys have a better prognosis than girls.
2. Prognosis is better in orbital and genitourinary tumours because they become symptomatic early and are detected before dissemination occurs.
3. Histologically embryonal types of tumour have a better prognosis.
4. Of patients with resectable tumours 80−90 per cent can be expected to have disease-free long-term survival.

Central nervous system tumours

Next to leukaemias CNS tumours rank highest in the incidence of neoplasms in children. Infratentorial tumours are relatively more common than suprasellar and cerebral neoplasms. Of the posterior fossa tumours, cerebellar neoplasms account for the majority. Central nervous system tumours have a peak among school age children (5−10 years). There are important differences between children and adults with regard to localization and morphology of brain tumours.

Approximately 80 per cent of tumours in children are gliomas compared with 45 per cent in adults whereas in adults most tumours are supratentorial, 55−60 per cent of childhood tumours are infratentorial. Approximately three-quarters of all tumours in children are in the midline. Craniopharyngiomas and optic gliomas are almost exclusively seen in children. The most common tumours in adults are meningiomas, pituitary adenomas, acoustic neuromas and metastatic malignancies. Common CNS tumours in children are listed in Table 14.8.

Clinical presentation
Infants generally present with head enlargement and hydrocephalus. Evidence of raised intracranial pressure is less likely and papilloedema seldom occurs.

Table 14.8 *Brain tumours*

1. Infratentorial (55—60 per cent):
   - cerebellar astrocytoma
   - cerebellar medulloblastoma
   - brain stem glioma
   - ependymoma of IV ventricle
2. Supratentorial:
   a. suprasellar:
      - craniopharyngioma
      - glioma of the optic pathway
      - hypothalamic glioma
   b. Cerebral hemispheres:
      - astrocytoma
      - oligodendroglioma
      - ependymoma
      - glioblastoma
      - sarcoma

In older children also some expansion of the skull is possible because the sutures are not closed, so evidence of raised intracranial pressure may be delayed. However, since the majority of tumours are in the midline, most children present with features of raised intracranial pressure.

Headache is the most frequent symptom. It is not present constantly and tends to increase with coughing, sneezing, change of posture etc. In posterior fossa tumours it localizes in the suboccipital area and in supratentorial tumours on the side of the lesion.

Other features include vomiting and slow pulse due to compression of vagal nuclei in the medulla, papilloedema, visual disturbances, VI nerve palsy and other false localizing neurological signs. In infratentorial tumours tonsillar herniation may take place through the foramen magnum, when the patient presents with neck stiffness, tilting of the head to the same side and features of medullary compression.

Focal neurological signs depend upon the location of the tumour and are most frequently associated with supratentorial tumours and midline brain stem glioma.

Seizures are an uncommon presenting feature.

Diagnosis
An infant presenting with hydrocephalus, or an older child presenting with raised intracranial tension, cerebellar symptoms or a focal neurological deficit must be investigated for the presence of a tumour. A skull X-ray may show evidence of raised intracranial tension and calcification. Angiography, CT scan and radionucleotide scans are important diagnostic aids.

Management
Raised intracranial pressure must be relieved. Initially medical measures using mannitol, acetazolamide and dexamethasone (in selected cases) may be necessary. Surgical decompression should be performed as early as possible. Treatment modalities include surgical excision, irradiation and chemotherapy. Most anti-cancer drugs do not effectively cross the blood—brain barrier. Nitrosourea compounds cross the blood—brain barrier and have been used. Methotrexate may be used intrathecally. Treatment plans depend upon the type and location of the tumour.

Cerebellar astrocytoma

This accounts for 25 per cent of all brain tumours. Most often it arises in the midline and tends to be cystic. The highest incidence is in the 2—8 years age group. It is a slow growing tumour.

Clinical manifestations
Raised intracranial tension develops early and most patients present with headache, vomiting and visual disturbances. Extension of the tumour into one of the cerebellar hemispheres is common. This results in lateralized cerebellar features. Pressure on the brain stem results in dilatation of the pupils, neck retraction, episodic extensor posturing and loss of consciousness and irregular breathing.

Management
Surgical excision of the tumour leads to long-term survival in 90 per cent of cases. Cystic tumours are easier to remove. Solid midline tumours may infiltrate into vital structures and may not be accessible. Post-operative radiotherapy is recommended if the solid portion of the tumour cannot be excised completely.

Cerebellar medulloblastoma

This is the most common posterior fossa tumour. The peak incidence is in the 2—6 years age group. The tumour is twice as common in boys as in girls. It is very rapidly growing tumour which arises from the cerebellum in the midline and then seeds along the entire cerebrospinal axis in the subarachnoid space. It may also metastasize into extraneural structures.

Clinical features due to raised intracranial pressure and localized cerebellar features are similar to those of an astrocytoma. Additionally a peripheral neuropathy and root pains develop because of extension into the spinal subarachnoid space.

Management includes surgical excision and irradiation. Chemotherapy with vincristine and cyclophosphamide may be given for a period of 12—18 months. The prognosis is quite poor and long-term survival after surgery and irradiation is likely in only 20—30 per cent of patients.

Ependymoma

This is the third most common infratentorial neoplasm in children. It is twice as common in boys as in girls. The tumour arises from the ependymal lining of the floor of the IV ventricle. Upward extension into the IV ventricle leads to obstruction and raised intracranial pressure. Brain stem infiltration causes cranial nerve palsies and an extensor plantar response. Calcification in the tumour may be seen on a plain X-ray.

Total surgical excision is generally not possible and a combination of surgery and irradiation is the recommended therapy. The long-term prognosis is very poor.

Brain stem glioma

It is seen almost exclusively in children and accounts for about 10 per cent of brain tumours in them. The peak incidence is in the 6—8 years age group. The classical clinical presentation is with a combination of cranial nerve palsies, pyramidal signs and ataxia. There may be no evidence of raised intracranial pressure. The tumour is not accessible to surgery and irradiation is the only treatment recommended. The prognosis is very poor and most patients die within 18 months of presentation.

Craniopharyngioma

This is the most common suprasellar tumour of childhood. It arises from squamous cell rests of the pouch of Rathke. It has a tendency to become cystic.

Clinical manifestations

Symptoms are due to raised intracranial tension, pressure on the optic chiasma and hormonal disturbances.

Headache, vomiting, visual impairment characteristically with bitemporal hemianopia, failure to thrive and diabetes insipidus may occur. Fundus examination may show optic atrophy or papilloedema.

Skull X-rays show suprasellar calcification in 80 per cent of cases. The sella turcica is distorted or ballooned, and clinoid processes may be eroded.

Surgical excision is the treatment of choice. Prednisolone $40\,mg/m^2/day$ is started on the day before surgery and is given for 2 weeks postoperatively. Hydrocortisone is given on the day of operation. Postoperatively, panhypopituitarism is very common and full hormanal replacement therapy is necessary.

Table 14.9 *Anticancer drugs*

Drug	Main action	Dosage	Main side effects
I. *Antimetabolites*	Interfere with purine and pyrimidine metabolism		
1. Methotrexate	Interferes with folate metabolism	$7.5\,mg/m^2/$daily, orally for 5 days every 3—4 weeks Intrathecal: $12\,mg/m^2/$dose	Oral and gastrointestinal ulceration, diarrhoea, hepatotoxicity, pneumonitis, bone marrow suppression
2. 6—Mercaptopurine (6—MP)	Interferes with hypoxanthine metabolism	$70\,mg/m^2/$daily orally	Marrow depression, vomiting

184

Table 14.9 *Anticancer drugs (continued)*

Drug	Main action	Dosage	Main side effects
3. Cytosine arabinoside (ara-C)	Interferes with cytidine metabolism	2 mg/kg/day i.v. increase to 4 mg/kg/day	Severe bone marrow suppression, fever, rash, keratitis, urinary retention, hepatotoxicity
4. 6−Thioguanine (6-TG)	Purine analogue. Inhibits purine synthesis	60−75 mg/m^2 orally 100 mg/m^2 i.v.	Marked granulocytopoenia, thrombocytopoenia, nausea, vomiting, cholestasis, oral ulceration
5. 5−Flurouracil (5-FU)	Inhibits DNA synthesis	500−1000 mg/m^2 i.v.	Marked bone marrow suppression, mild gatrointestinal upset, ataxia, conjunctivitis
II. *Alkylating agents*	Interfere with nucleic acid replication		
1. Cyclophosphamide	− as above −	80−90 mg/m^2 orally, i.v.	Severe bone marrow depression, gastrointestinal upset, alopecia, haemorrhagic cystitis
2. Busulphan	− as above −	2.3−4.6 mg/m^2 orally	Marrow depression, skin pigmentation, gynaecomastia, glossitis, pulmonary fibrosis
3. Chlorambucil	− as above −	4.5 mg/m^2 orally	Marrow depression, nausea, vomiting, diarrhoea
4. Carmustine (BCNU)	Causes breaks in DNA strands and cross links	200−225 mg/m^2 i.v.	Marrow suppression, gastrointestinal disturbances, pulmonary fibrosis, neuropathy
5. Lomustine (CCNU)	Same as carmustine	100−150 mg/m^2 orally	As for carmustine
6. Cisplatin	Inhibits formation of DNA cross strands	50−100 mg/m^2 i.v. infused over 6 hours	Bone marrow suppression, severe GI upset, renal failure, Mg^{++} wasting, peripheral neuropathy
III. *Plant alkaloids*			
Vincristine	Arrests mitosis and inhibits RNA polymerase	1.5 mg/m^2 i.v. weekly	Constipation, alopeica, neuropathy
Vinblastine	Same as vincristine	5 mg/m^2 i.v. weekly	Nausea, vomiting, stomatitis, alopecia, peripheral neuropathy, marrow suppression

Table 14.9   *Anticancer drugs (continued)*

Drug	Main action	Dosage	Main side effects
VM 26	Arrests cells in G2 phase of mitosis. Produces breaks in DNA	70 mg/m^2 i.v.	Bone marrow suppression, gastrointestinal upset, peripheral neuropathy
IV. *Antibiotics*	Cause breaks in RNA and inhibits RNA polymerase		Cardiotoxic, effects on heart are irreversible, → cardiomyopathy
Doxorubicin	– as above –	Induction: 45 mg/m^2 i.v. weekly Maintenance: 30 mg/m^2 i.v. every 3–4 weeks Maximum cumulative dose 500 mg/m^2.	– as above –
Daunorubicin	– as above –	Induction: 60 mg/m^2 i.v. weekly Maintenance: 30 mg/m^2 every 3–4 weeks	– as above –
Actinomycin D	Anti-DNA	Total of 2250 μg/m^2 divided into 7 daily doses i.v. Course every 8–12 weeks	Nausea, vomiting, alopecia, stomatitis, flare reaction over irradiated areas, bone marrow suppression
Bleomycin	Anti-DNA	5 mg/m^2 i.v.	
Mitomycin	Inhibits DNA	2 mg/m^2 i.v.	Mild gastrointestinal toxicity, uncommonly bone marrow suppression, skin pigmentation, allergic rash, pulmonary fibrosis
V. *Miscellaneous* l-Asparaginase	Inhibits protein synthesis	50 000 – 100 000 units/m^2 i.v.	Nausea, vomiting, fever, chills, hypersensitivity, pancreatitis, liver dysfunction, renal impairment, CNS symptoms
Dacarbazine	Kills cells in mitosis cycle. Acts like alkylating agents	375 mg/m^2 i.v.	Mild bone marrow suppression, marked gastrointestinal toxicity, 'flu-like syndrome

15

Central Nervous System Disorders

Seizure disorders in children

Seizure disorders refers to recurrent paroxysmal episodes of central nervous system (CNS) dysfunction manifested clinically by stereotyped sensory, motor or autonomic activity either singly or in combination.

Seizures may occur in children with or without recognizable brain disease. Secondary epilepsy is the term used when the seizures are a part of underlying brain disease. Idiopathic epilepsy refers to seizures where no brain disease is found. The terms seizures, fits and convulsions have the same meaning and can be interchanged.

Pathophysiology

All seizures result from the synchronous discharge of a large number of neurones from an epileptogenic focus. The neurones of such an area are functioning abnormally and show high-amplitude prolonged depolarization with superimposed high frequency bursts of action potential. The activity is present even in the interictal period and can be recorded in the EEG. During a seizure the neurones show even greater activity. In focal epilepsies the abnormal neuronal behaviour remains confined to localized cortical areas, but when a seizure becomes generalized the activity spreads to wider cortical areas bilaterally.

Clinical classifications of seizures

A varying nomenclature has been used to designate different types of seizures. The following simplified adaptation of the International League against Epilepsy Classification includes the common seizure disorders; the old nomenclature is given in parenthesis:

1. Generalized seizures:

tonic-clonic (grand mal)
absence (petit mal)
atonic, akinetic (minor motor)
myoclonic epilepsy
infantile spasms
2. Partial (focal) seizures:
    (a) simple partial:
        focal motor (Jacksonian)
        sensory
        autonomic
        benign partial
    (b) Complex partial seizures:
        psychomotor
        compound forms
    (c) partial seizures with secondary generalization

Tonic-clonic seizures

Pre-ictal phenomena may be present. These include localized muscular twitching, irritability, headache, abdominal pain, strange sensations in the epigastrium or odd behaviour.

The attack itself starts abruptly with loss of consciousness. The tonic phase with gross, sustained contraction of body muscles and upward deviation of the eyes lasts for 10 to 20 seconds. An epileptic cry due to forced expiration through contracted vocal cords may be heard. Pupils are dilated, blood pressure and heart rate rise and urinary and faecal incontinence may occur. The clonic phase lasts for 20 to 30 seconds, during which rhythmic, forcible contractions of major muscle groups are observed. There may be frothing from the mouth. Postictal manifestations include muscular relaxation, drowsiness or sleep, headache, bodyaches, etc. There is complete amnesia of the seizure events. Classical attacks are uncommon before adolescence and many variations occur clinically.

Transient paresis (Todd's paralysis) or permanent focal lesions due to hypoxic damage may occur.

Chronic seizures may lead to personality changes and intellectual deterioration.

Absence seizures

These are seldom seen before 3 years of age and are common in the age group 4—12 years. Absence seizures tend to have a familial occurrence. The characteristic spike-wave pattern of the EEG is due to an autosomal dominant gene with age-dependent expression. There is an 8—12 per cent chance of seizures occurring in the offspring of a patient. Most children have normal intelligence and one-third to one-half patients are likely to have grand mal seizures.

Clinically the attack consists of a brief interruption of consciousness, sometimes accompanied with flickering and deviation of eyes, clonic jerks of limbs, increase or decrease in postural tone, autonomic phenomena such as pupillary dilatation, change in skin colour, tachycardia, piloerection and automatism.

Myoclonic seizures

These are a feature of hereditary myoclonic epilepsy and a number of degenerative diseases of the CNS. Myoclonic seizures may also occur in retarded children with non-progressive brain damage.

Clinically the attack consists of bilaterally symmetrical brief, rapid muscular contractions, occurring singly or repetitively. Generally there is no alteration of consciousness. Associated absence or tonic-clonic seizures may occur.

Infantile spasms (hypsarrhythmia; salaam attacks)

The onset of infantile spasms is almost always below the age of 1 year and the seizures seem to represent an age-specific reaction of the immature CNS. The disorder may be idiopathic in nature or secondary to underlying disorders including congenital malformations, intrauterine infections, birth asphyxia and trauma, encephalitis and metabolic disorders. There may be a genetic predisposition.

The natural history varies according to the presence or absence of underlying brain disease:

1. Infants who have never been developmentally normal — these infants are likely to have underlying brain disease.

2. Infants who have been developmentally normal until about 6 months of age — these infants are likely to belong to the idiopathic group but an undiagnosed metabolic disorder, e.g., phenylketonuria or encephalitis may be responsible.

Clinically the patient presents with 'salaam' attacks consisting in sudden flexion of head and trunk simultaneously with flexion and adduction of limbs. The number of attacks may vary from a few to several hundred per day.

Seizures and EEG abnormalities tend to disappear by 2—5 years of age even without treatment. However, severe mental retardation is likely to ensue and other types of seizure may reappear later. Infants in the idiopathic group and those with normal development before the onset of seizures tend to have a relatively better prognosis. However, only 10 per cent of this group are likely to grow with normal intelligence.

Focal (partial) seizures

These represent a group of seizure disorders which result from focal epileptogenic discharges due to localized brain dysfunction.

Various neurological disorders such as subdural haematoma, arterio-venous malformations, Sturge—Weber syndrome, cerebral embolism, cerebral atrophy, porencephaly and space-occupying lesions, as well as metabolic disturbances such as hypoglycaemia, hypocalcaemia and water intoxication may be responsible for partial seizures. However, all these causes as a group are responsible for only a small percentage of cases and in the majority there is no recognizable underlying cause.

Partial seizures are distinctly less common in children as compared with adults. The seizures may be sensory, motor (Jacksonian) or autonomic. Sensory partial seizures are uncommon in children.

Focal motor seizures (Jacksonian seizures)
The seizure is typically clonic though it may be preceded by a transient tonic phase. Muscles with highly specialized functions are generally involved, with muscles of hand and face more commonly affected. The attack classically starts with twitching of a small group of muscles, e.g., of the thumb and then gradually progresses to involve the hand, wrist, arm, face, etc. (Jacksonian march). Occasionally a seizure may become generalized with loss of consciousness. When this happens, it cannot be

clinically differentiated from a grand mal seizure.

Focal seizures, irrespective of type, may become generalized.

Benign focal epilepsy of childhood (Rolandic epilepsy)

This is a seizure disorder which starts between the ages of 4 and 13 years in a previously healthy child. Attacks are clearly more common during sleep, have a focal onset with twitching of one side of the face, anarthria, drooling, paraesthesiae on the face, tonic posture or clonic movements of one half of the body. Attacks may become generalized or be followed by Todd's paralysis. There is a characteristic EEG abnormality (see Table 15.1). The trait is inherited through an autosomal dominant gene with age-dependent penetrance. Prognosis is good and anticonvulsants are very effective.

Seizures and EEG abnormalities disappear by mid or late adolescence.

Complex partial seizures (psychomotor epilepsy)

The temporal lobe is a vulnerable part of the brain that is particularly liable to damage from cerebral oedema. This may occur after head injury, status epilepticus and in various encephalopathies. Cerebral oedema leads to tentorial herniation of the inner aspect of the temporal lobe.

This type of seizure is uncommon before adolescence. Visual, auditory and olfactory hallucinations, the déjà-vu phenomenon, alterations of consciousness, unresponsiveness and automatism are the characteristic manifestations.

Clinically the patient presents with purposeful but inappropriate motor acts which are repetitive and often complicated. Pre-ictal aura may be in the form of a shrill cry or a short run for help. Simultaneously there is a gradual loss of postural tone and the patient may fall to the ground. Often there are vasomotor changes, such as circumoral pallor. The seizure may last from 30 seconds to 5 minutes and is usually followed by a period of drowsiness or sleep.

Lennox—Gastaut syndrome

This includes a group of children with a severe seizure disorder, mental retardation and a characteristic EEG pattern. One third of the patients are without apparent cause, the rest have a diverse aetiology including trauma, anoxic damage, infections and post-vaccinial encephalopathies and degenerative brain disease.

The seizures are very difficult to control and combinations of drugs may have to be tried. Sodium valproate or clonazepam in combination with other drugs may help to control seizures. A ketogenic diet may have a place in some.

Diagnosis

Clinical diagnosis of seizure disorders depends upon a detailed description of the fit including the pre-ictal and post-ictal phenomena. Preferably a seizure should be observed.

Two non-seizure disorders which may present with episodic manifestations are syncope and breath-holding spells; these need to be differentiated.

The EEG is the single most useful investigation for the diagnosis and classification of seizures. However, interpretation of the EEG is more complicated in children and a considerable number of patients with seizure disorders may have normal interictal records. Table 15.1 gives some classical patterns.

Patients must be screened for inborn errors of amino acid metabolism as well as for other metabolic disorders, if clinically suspected. The presence of café au lait patches suggests either tuberose sclerosis (epiloia) or neurofibromatosis.

Skull X-rays are helpful in only a minority of cases. Computerized tomography (CT scans) are

Table 15.1 *Characteristic EEG appearances in seizure disorders*

Seizure type	EEG appearance
Tonic-clonic	Interictal generalized bursts of spikes and irregular spike-wave complexes in 4–6 /sec range
Myoclonic	Generalized bursts of multiple spikes
Absence	Characteristic 3–4 /sec spike-wave activity, can be induced by hyperventilation
Infantile spasms	High voltage irregular slow waves occurring asynchronously and randomly, mixed with spikes and polyspikes – hypsarrhythmia
Complex partial	Spiking over one or both temporal lobes

useful in selected cases when an underlying abnormality of the brain is suspected, but in uncomplicated idiopathic epilepsy, it is likely to be normal.

Therapy

Although control with drugs is the mainstay of treatment in seizure disorders, general aspects of management are equally important.

Principles of drug therapy

1. A single isolated uncomplicated seizure, if accompanied by a normal EEG and a negative family history does not require drug treatment.
2. Therapy should begin with minimum recommended dosage of a single agent. The dose should be gradually increased, if there are no major side effects, until seizure control is achieved or the maximum permissible dose is reached. Drugs of choice are listed in Table 15.2.
3. A second drug should only be added if maximum recommended dosage of a single agent fails to control seizures. More than two drugs are seldom required and if used, may cause serious side effects due to drug interactions.
4. Younger children require relatively larger doses and more frequent dosage schedules to maintain therapeutic blood levels.
5. Patients receiving phenobarbitone and phenytoin on long-term therapy develop decreased serum calcium and 25-hydroxycalciferol levels; such patients require vitamin D supplements of 10 000 i.v. weekly.
6. Ideally drug levels should be monitored.
7. Anti-epileptic drugs should be withdrawn slowly over a 3 to 6 month period, as sudden abrupt withdrawal may precipitate status epilepticus.
8. There are no clear-cut rules regarding withdrawal of anti-epileptic drugs after seizure control. Certain types of seizures such as absence seizures and benign focal epilepsy have good prognosis. In these types therapy may be gradually withdrawn over 3 to 6 months after a 1 to 2-year seizure-free period.
   A history of prolonged convulsions before onset of treatment, the presence of underlying brain disease and gross EEG abnormalities are bad prognostic signs. In generalized convulsive seizures and in partial seizures a 2-year seizure-free period with a normal or near-normal EEG are

Table 15.2 *Drugs of choice in seizure disorders*

Seizure type	Drugs of choice
Tonic-clonic	Sodium valproate
	Carbamazepine
	Phenytoin; phenobarbitone
Myoclonic	Benzodiazepines: clonazepam,
	Nitrazepam
	Sodium valproate
Absence	Sodium valproate
	Ethosuximide
Infantile spasms	1. Corticotrophin and prednisolone
	2. Benzodiazepines: nitrazepam
	clonazepam
Focal motor	Carbamazepine
	Sodium valproate
Complex partial	Carbamazepine
	Primidone (or phenobarbitone);
	Phenytoin

pre-requisites for drug withdrawal. In some patients a 4-year seizure control is desirable before stopping treatment.

9. Proper compliance should be assured. Non-compliance is a common reason for uncontrolled seizures.

Dosage, prescribing instructions and major side effects of commonly used anti-epileptic drugs are given in Table 15.3.

General measures

General measures include parental guidance on the management and care of a child with chronic illness; dealing with behaviour and personality problems secondary to epilepsy and accident prevention.

Children with poorly controlled epilepsy often have behaviour problems and learning difficulties at school which improve, sometimes dramatically, once the seizures are adequately controlled.

In most communities epilepsy is a dreaded disease. There are many different beliefs and superstitions about the aetiology and to have the disease carries a great stigma, so that it is not surprising that relatives may keep the existence of the disease a closely guarded secret within the family and patients go untreated.

There is an urgent need to educate parents and school teachers especially about the nature of epilepsy and how proper treatment can help the child.

Table 15.3 *Maintenance dosage of anti-epileptic drugs*

Drug	Dosage range (oral)	Dosage internal	Therapeutic range	Major side effects
Phenobarbitone	2−8 mg/kg/day	Once or twice daily	10−25 µg/ml	Drowsiness or hyperkinetic behaviour, skin rash, fever
Phenytoin	Infants: 5−15 mg/kg/day Children: 5−10 mg/kg/day	Twice daily	5−20 µg/ml 10−20 µg/ml (adults)	Gingival hyperplasia, hypertrichosis, coarsening of facial features, ataxia, nystagmus, extra pyramidal movements; chronic intoxication may cause cerebellar damage and dementing encephalopathy; fetal hydantoin syndrome; rickets
Primidone *	10−25 mg/kg/day	Twice daily	Judge by phenobarbitone levels.	Drowsiness, ataxia, dermatitis; may cause megaloblastic anaemia
Carbamazepine	10−20 mg/kg/day	Two or three times daily	4−10 µg/ml	Headache, dysequilibrium, diplopia, blurred vision, jaundice, rash, aplastic anaemia, increases ADH secretion
Clonazepam	0.01−0.03 mg/kg/day (Max 0.2 mg/kg/day)	Two or three times daily		Toxicity dose-related; lethargy or hyperactive aggressive behaviour, hypersalivation, increased bronchial secretions, ataxia, increased seizures; thrombocytopenia
Ethosuximide	20−40 mg/kg/day	Two or three times daily	40−100 µg/ml	Nausea, dizziness, drowsiness, skin rash, hiccups; may cause blood dyscrasias; caution in liver and renal disease
Sodium valproate	20−30 mg/kg/day	Twice daily	60−100 µg/ml	Anorexia, nausea, vomiting (usually transient), raised liver enzymes, hepatocellular failure (infrequent), abnormal platelet function, hair loss, fine tremor, rarely fatal, pancreatitis, increases sedative effects of phenobarbitone

* The dose of primidone is approximately five times that of phenobarbitone to produce an equivalent blood level.

Successful treatment should aim to integrate the child back into his community as completely as possible. This starts with allowing the child back to school and a letter of explanation to the teacher or headmaster is often helpful. There is still much fear, mistrust and prejudice but if teachers treat the child as normal then other children will do so too. Children who have only occasional seizures should not have their school careers stopped because of the label of epilepsy. Epileptic children should not be allowed to feel 'different'. Their activities should not be restricted and they should not be prevented from playing games or doing PE at school though swimming might have to be restricted. Epilepsy is not a bar to employment, marriage or having children, except of course in the more severe and intractible cases or with severely disturbed behaviour. There is, therefore, a considerable onus on doctors to educate their paramedical staff and nurses and teachers and parents especially about the nature of epilepsy.

Febrile seizures

A febrile seizure is an event in infancy or early childhood, usually occurring between the ages of 6 months and 5 years, associated with fever, but without evidence of intracranial infection, underlying brain disease or other defined cause. Siezures with fever in children who have suffered a previous non-febrile seizure are excluded from this definition.

Various studies suggest that between 3 and 7 per cent of all children are likely to have seizures during infancy and pre-school years, and half of these will be febrile seizures. Most attacks occur in the age group 6 months to 2 years. Some families have an increased susceptibility, and the disorder may be transmitted through a dominant gene with incomplete penetrance.

A simple uncomplicated seizure has the following characteristics:

1. Seizures are most commonly associated with upper respiratory and ear infections, although any infection may be associated with a febrile seizure. Certain organisms such as *Shigella* have a particular association.
2. Convulsions generally occur during a sudden rise in temperature, often to 39°C or more and at the onset of an illness or infection.
3. The seizure is generalized and lasts for less than 15 minutes.
4. Seizures are unlikely to recur during the course of an illness, if they do, it is usually within the next 24 hours.
5. There is no residual neurological damage.
6. The interictal EEG is normal.
7. There may be a positive family history of febrile seizures.

The following characteristics suggest a complex (complicated) seizure:

1. Duration of the seizure is more than 15 minutes.
2. Seizures are focal.
3. There is more than one episode of convulsions during a 24 hour period.

4. There is a transient or permanent neurological deficit.
5. The interictal EEG is abnormal.
6. There is a family history of non-febrile seizures.

Febrile seizures have two associated risks:

1. About one-third of children with a febrile seizure are likely to have a recurrence, the risk being greatest in the younger age group.
2. The subsequent risk of developing epilepsy is slightly increased being 1.6 per cent as compared with 0.5 per cent in the general population. The risk is greater in children who have had a complicated seizure (13 per cent).

Risk factors for epilepsy include:

- a family history of epilepsy in a first degree relative
- prolonged or focal seizures
- neurological abnormality after the first seizure.

A complete history with physical examination should be carried out, to exclude neurological, metabolic, infective or traumatic causes for the seizure. Examination of the fundus is mandatory. Although viral upper respiratory infections are much the commonest cause of febrile seizures, in the absence of signs such as a runny nose, congested throat or inflamed ears, the urine should be carefully examined to exclude an unsuspected urinary tract infection. Other laboratory investigations should include an infection screen, a thick blood film for malarial parasites in endemic areas, blood sugar, serum calcium, electrolytes and blood urea. A lumbar puncture is not necessary in all cases, when the history and findings clearly point to a simple uncomplicated febrile seizure, but if there are any doubts at all about the possibility of meningitis or CNS infection a lumbar puncture must be done. It is not necessary to perform an EEG unless:

- There is doubt as to whether the seizure was associated with fever.
- There is a strong family history of epilepsy (not febrile seizures).
- The seizure was complicated.
- The child has had repeated previous febrile seizures.

Management

Many parents especially with the first convulsion are convinced that their child will die. They must be reassured that their child will not die.

Treatment of the acute seizure is the same as for any convulsion (see below).

First aid measures include control of the convulsion with intravenous diazepam; antipyretics such as paracetamol and tepid sponging and fanning to bring the temperature down. Care must be taken not to chill the child, however. Parents should be advised on the above measures, and also on the prompt use of rectal diazepam (0.3 mg/kg) in controlling and stopping convulsions when they occur at home. Given at the onset of a high fever, rectal diazepam may also prevent a seizure developing in susceptible children.

Continuous anticonvulsant therapy is only recommended when:

- The seizures are so frequent as to make life intolerable for the parents.
- The child has had at least three or four within a short time.
- The parents demand treatment because of the frequency.
- The EEG is abnormal.

The drug choice for continuous prophylactic therapy is phenobarbitone (4 or 5 mg/kg/day); treatment will prevent recurrence of seizures in most cases, but does not alter the ultimate risk of epilepsy. Treatment should be continued until the child is about 5 years old, or has been free of seizures for 2 years, but can be stopped earlier if parents can be persuaded to use rectal diazepam instead when the child is febrile. Sodium valproate is an alternative to phenobarbitone, but carries the slight risk of hepatic toxicity.

Management of the child with convulsions

A child with acute convulsions is one of the commonest problems presenting in the paediatric emergency room. The majority are febrile convulsions but meningitis must always be considered in young children, especially under 2 years of age, and if there are any doubts at all about the diagnosis, a lumbar puncture must be carried out. Convulsions may also be manifestations of other CNS infections such as viral meningitis or encephalitis; anoxic damage, toxic causes (lead or tetanus); metabolic causes (hypoglycaemia, hypocalcaemia, hypomegnesaemia); hypertensive disease, or post-traumatic.

1. Irrespective of the cause or diagnosis, the first priority is to stop the convulsions because continued convulsions (status epilepticus) may cause and/or aggravate CNS damage.
2. Status epilepticus is a condition in which seizures recur before the patient has recovered from the effects of the previous one. It occurs most often in epileptic children in whom therapy has suddenly been withdrawn, and severely brain-damaged children, although occasionally from any of the above causes. It is a life-threatening situation, complicated by hyperpyrexia, hypoxia and peripheral circulatory failure if convulsions are not controlled promptly. Fifteen to twenty per cent of patients may be left with neurological damage.
3. Treat the child as for the unconscious patient. Place the child on his side with the head slightly lower than the rest of the body.
4. Place a padded spatula between the teeth to prevent the tongue from being bitten. It is essential to pad the spatula to prevent it from breaking the teeth. Ensure that the tongue does not fall back and block the posterior pharyngeal airway. If possible place an appropriate sized Guedel airway in the child's mouth.
5. Aspirate any secretions.
6. Insert an intravenous line.

Any of the following drugs may be used:

1. Intravenous diazepam 0.2 mg/kg is the drug of choice. It must be given slowly while watching the child carefully for evidence of respiratory depression. The injection can be repeated after a short interval, but the dose is cumulative so watch for signs of respiratory depression especially if other anticonvulsant drugs have been given already. Tolerance develops after three or four injections.
2. Paraldehyde 0.15 ml/kg as deep intramuscular injection. An alternative dosage is 1 ml per year of age to a maximum of 10 ml, a dose as large as this should be divided and given into two sites. Injections are painful, and may cause tissue necrosis and sterile abscesses, so should always

be given into the lateral aspect of the thigh to avoid damage to the sciatic nerve. Injections are effective within 15 to 20 minutes of administration. Paraldehyde should be given in glass syringes.

3. Both diazepam and paraldehyde are well absorbed rectally and effective within 10 to 20 minutes by this route. Dosage: diazepam 0.6 mg/kg (available in 5 mg and 10 mg single disposable units). Paraldehyde dose as for i.m. injection but dilute with an equal volume of arachis, olive or other oil.

4. Phenobarbitone is too slowly acting to stop convulsions immediately, but may be given in a dose of 10 mg/kg by intramuscular injection to prevent further convulsions.

5. In severe intractible convulsions, failing to respond to the above measures, one of the following may be tried:
   - Diazepam infusion. Dilute 50 mg diazepam in 500 ml 5 per cent dextrose and infuse slowly at eight to ten drops per minute to control seizures. Maximum infusion over 24 hours should not exceed 3 mg/kg. *Caution*: there is a risk of apnoea especially if the patient is already receiving phenobarbitone.
   - Chlormethiazole infusion, as 0.8 per cent solution (8 mg/ml). Give 30 ml and infuse slowly at 1 ml/minute, then continue on a reducing dose of 0.5−0.25 ml/minute for not longer than 24 hours.

As a last resort, with failure to respond to any of the above measures, the patient should be intubated and ventilated by an anaesthetist and given an infusion of thiopentone.

Other measures:

1. If the child is febrile, tepid sponge and cool with fanning, checking the rectal temperature from time to time to avoid chilling. Give paracetamol as a suppository.

2. Carry out appropriate laboratory investigations. In non-febrile convulsions, check the blood sugar by fingerprick method (Dextrostix or BM-stix) to exclude hypoglycaemia.

3. Do not forget to treat the parents. Nothing is more frightening to parents than a convulsing child; they panic and fear the child will die. Many are only too well aware of the disastrous consequences that sometimes follow convulsions. Reassure and calm them sympathetically.

The unconscious child

One of the most dramatic and challenging problems in paediatrics is the emergency admission of an unconscious child. Disturbances of consciousness complicate many childhood illnesses and some are listed in Table 15.4, though the cause may sometimes may be difficult to determine or indeed may never be determined. The attendents or witnesses

Table 15.4   *Common causes of unconsciousness*

Head injuries	— Road accidents; falls from trees, etc
Other accidents	— Near drowning
Infections	— Meningitis; encephalitis and encephalopathies — Cerebral malaria — Septicaemia
Central nervous system disease	— Haemorrhage; thrombosis; tumours
Hypertensive encephalopathy	
Epilepsy	— Postictal state
Accidental poisoning	— Drugs and medicines — Household and industrial poisons; lead — Plants — Indigenous and traditional medicines — Solvent and drug abuse
Metabolic causes	— Severe dehydration and electrolyte imbalance, e.g., hypernatraemia — Hypoglycaemia (traditional medicines and alcohol) — Hypoglycaemic and hyperglycaemia diabetic coma — Uraemia and renal failure — Hepatic failure — Reye's syndrome

Hysteria may simulate a state of unconsciousness

must be closely questioned as to the circumstances in which the child was found. For instance it is important to know if the child suffered from epilepsy or diabetes, or if he was found unconscious under a tree or near an empty bottle or other toxic substance. This can be done while making an initial rapid examination and assessment of vital functions and signs. There may be a characteristic smell of drugs, household products, kerosine or ketones. Deep rapid breathing (Kussmaul respiration) is indicative of a metabolic acidosis due to salicylate intoxication, electrolyte disturbances, diabetic keto-acidosis or renal failure, while irregular periodic respiration is suggestive of brain stem dysfunction. Blood pressure is elevated when intracranial pressure is raised, as well as in hypertensive encephalopathy. Pupil size and reaction is important. Dilated pupils may be due to atropine (*Datura*) poisoning, follow installation of mydriatics, or after a grand mal seizure. Dilated non-reacting pupils may indicate irreversible coma. A unilateral sluggishly reacting pupil may be due to a III cranial nerve palsy. Pinpoint pupils may be due to narcotic (opioid) poisoning or lesions of the pons. Absence of the 'doll's eye movement' (conjugate deviation of the eyes to the opposite side when the head is quickly turned) suggests a brain stem lesion. In III cranial nerve palsy, the eye is deviated downwards and outwards, and the pupil dilated.

A classification of the grade or depth of coma is shown in Table 15.5.

Table 15.5 *Classification of grade of coma*

Grade 0	Patient drowsy but can be aroused to answer questions rationally.
Grade 1	Comatose. May be roused very briefly; withdraws from painful stimuli; reflexes intact.
Grade 2	Comatose. Cannot be roused by painful stimuli; may make semi-purposeful avoidance movements. No respiratory or circulatory depression.
Grade 3	Comatose. No response to painful stimuli; decerebrate posturing (extension and pronation of arms); almost all reflexes absent. No respiratory or circulatory depression.
Grade 4	Comatose. Reflexes absent; hypotonic; respiratory depression (apnoea) and circulatory failure.

Management

1. Place on a bed in the semi-prone position on the side with the head slightly lower than the rest of the body.
2. Maintain an adequate airway by inserting an oral airway; this will prevent the tongue from falling backwards and so choking the child.
3. Suck out secretions gently, taking aseptic precautions to avoid trauma to the mouth. Repeat as often as necessary.
4. Give oxygen if required by face mask or nasal catheter.
5. Insert a nasogastric tube and aspirate the stomach. Leave the tube in for future feeding.
6. Set up an intravenous drip using one-fifth isotonic saline in 4.5 per cent dextrose at maintenance rates. Restrict fluid intake to about 60 per cent of normal requirements if cerebral oedema is suspected, and in conditions associated with inappropriate ADH secretion.
7. Catheterize the bladder to measure urinary output. Record carefully all fluid intake and output.
8. General measures include care of the mouth and eyes, turning the child every 2 hours from side to side and physiotherapy with postural drainage and passive limb movements.
9. Antibiotics should only be given if there are appropriate indications.
10. Laboratory investigations include a full blood count; estimation of electrolytes, calcium, urea, glucose; blood culture and a thick blood film for malarial parasites in endemic areas. Samples of blood, urine and gastric aspirate should be preserved in cases of suspected poisoning for further analysis. Other investigations should be performed as indicated by the history and examination.
11. A lumbar puncture may be carried out in selected cases to exclude meningitis after examining the fundi to ensure there is no papilloedema.

Monitoring of vital signs

A head injury or neurological observation chart should be used to record:

- the level of consciousness (see Figure 15.1)
- pupil size and reaction
- pulse rate

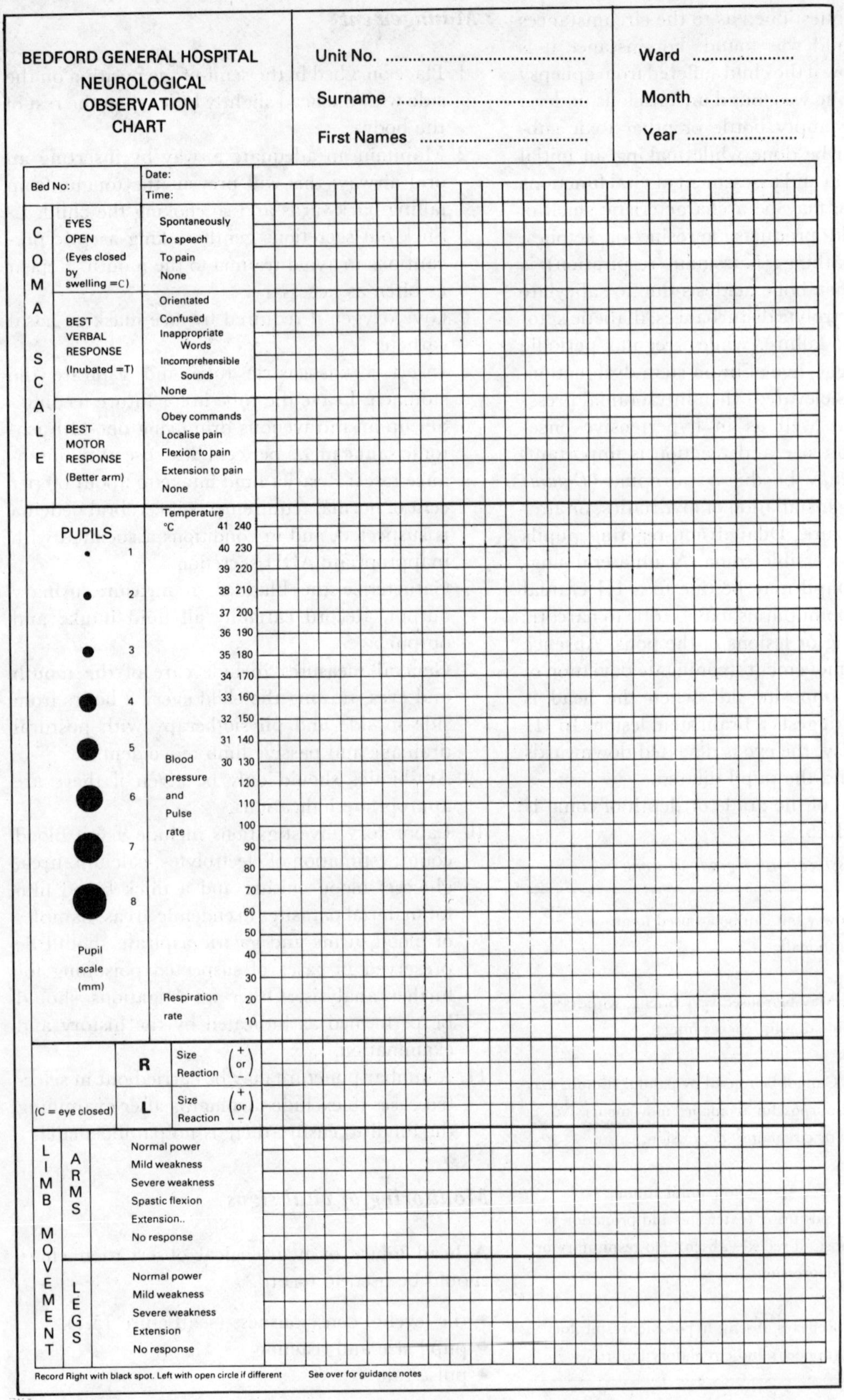

BEDFORD GENERAL HOSPITAL	Unit No.	Ward ....
NEUROLOGICAL OBSERVATION CHART	Surname	Month ....
	First Names	Year ....

Figure 15.1 An example of a neurological observation chart

- respiratory rate
- blood pressure

The frequency at which these observations are made depends on the state of the child, but in a seriously ill child should be carried out every 15 minutes.

Raised intracranial pressure and cerebral oedema

This may, ultimately, require neurosurgical intervention. The early signs are:

- dilatation of the pupils
- unequal pupils
- slowing of the pulse rate
- an increase or decrease in respiratory rate, or an alteration in the pattern of breathing
- sudden development of paralysis of a limb
- convulsions

The first line of management is medical decompression using the following regimes:

1. Restriction of fluid intake.
2. For transient but rapid action give mannitol 20 per cent solution, 1−2 g/kg (or 5−7 ml/kg) infused over 20−30 minutes intravenously. The effect lasts up to 6 hours, but may be associated with rebound effects and repeated infusions may result in metabolic disturbances.
3. For a more sustained effect give dexamethasone 0.2−0.4 mg/kg i.v. followed by 0.1−0.2 mg/kg 6-hourly i.m. Dexamathasone should not be used in the presence of raised blood pressure.

Cerebral palsy

Cerebral palsy is a non-progressive neurological disorder due to a variety of prenatal, natal or postnatal causes (Table 15.6). Even though the disorder is non-progressive by definition, many children tend to improve with regard to motor function as they grow. On the other hand disuse atrophy, contracture formation, the psychological sequelae of chronic disease and possibly parental neglect may give an impression of a progressive disease.

Although motor disability is the major clinical problem, several associated disturbances including various grades of mental and intellectual retar-

Table 15.6 *Aetiology of cerebral palsy*

Prenatal:	Developmental anomalies
	Intrauterine infections
	Maternal exposure to X-rays
	Disorders of pregnancy − toxaemia
Perinatal (often multiple):	Bad obstetric history
	Difficult labour: birth trauma: asphyxia
	Hypoglycaemia: neonatal jaundice
	Low birth weight
Postnatal:	CNS infections
	Uncontrolled seizures
	Hypernatraemia and dehydration
	Vascular accidents
	Trauma
	Malaria

Table 15.7 *Clinical classification of cerebral palsy*

1. Spastic:
   Diplegia
   Tetraplegia (or quadriplegia)
   Hemiplegia (and double hemiplegia)
   Paraplegia
   Monoplegia
   Triplegia
2. Ataxic
3. Dyskinetic
4. Atonic
5. Mixed

dation, speech and hearing disability, squint and seizures may be present. Localized atrophy of the affected part may occur.

Clinical types

The disorder has been classified into various clinical types depending upon the topographical distribution of the defect as well as the type of motor deficit (Table 15.7).

Spastic cerebral palsy

Major involvement is of the upper motor neurone, and so it is characterized by hypertonia, exaggerated tendon reflexes and an extensor plantar response. It has various sub-types:

Cerebral diplegia
This is often referred to as Little's disease. There is involvement of all the four limbs with maximum disability in the lower limbs. It is mainly due to prenatal causes, and birth trauma and asphyxia. The child has a characteristic posture with hips and knees partially flexed, legs internally rotated and the weight taken on the toes. The upper limbs are adducted at the shoulders, flexed at the elbow and pronated at the wrists.

Tetraplegia (quadriplegia)
In this all the four limbs are equally involved.

Hemiplegia
This is the most common type of acquired cerebral palsy and the causes include CNS infections, trauma and vascular accidents. There may be an associated seizure disorder. The arm is affected more severely. The hand is fisted with thumb clenched in the palm of hand, wrist flexed and pronated, elbow flexed and shoulder adducted.

Double hemiplegia is the most crippling type leading to grossly delayed development. Perinatal and postnatal causes are important.

Paraplegia
This is more commonly a manifestation of spinal cord lesions and CNS disease is rarely the cause. Both lower limbs are involved and the deformity is similar to that in diplegia.

Ataxic cerebral palsy
Clinical features include generalized hypotonia, weakness and cerebellar signs. Perinatal hypoxic damage and cerebellar damage during breech delivery are important factors.

Dyskinetic cerebral palsy
This is due to lesions of the extra-pyramidal system resulting from either prenatal causes or kernicterus. The latter is usually associated with nerve deafness. The child presents with delayed motor development, hypotonia with brisk reflexes and choreo-athetosis. Dystonia develops later. This group of children are usually not retarded.

Atonic cerebral palsy
The muscles, particularly in the lower limbs are markedly hypotonic but the tendon reflexes are exaggerated. As the child grows hypotonia gives way to spasticity. This group of children is often severely retarded.

Mixed cerebral palsy
This has the combined features of various other types. It has the highest incidence of associated mental retardation.

Management

Proper management requires an accurate assessment of not only the physical disability but also any other associated defects. Full testing of vision and hearing are important; speech and language development must be assessed, and psychological and intelligence testing carried out. Full discussion with the parents is necessary, to assess their attitude towards the child, their understanding of the nature of his illness and problems and to give them guidance on how best he can be managed.

Management requires a multidisciplinary approach which should include, besides the paediatrician, a physiotherapist, child psychologist, speech therapist, occupational therapist, social worker and teachers specially trained in the management of handicapped children. The medical side of the team includes an orthopaedic surgeon, ear, nose and throat surgeon and eye surgeon.

The physiotherapist is the mainstay of the team. Treatment is directed towards the prevention of contractures and deformities, encouraging active movements and improving motor function. It must be emphasized that surgery has a very limited role in treatment and is confined mainly to tendon lengthening procedures for severe contractures, to ease nursing care.

Parents must be encouraged to take an active part in the management of their child; they must also be given a realistic expectation of what can be achieved and discouraged from taking the child from doctor to doctor in the hope that useless tablets and medicines will provide a cure.

Hydrocephalus

The term hydrocephalus implies an absolute increase in circulating cerebrospinal fluid (CSF). It is due to an imbalance between CSF production and absorption and results in enlargement of the ventricular system with or without a rise in intracranial tension.

Pathophysiology

Cerebrospinal fluid circulation

CSF is largely produced in the choroid plexuses of the ventricles. The choroid plexus consists of villous folds lined by epithelium with a central core of highly vascular connective tissue. The CSF is formed by an active transport of ions (mainly sodium) across the plexus into the ventricular cavity, with passive diffusion of water.

Once formed, the CSF follows a course of circulation in the subarachnoid space of the brain and spinal cord (Figure 15.2). From the lateral ventricles the foramina of Monro carry it into the third ventricle, from where it reaches the fourth ventricle via aquduct of Sylvius. It flows out of the ventricular system into the basal cisterns through foramina of Luschka and Magendie. The basal cisterns in the posterior fossa communicate with the subarachnoid space over the cerebral hemispheres through pathways that traverse the tentorium; the cisterns also communicate with the spinal subarachnoid space.

Absorption takes place mainly into the venous circulation through the arachnoid villi which project into the sagittal sinus. Some absorption also occurs across the ependymal lining of the ventricular system and from spinal subarachnoid spaces.

Pathogenesis

Excess of CSF in the circulation can result from increased production, obstruction to circulation or decreased absorption. Excessive production is exceedingly uncommon and can only result from papilloma or hypertrophy of the choroid plexus. Decreased absorption may result from alteration in absorptive surfaces in certain inflammatory conditions as well as in sagittal sinus thrombosis.

Obstruction to flow accounts for the majority of cases. This may occur at any level starting from the foramina of Monro to the openings of the fourth ventricle and the basal cisterns, though the aquduct of Sylvius is the commonest site.

Hydrocephalus is designated obstructive or noncommunicating if the obstruction is within the ventricular system. If the block is at the level of the basal cisterns, tentorium or the arachnoid villi, with a free communication between the ventricular system and the spinal subarachnoid space, it is termed communicating (or external).

In obstructive hydrocephalus the ventricles begin to enlarge and compress the surrounding nervous tissue, which begins to atrophy. The white matter is selectively affected, the cerebral cortex and deep nuclei being relatively spared.

In the infant and the young child the sutures are not fused with the result that head begins to expand. Papilloedema is rare in this situation, but can occur due to compression of retinal vein in the optic nerve sheath.

Aetiology

A number of congenital anomalies are associated with hydrocephalus. In the Arnold—Chiari malformation, in which the medulla and cerebellum are displaced downwards, there is obstruction of subarachnoid pathways around the brain stem. In the

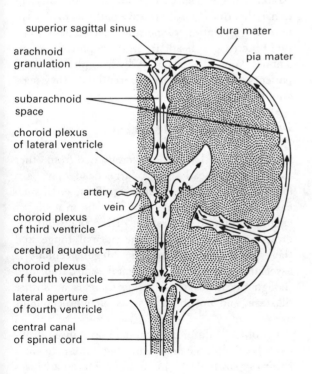

superior sagittal sinus

dura mater

arachnoid granulation

pia mater

subarachnoid space

choroid plexus of lateral ventricle

artery

vein

choroid plexus of third ventricle

cerebral aqueduct

choroid plexus of fourth ventricle

lateral aperture of fourth ventricle

central canal of spinal cord

Figure 15.2 Circulation of cerebrospinal fluid

Dandy–Walker malformation the defect is in the midline cerebellar structures and the obstruction is at the level of foramina of Luschka and Magendie. In Hurler's syndrome there is fibrosis of the subarachnoid space and in achondroplasia a small posterior fossa interferes with CSF circulation.

Congenital stenosis of the aqueduct of Sylvius may be an isolated anomaly. In a few cases it is transmitted as an X-linked recessive condition. Mumps infection during fetal life has been implicated.

Several intrauterine infections including rubella, cytomegalovirus infection, toxoplasmosis and syphilis may cause an inflammatory reaction in the ventricular system and the meninges resulting in hydrocephalus.

Birth trauma may lead to intraventricular and subarachnoid haemorrhage, which organizes to cause obstruction. A subdural haematoma in the posterior fossa may compress the aqueduct from outside and lead to hydrocephalus in neonatal period.

In acquired hydrocephalus, inflammatory diseases such as meningitis, encephalitis, as well as subarachnoid haemorrhage and space-occupying lesions, particularly of the posterior fossa, are the most important causes.

Clinical features

Presentation depends upon the age of onset and the rapidity with which hydrocephalus develops.

In congenital hydrocephalus the head size may be so big that normal vaginal delivery is not possible. On the other hand the head size may be near-normal at birth, enlargement developing soon afterwards.

Head enlargement, prominent in the frontal region, is an essential feature of congenital hydrocephalus and with onset in infancy. If the progress is slow there may be no other symptoms and signs until a late stage. In rapidly progressive disease the infant is irritable, has vomiting and fails to thrive. The anterior fontanelle is large, bulging and tense and the skin of the scalp is shining with prominent veins. Suture separation gives rise to a positive MacEwen sign ('cracked-pot' sounds on percussion of the skull). Pressure on the midbrain impaires upward gaze so that the upper part of sclera is visible when the eyes are open (setting-sun sign).

Spasticity, more obvious in the lower limbs,

along with exaggerated reflexes and a positive Babinski response, all indicate brain dysfunction secondary to pressure effects. A dilated third ventricle may press on the hypothalamus causing disturbances in growth, precocious sexual development and fluid and electrolyte disturbances.

In toddlers an occasional feature of hydrocephalus is a peculiar language disorder in which the child appears to be disinhibited and precocious; the exact mechanism is not known. It has been given an exotic designation, 'the cocktail party syndrome'.

In the Dandy–Walker malformation the occipital area may be transilluminated due to expansion caused by a hugely dilated fourth ventricle.

In hydrocephalus with onset in late childhood there is little scope for head enlargement. Raised intracranial tension, papilloedema and secondary brain damage develop, sometimes very rapidly. Higher cortical functions are disturbed and pyramidal signs appear.

Arrested hydrocephalus

In some patients with hydrocephalus a balance is established between CSF production and absorption, either due to an alternative pathway of absorption or restoration of normal mechanisms. The rapid increase in head size in these patients stops. This is known as arrested hydrocephalus. Such patients do not require active treatment; they need only follow-up.

Differential diagnosis

Hydrocephalus has to be differentiated from other causes of big head size. A large head may be a familial trait without clinical significance. In such cases the head circumference may be in a higher centile compared to the rest of the body but the growth velocity is within the normal range and there is no suture separation. Megalencephaly is associated with profound mental retardation and though the head size is large, there is no suture diastasis and no physical signs of hydrocephalus are present.

Chronic subdural haematoma may cause significant head enlargement with big fontanelle and suture separation. A unilateral haematoma causes an irregular head enlargement, though subdural haematomata are usually bilateral. Unlike hydrocephalus, the head enlargement in this disorder is in the parietal region predominantly, and trans-illumination is generally positive.

Diagnosis

Presence of the 'setting sun sign', dilated scalp veins and a large bulging fontanelle with suture separation are suggestive of progressive hydro-cephalus. However, a definite clinical diagnosis can only be established by demonstrating in-creased growth velocity of the head by serial head circumference measurements.

Ultrasound or computerized tomography are reliable non-invasive procedures which confirm not only the presence of hydrocephalus but also help to locate the level of obstruction or the presence of any space-occupying lesion.

Pneumoencephalography and angiography are occasionally useful. Cerebrospinal fluid examin-ation is indicated when an inflammatory cause is suspected.

Management

Primary management of progressive hydrocephalus is surgical; medical measures can, at best, be used temporarily.

Medical decompression

It is aimed at decreasing CSF production. Acetazo-lamide, isosorbide, furosemide and glycerol are some of the agents occasionally used.

Surgical removal of the obstruction is generally not possible and most procedures aim at draining the CSF into a body cavity. Ventriculo-peritoneal and ventriculo-atrial shunts are the two most com-monly used surgical procedures. A valve such as Spitz-Holter or Pudentz valve, is placed in the shunt pathway to control flow, regulate pressure and avoid excessive drainage.

Constant medical supervision is necessary after the shunt operation since several complications may arise. Valve infection particularly involving *Staphylococcus albus*, a low grade ventriculitis, shunt failure and subdural haematoma due to low intra-cranial pressure are some of the complications. Up to 20 per cent of shunts require revision or replacement ultimately.

Acute shunt failure and blockage of a valve causes an acute rise in intracranial pressure with vomiting, loss of vision, coma and death unless the pressure can be relieved and drainage of CSF re-established promptly. Immediate referral to a neurosurgical unit is necessary.

Even after surgery less than half the children are likely to survive, and of the survivors less than half are expected to have a normal intelligence.

Mental retardation

'The genius is notoriously deficient in some as-pects of life'

Neil Gordon, 1976

Mental retardation signifies sub-average general intellectual functioning. It is classified into severe subnormality, implying severe retardation, and subnormality which includes mild and moder-ate retardation. The terms idiocy, imbecility and feeble-mindedness are aesthetically undesirable and should not be used.

Severe subnormality is defined as a state of arrested or incomplete development of mind which includes subnormality of intelligence and is of such a degree and nature that the patient is incapable of living an independent life, or of guarding him-self against serious exploitation. The mildly and moderately retarded child can be trained to be independent in needs related to personal and social requirements. A general assessment of intellectual function can be made from an assessment of devel-opmental achievements in the pre-school child, from learning abilities in the school child and social behaviour after the school years. A more objective assessment can be made from the intelligence quo-tient *(IQ) or development quotient †(DQ). Sub-jects who have an IQ of 70 or less are classified as mentally handicapped. Those with scores between 50 and 70 have mild retardation, those in the range of 30 to 50 are moderately severely retarded and those below 30 are very severely or profoundly retarded.

A large number of aetiological factors (Table 15.8) can result in mental retardation. However, the majority of mildly retarded children have no

* $\text{IQ} = \dfrac{\text{Mental age of the child}}{\text{Chronological age}} \times 100$

† $\text{DQ} = \dfrac{\text{Developmental age of the child}}{\text{Chronological age}} \times 100$

Table 15.8 *Aetiological factors in mental retardation*

1. Environmental factors:

   – lack of proper stimulation
   – ignorant, uneducated parents
   – malnutrition
   – emotional deprivation

2. Organic causes:

   a. Prenatal:
      – genetic and chromosomal disorders
      – intrauterine infection – toxoplasmosis, rubella, cytomegalovirus and syphilis
      – placental dysfunction (pregnancy toxaemia, maternal diabetes, chronic diseases) especially if there is associated intrauterine growth retardation
      – severe maternal malnutrition
      – anticonvulsant drugs: drugs of addiction
      – inborn errors of metabolism
   b. Perinatal:
      – birth asphyxia
      – birth trauma
      – jaundice (kernicterus)
      – hypoglycaemia
      – hypernatraemia
      – impaired temperature regulation
      – infections (meningitis, septicaemia)
   c. Postnatal:
      – CNS infections
      – head injury
      – toxic (lead)
      – uncontrolled seizures
      – degenerative brain disease

identifiable cause. Of all the causes environmental factors are more common than organic diseases. However, once a diagnosis is made, screening for the more common causes should be carried out. This should include screening for congenital ('TORCH') infections, karyotyping for chromosomal abnormalities, hormonal assays for hypothyroidism and urinary metabolic screening. A number of spot tests are now available for the screening of neonates for treatable causes of mental retardation, such as phenylketonuria. It is important to detect such diseases as soon as possible after birth because therapeutic results are satisfactory only if management is started early.

Management

Exact assessment of mental (and associated physical) handicap is necessary to plan proper management. Associated psychiatric disorders are common and must also be taken into account. Treatment has to be individualized, as also the decision to manage at home or in an institution. Some important aspects of management include:

1. measures to relieve anxiety and stress in the patient and the family
2. finding ways to circumvent the handicap
3. encouraging development of areas least affected

Preventive measures are more rewarding and include good antenatal and natal care, early management of treatable causes such as phenylketonuria and hypothyroidism, accident prevention and genetic counselling for inherited disorders.

The child with a handicap

Handicap is a disadvantage for a given child resulting from an impairment or a disability that limits or prevents the fulfilment of a role that is normal for a child of similar age, sex and socio-economic background.

There are nearly one hundred million disabled children in the world of whom 80 per cent are in the developing world. At the turn of the century these countries will have an estimated one hundred and fifty million handicapped children.

Handicap is conveniently divided into the following groups:

1. Physical – such as congenital deformities, e.g. talipes equino-varus, congenital or acquired heart disease, or paralysis following poliomyelitis.
2. Visual – resulting in partial or complete loss of sight.
3. Auditory – with partial or complete loss of hearing. If present from birth, or soon afterwards, it will result in failure of speech and language development – 'deaf mutism'.
4. Mental and intellectual handicap.

Physical handicap

Some physical disabilities such as hare lip and cleft palate, talipes and the more severe forms of congenital heart disease can be readily recognized at birth or in early infancy. Acyanotic heart disease and chronic renal disease may remain undetected for months or years, requiring careful physical examination and sometimes sophisticated investigations for diagnosis. Similarly, milder forms of hearing impairment may remain undetected until the child lags in school performance.

In developing countries, physical handicap of congenital origin contributes to only a small percentage of disabled children, the major problems being post-poliomyelitis paralysis and blindness, and to a lesser extent accidents. In spite of tremendous efforts by national organizations as well as international agencies such as WHO and UNICEF, poliomyelitis is still rampant in developing countries, and apart from the risk of death in the acute phase, many patients are left with lifelong crippling physical disabilities.

Blindness

Vitamin A deficiency is still highly prevalent in many developing countries. Infants and young children in the age group 6 months to 6 years are most frequently affected with severe blindness due to corneal destruction. Vitamin A deficiency and resulting complications are endemic in Africa, Asia, the Middle East, Caribbean and Latin America. Most of the 500 000 new cases of corneal lesions in pre-school children are from these areas.

Other important causes of preventable blindness include:

1. Trachoma — especially common in hot dry climates and estimated to affect up to four hundred million people.
2. Onchocerciasis or 'river blindness' — prevalent across West, Central and East Africa and Central America.
3. Measles — where secondary herpetic infection, especially in malnourished children, results in conjunctivitis and a staphyloma with scarring or rupture of the eye.
4. Penetrating eye injuries.
5. Inadequate treatment of conjunctivitis and gonococcal ophthalmia in the newborn.

Hearing loss: speech and language development

Impairment of hearing, whether partial or complete, if present from birth or from afterwards will interfere with speech and language development, and so any child in whom speech is delayed should have a hearing test and audiometric assessment. It is generally possible to make some assessment of a child's hearing by 8 months of age. Because of hearing loss, a child cannot communicate adequately with parents or siblings and is often mistakenly diagnosed as being either mentally defective or having behaviour problems and a psychological disturbance. Common acquired causes of hearing loss include recurrent otitis media and 'glue ear', chronic otitis media with perforation, discharge and mastoiditis, and following meningitis. Children with a cleft palate also have a higher incidence of hearing loss.

Mental handicap

Mental handicap may be of varying severity; the most severe forms often also have associated physical handicaps, such as cerebral palsy, visual and hearing impairment, speech and language disorders as well as behavioural and emotional problems.

In the developed countries, with improved obstetric and neonatal services, and better control of communicable diseases, a large percentage of mental handicap results from inherited and chromosomal disorders of which Down's syndrome and the recently recognized Fragile X syndrome are the commonest.

In the developing countries, on the other hand, infections during pregnancy, poor obstetric care and neonatal services resulting in birth asphyxia and injuries, nutritional and emotional deprivation and inadequate control of communicable diseases are much more important causes of mental handicap. Meningitis, febrile convulsions and hypernatraemic dehydration are especially common, while road traffic and other accidents are an increasing cause for concern. Lack of adequate medical facilities and treatment are also responsible for some.

The most severely handicapped children and those with specific syndromes can be detected early. In many, however, the handicap only becomes evident with the passage of time. Children with a mild handicap may only be identified when they lag behind in their school performance.

Epilepsy is a common associated disorder in children with mental handicap or brain damage from any cause. Epilepsy itself is commonly associated with a mild degree of mental handicap or learning difficulties. However, the impairment of mental and intellectual functions may increase with time if seizures remain uncontrolled.

Care and provision of services for handicapped children

Early detection of handicap is the key to proper management. Every newborn baby should be thoroughly examined for physical deformities before leaving the maternity hospital. Developmental screening of infants and young children in Well Baby Clinics is essential for the early detection and identification of mental handicap.

Physical disabilities that can be treated surgically, such as talipes and congenital dislocation of the hip, should be corrected at an early age to prevent secondary complications or permanent disability. Harelip and cleft palate not only cause feeding difficulties in infancy but if not repaired early may result in speech and learning difficulties. Post-poliomyelitis paralysis requires continuous physiotherapy to prevent secondary contractures.

The first need is to define the child's problems and then his needs, and finally to decide what, if anything can be done for him (Table 15.9). Management should not await a final medical diagnosis, which in some instances may only be possible after a period of observation. Intercurrent disease such as anaemia, malnutrition and tuberculosis will require treatment. An attempt should be made to identify the cause of the handicap, for example prenatal or perinatal or postnatal. Prolonged observation may be required if there is only developmental delay since classical signs of cerebral palsy, for example, may not appear until later.

Diagnosis and assessment are only the first though important, step towards management. More detailed assessment may involve the services of orthopaedic, ENT, eye and dental specialists whose co-operation and interest should be sought and stimulated at an early stage. Different attitudes and approaches must be developed for the care of handicapped children compared with those with acute illnesses. It is important for one doctor to be in overall charge on a long-term basis co-ordinating the management by other members of the team so that omissions or duplications of services do not occur, and parents are not confused by personnel sometimes working at cross purposes.

Table 15.9 *Scheme of management of the handicapped child*

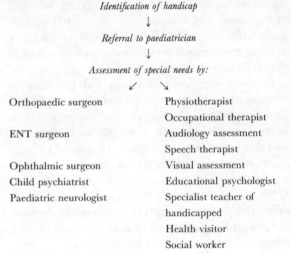

Identification of handicap
↓
Referral to paediatrician
↓
Assessment of special needs by:
↙ ↘

Orthopaedic surgeon	Physiotherapist
	Occupational therapist
ENT surgeon	Audiology assessment
	Speech therapist
Ophthalmic surgeon	Visual assessment
Child psychiatrist	Educational psychologist
Paediatric neurologist	Specialist teacher of handicapped
	Health visitor
	Social worker

↓

Case conference
1. Identification of major problems
2. Provision of appropriate treatment
3. Plan of long-term management and therapy
4. Nomination of key worker(s)
5. Provision of support to family

↓

Follow-up
1. Paediatrician − co-ordination and continuation of care
   − regular review of needs with key worker(s)
2. Key worker(s) − specific therapies

It is important to draw up a plan of action for each child after full assessment by members of the team, with as much involvement as possible by parents. We often underestimate their intelligence, interest and enthusiasm in helping with the child. It is important to explain clearly at the beginning that 'cure' is not possible and that only a degree of improvement is to be expected, how much improvement can be expected and over what period of time. They must be encouraged to do as much as they can for the child and given explicit guidance on everyday matters and simple care. They must not be confused by being told too much at once. All families of handicapped children are under some stress, especially the mother who may have to devote time to the child at the expense of her husband and other children. In a large family an older child may take on this role. The services of a medical social worker are of special help here.

The provision of services for handicapped children in most developing countries is virtually non-existent. Such services are expensive and where health budgets are severely limited, priority must understandably be given to more pressing problems and preventive services. A modest start can be made in many centres by providing outpatient and physiotherapy facilities by interested and motivated staff. It must be realized from the outset that management is a team affair with, usually, a paediatrician or other interested health professional at the head of the team and a physiotherapist, preferably trained in the problems of the handicapped child, as his key colleague. The facilities will depend on what is available locally and how much enthusiasm can be generated in the local community for voluntary help. All religious bodies and international service organizations have a keen interest in services for the handicapped. Though facilities should be closely linked with the hospital, day care centres for handicapped children need not necessarily be on a hospital site. Day care should be run on an outpatient basis. Distance and cost will prevent many parents from regular visits, and there may be a need for temporary hostel ac-

commodation where parents and children can stay for a short while to be taught the basis techniques of home physiotherapy.

Very severely affected children are unlikely to survive much beyond infancy, others with considerable physical and mental handicaps may require institutional care, especially if abandoned by parents. The present trend, however, is against institutionalization whenever possible and the concept of 'normalization' of care, which implies management in a home setting with participation and involvement of the family and community is now being widely accepted.

The aim of treatment should be to select children who are most likely to benefit from help — that is mild to moderate cases who can be rehabilitated. Treatment need not necessarily be expensive, a simple piece of equipment can often be made or adapted to suit the special needs of an individual. For the more severely handicapped, it may not be possible to do very much, but nevertheless, in children with multiple handicaps attempts to help in one sphere are often rewarding because reduction of one disability often helps to reduce the overall burden, making management for the mother much easier and simpler. Later, it may be possible to provide special schooling for educable children, although this is not yet available in most developing

Table 15.10   *Measures to prevent childhood handicaps*

Area	Important handicaps	Preventive measures
1. Communicable diseases	Post-polio paralysis Rubella syndrome	Immunization of children, safe water supply and waste disposal
2. Child labour	Physical handicaps from industrial accidents	Legislation, economic growth, population control
3. Nutrition	Impaired physical and mental development	Nutritional supplementation, active promotion of breast feeding, health education, agricultural production, iodinization of salt.
4. Accidents and poisoning	Physical handicaps Mental impairment	Legislation, traffic regulation, control of distribution of drugs, community health education — schools, TV, radio, newspapers.
5. Pregnancy and childbirth	Cerebral palsy, mental retardation Physical handicaps	Improved mother and child health services as part of primary health care, immunization of girls and pregnant women, improved obstetric services, early management of congenital anomalies

countries. The aim should be to try and integrate children, especially those with mild handicaps, back into the normal school and community, though some may require special care or facilities, e.g. physiotherapy. These children tend to improve both psychologically and intellectually with stimulation and adequate support in their special needs.

Special provision will be needed for children who are blind or partially sighted, deaf or partially deaf and who have speech problems. Facilities for many of these children are not yet available, and depend to a large extent on the availability of skilled therapists.

Prevention of handicap

Preventive measures to reduce the incidence of handicap are less costly and much more cost effective than curative medicine and yield rich dividends. A broad plan of preventive measures is given in Table 15.10.

Proper maternal and child health services at primary level with good antenatal and obstetric care, primary immunization, and health and nutritional education of young mothers (including the value of family spacing) constitute the most effective measures of disease prevention in developing countries. A more vigorous approach to the importance and value of breast feeding, including stricter implementation of the WHO Code on the Marketing of Breast Milk Substitutes by governments, would go far towards reducing the ever increasing amount of marasmus and chronic illness resulting in handicap caused by artificial feeding in many countries. Prevention of much disease and handicap, however, lies in improving environmental and public health services, such as provision of pure water supplies, proper sanitation and sewage disposal, and other non-medical measures such as better housing, less overcrowing, and prevention of road accidents by better traffic regulation and use of seat belts.

16

Endocrine Disorders

Diabetes mellitus

Diabetes mellitus is the commonest metabolic disorder of children and young adults. It results from failure of the pancreas to produce adequate amounts of insulin, almost always due to irreversible destruction of the islet (beta) cells of the pancreas. Lack of insulin causes impairment of peripheral utilization of glucose at cellular level, resulting in hyperglycaemia and glycosuria which in turn produce more generalized metabolic disturbances.

Diabetes in children is always insulin dependent or type I (juvenile onset).

Aetiology

The aetiology of diabetes is still poorly understood but present evidence suggests that it is due to both genetic and environmental factors. Genetic factors are much more important in non-insulin dependent diabetes (type II).

1. Only 50 per cent of identical twins will develop diabetes when the other has insulin dependent diabetes, whilst nearly 90 per cent of identical twins will develop diabetes when the other has non-insulin dependent (type II) diabetes.
2. The incidence of non-insulin dependent diabetes is the same amongst parents of diabetic children as in the general population.
3. There is a close association between insulin dependent diabetes and inheritance of HLA antigens B8, B15 and B18 and an even stronger association with DW3 and DW4 antigens, but not with type II diabetes. DW3 is also associated with many other autoimmune disorders.
4. Environmental triggers are still not known.
5. Viral infection has long been suspected but is still far from proven. It is suggested by:
   - a seasonal incidence with a peak in autumn

and winter, recognized in many parts of the world
   - transient (or occasionally permanent) damage to islet cells by some viruses
   - diabetes following mumps is uncommon but has long been recognized
   - high levels of Coxsackie B4 antibodies in some newly diagnosed children
   - an increased susceptibility to insulin dependent diabetes in infants with congenital infections, e.g. rubella and cytomegalovirus

   Attempts, however, to establish a firm link between diabetes and common human viruses − mumps and Coxsackie B4 − have so far failed.
6. Islet cell antibodies are almost always present and often long before clinical diabetes is apparent. They may destroy the islets or inhibit insulin release, or sometimes be an indication of islet cell damage. One suggestion is that a virus infection initially damages islet cells and further destruction is then continued by autoimmune induced antibodies.
7. Diet − studies from several parts of the world show that a Western European type diet high in sugar and carbohydrate has a diabetogenic effect on a population in whom diabetes was previously uncommon. In parts of tropical Africa and amongst American Indians the rise in diabetes has coincided with the ready availability of refined sugar (sucrose).

Clinical presentation

Diabetes is rare in infancy but the incidence increases with age throughout childhood with a peak around early puberty and a smaller peak at 4−6 years. Boys and girls are equally affected.

The onset is usually acute, with symptoms appearing over a few days or at the most over a few weeks, though occasionally present for much longer. Family studies have shown a subclinical derangement of glucose tolerance may exist for a long time, however, before symptoms appear.

The classical presentation is with:

- thirst and polydipsia (excessive drinking)
- polyuria, day and night, causing onset of nocturnal enuresis
- weight loss and muscle wasting
- tiredness, lethargy and decreased activity
- increased appetite, later followed by anorexia

Less often, other symptoms may include:

- abdominal pain and tenderness, sometimes severe enough to mimic an acute surgical abdomen
- recurrent attacks of thrush, especially on the perineum

A mild infection may precede the onset of symptoms. Many children have already progressed to diabetic ketoacidosis when first seen, with additional symptoms of:

- vomiting, progressing to dehydration, hypotension and shock
- severe abdominal pain
- sweetish smell of ketones in the breath, and ketones in the urine
- drowsiness
- Kassmaul respiration − or air hunger − deep sighing respiration due to the acidaemia − in very severe acidosis, respiration becomes depressed.

Diagnosis

Is simple. Any child with the above symptoms, and with glucose and ketones in the urine has diabetes. The diagnosis is confirmed by finding a raised blood glucose, usually within the range 400−800 mg/100 ml. It is rarely necessary to perform a glucose tolerance test, and no other investigation is necessary.

Treatment of diabetic ketoacidosis

Diabetic ketoacidosis is a paediatric medical emergency. The principles of treatment are:

- rehydration, with correction of fluid and electrolyte losses
- maintain serum potassium at 4.0−5.0 mmol/l

- correction of insulin deficiency and restoration of normal blood sugar
- treatment of any intercurrent infection

Management

1. Weigh the child. Assume that at least 10 per cent body weight has been lost through dehydration (see page 30 for assessment of dehydration).
2. Pass a nasogastric tube and empty the stomach. Continue aspiration hourly. *Do not* give anything by mouth.
3. Set up an intravenous drip.
   - Rate and volume are the same as for correction of dehydration.
   - Calculate the deficit and add to the maintenance requirements for the next 24 hours. Give ⅓ in first 6 hours
     ⅓ over next 6 hours (7−12 hours)
     ⅓ over next 12 hours (13−24 hours)
   - After the first 24 hours, or correction of dehydration, maintenance is at following rates per 24 hours:

Weight of child (kg)	Water (ml)/kg
4	120
10	100
20	80
40	60
65 (adults)	45

   - In young children 10 per cent dehydration is equal to a loss of approximately 100 ml per kg.

     Example:
     18 kg child with ketoacidosis. Deficit is 10 per cent; thus expected weight = 20 kg
     Deficit = 2000 ml
     Maintenance requirements are 20 (kg) × 80 (ml) = 1600 ml
     Total replacement = 2000 + 1600 = 3600 ml
     Volume in first 6 hours = ⅓ × 3600 = 1200 ml
     Rate = 200 ml/hour

   - NB Assess clinical state at regular intervals to avoid overhydration.

Type of fluid

Use 0.9 per cent (isotonic) saline initially. If child is in peripheral circulatory failure and shocked, use plasma (or a substitute) and infuse at 20 ml/kg over the first hour.

Change to 0.18 per cent saline in 4.3 per cent

dextrose when the blood sugar falls below 250 mg/100 ml (14 mmol/l).

Intravenous fluids should be continued at maintenance rates for 24–36 hours until the child is no longer vomiting, is drinking normally and eating a light diet.

Oral feeds can be started at 12–18 hours depending on the clinical condition. These must include adequate potassium supplements – from fresh fruit juice or potassium chloride 0.5–1 g 6-hourly for at least a week to replace body losses.

Insulin

Use only soluble (regular) insulin. It can be given either intramuscularly or intravenously (see below). Both regimes are equally effective and result in a smooth fall in blood sugar over about 6 hours. Too rapid a fall in blood sugar should be avoided. Subcutaneous insulin should *not* be used in this situation as absorption is very irregular and unpredictable.

Intramuscular

Give an initial stat dose of 0.25 units/kg followed by 0.1 units/kg hourly until the blood sugar falls to approximately 200 mg/100 ml (10 mmol/l). Use the arms or thighs and not the buttocks.

Intravenous

Do not use this route unless an intravenous infusion pump is available to deliver insulin continuously at an even rate. It should be given into the drip tubing through a Y connection, from an infusion pump containing 30 units of soluble insulin in 30 ml isotonic saline – insulin should not be put directly into the i.v. infusion bottle. Give 0.1 units/kg as stat. dose followed by 0.1 units/kg per hour until the blood sugar falls to approximately 200 mg/100 ml (10 mmol/l).

Potassium

In ketoacidosis, potassium leaks into plasma from the cells and considerable amounts are lost in the urine. Initially, serum potassium levels may appear normal in spite of an overall body deficit. Insulin causes a shift of potassium (and glucose) back into the cells, so after starting treatment serum potassium falls progressively and can reach dangerously low levels, below 2 mmol/l unless supplements are given.

After the first hour when rehydration is well under way or after the child has passed urine, add potassium chloride to the replacement fluid, 1 to 1.5 g (13 to 20 mmol) to 500 ml.

Glucose and electrolyte monitoring

Good biochemical control depends on the availability of laboratory facilities. Ideally, blood glucose should be measured hourly, and electrolytes 2-hourly until a stable state has been reached. Glucose should then be measured 6-hourly or before main meals, depending on clinical circumstances, and electrolytes twice daily. All urine specimens should be tested for glucose and ketones. If laboratory facilities are inadequate or not available:

1. Do hourly finger prick blood sugars (using Dextrostix or BM Glycemie 20–800) until the blood sugar has stabilized.
2. Check urine glucose and ketone levels hourly or 2-hourly. In this situation an indwelling catheter (or urine bag) is essential.
3. Monitor potassium levels with an ECG.
   - Hypokalaemia – below 2.5 mmol/l – produces ST depression. Flat or biphasic T waves prominent U waves (may merge into T waves).
   - Hyperkalaemia – over 6.0 mmol/l – produces tall peaked T waves followed by an increasing PR interval. Widening of QRS waves.

If neither biochemical or ECG facilities are available:

1. Add 20 mmol (1.5 g) potassium chloride to 500 ml saline after the first hour or after the child has passed a good volume of urine. Stop intravenous potassium when the blood sugar reaches 200 mg per 100 ml and change to oral supplements.
2. Rehydrate and lower the blood glucose more slowly to avoid the risks of overhydration and cerebral oedema, and hypoglycaemia.

Correction of acidosis

Use of sodium bicarbonate is not necessary and is potentially dangerous unless the child is severely shocked. When adequate rehydration and replacement of electrolytes is under way, using the above regime, the kidneys cope very efficiently in correcting the acidosis, and no other treatment is required.

General measures

1. Record pulse, respiration and blood pressure every half-hour for first 6 hours, then hourly. Record temperature 2-hourly.
2. Keep a careful record of fluid balance:
   - input − intravenously
   - output − urine and gastric aspirate

   Pass an indwelling urinary catheter, or attach a urine bag. Test the urine hourly for glucose and ketones.
3. Search for any source of infection − including throat and other swabs, blood culture, chest X-ray, urine and stools for microscopy and culture. A full blood count should also be done.
4. Watch for hypoglycaemia.

Management after initial resuscitation

Many children relapse after initial resuscitation because of a failure to continue adequate follow-on treatment.

It is essential to continue i.v. fluids until the child is eating and drinking normally.

Continue with subcutaneous soluble insulin at 6-hourly intervals, including during the night, for the next 24−48 hours on a sliding scale when hydration has been corrected. The sliding scale is particularly useful when frequent blood glucose estimations are not readily available.

A suitable scale is shown in Table 16.1.

Long-term management

There is probably no other disorder in medicine which requires so much patient or parental participation as diabetes, since all of the day-to-day management is done by them, not the doctor. From the time of initial diagnosis, the child should be involved as much as possible in the management of his diabetes − giving his own injections and testing his own urine − while parents take on a more supervisory role, depending on the child's age.

Parents are shocked and anxious and need a period of adjustment and reassurance as well as education about diabetes while their child is stabilized. It has to be emphasized that their child:

- will recover normal health,
- will have no physical or mental handicap, and can ultimately marry and have children, and
- can lead a normal life with no restrictions and with involvement in all school and life's activities.

On the other hand it must be made clear that:

- the disease is here to stay for life, and
- insulin injections will be needed twice daily.

Several pharmaceutical companies involved in diabetic care have produced excellent handbooks explaining diabetes and its management in simple easily understood terms for patients and are available free on request.

The three main aspects of management are

1. diet
2. insulin injections
3. urine/blood glucose testing and regulation of insulin dosage

Diet

The help of a dietitian is invaluable both in the construction of a diet suitable for an individual patient and for parental education.

Recent advances have shown that the best diabetic diet is one in which carbohydrate intake

Table 16.1 *Amounts of insulin to be given during follow-on treatment*

Urine glucose	Ketones	Blood glucose		Soluble insulin
		mg/dl	mmol/l	
2% glucose	with ketones	⩾400	⩾20	0.5 units/kg
2% glucose	no ketones	300−400	15−20	0.4 units/kg
1% glucose	with ketones	200−300	10−15	0.3 units/kg
1% glucose	no ketones	100−200	5−10	0.2 units/kg
½% glucose	no ketones	⩽100	⩽5	0.1 units/kg
no glucose	no ketones	⩽100	⩽5	none

provides 50–55 per cent energy (calories), combined with high fibre foods (pulses, vegetables, fruit, wholegrain cereals) and reduced fat intake (not more than 25–30 per cent energy). The main restriction is on the intake of highly refined carbohydrates – sugars, sweets, syrups, cakes and high energy fatty foods. There is no restriction on protein. A high fibre diet gives smoother control, avoids wide swings of peaks and troughs in blood sugar after main meals, and a lower average blood sugar.

Children's energy requirements vary considerably; an estimate of an individual child's needs can be made by the dietitian by assessing the diet before the onset of diabetes. An approximate guide to the carbohydrate allowance can be calculated from the formula:

Carbohydrate allowance (g/day) = 100 + (age in years × 10)
i.e. for a 7-year-old, allowance = 100 + (7 × 10) = 170 g/day

The dietitian will provide a list of the carbohydrate content of usual foods and the diet is constructed from 10 g exchanges or portions. An attempt is made to ensure that the carbohydrate allowance is spread out as evenly as possible so that there is a steady intake of carbohydrate throughout the day, thus the diet for a 7-year-old child on 170 g could be distributed as follows:

Breakfast	30 g
Mid-morning snack	15 g
Lunch	50 g
Mid-afternoon snack	15 g
Evening meal	50 g
Bed-time snack	10 g

It must be recognized that these are guidelines, and can be increased or decreased to suit individual needs. Cultural and family patterns of eating vary considerably in different countries. Some families eat little or no breakfast; the main meal may be taken in the afternoon or late evening, necessitating adjustments in insulin regimes and dosage. It is important, however, that the child should eat regularly, but, as far as is practical, with the rest of the family and that his regime is incorporated in the routine life of the family.

Insulin

Twice daily injections, given before breakfast and the evening meal, provide the best control, though young children under 5 or 6 years (and some older children) can be managed well on a single daily dose.

Most paediatricians prefer isophane insulin whose duration of action is ideally suited for twice daily control. The longer acting insulin zinc suspension requires careful control and a high evening dose may cause nocturnal hypoglycaemia. It is, however, the insulin of choice if once daily injections are preferred. An additional small dose of soluble insulin, may be necessary in the morning or before the main meal if blood sugar levels are consistently high. Insulins can be mixed in the same syringe but parents require adequate instruction. Avoid complicated regimes with other insulins which parents will not understand.

Use human insulin or a highly purified mono-component insulin. These are the least antigenic and cause fewer local reactions e.g. atrophy of fat. Human insulins are now widely available and cheap and are replacing those of bovine and porcine origin. There may be cultural or religious objections to the use of porcine or bovine insulins although most patients are usually unaware of the origin of their insulin.

Children over the age of 6 or 7 years can be taught to give their own injections under the supervision of parents who should carefully check the dose of insulin.

Both parents, or two adults in the household, should be taught how to give the child injections, in the event of one parent being unable to do so.

After correction of ketoacidosis, start with 0.5 units/kg of medium acting insulin, giving about two-thirds in morning dose and one-third in evening dose, and adjust as necessary. Parents should be taught to make small changes in dosage if blood sugar is consistently high or low.

Insulin can be kept in a cool room, or refrigerator (but *not* in the freezer compartment) but should never be left in a hot room or direct sunlight.

Use 1.25 cm (half inch) gauge 25 needles and inject subcutaneously through the full thickness of the skin, not directly into the skin or fat. The preferred site is the lateral or anterior aspect of the thigh, alternatively use the lower abdominal wall. Do not use the buttocks, as injections may go into the fat, or, in thin children, the upper arm because of the risk of damage to the circumflex nerve.

Control of blood sugar

Good diabetic control aims to produce a blood glucose pattern throughout the day resembling, as near as is possible, that of the normal non-diabetic. Parents, and patients, must understand the need to monitor urine or blood regularly, every day, with the aim of keeping blood sugar within the range 60—160 mg/100 ml (3—8 mmol/l) and below 200 mg/100 ml (10 mmol/l). Urine tests should show glucose ranging from none to ½ or 1 per cent with occasional 2 per cent. Persistently negative tests indicate a risk of hypoglycaemia and the need for a reduction of insulin, or falsification of results. Persistent 2 per cent glycosuria for 2 or more days indicates a need for more insulin or an impending infection. Wide swings of urine or blood glucose indicate poor control and a need to review diet, activity and insulin dosage with perhaps addition of soluble insulin.

Routine testing for ketones is unnecessary but should be done at times of stress, infection or when glycosuria is persistently above 2 per cent.

Remember that urine tests do not accurately reflect present blood sugar levels, but merely indicate the range of levels over the past few hours since the last test, nor do they warn of impending hypoglycaemia.

The advantages of home blood glucose monitoring, giving an instant indication of blood glucose level are obvious. A drop of capillary blood from a finger prick is placed directly on to a glucose oxidase strip (e.g. Dextrostix or BM Glycemie 20—800) and the resulting colour changes indicate the approximate blood sugar level, within a range of values. Alternatively, the strip may be inserted into a colorimeter or reflectance meter which gives a more accurate and direct reading in figures.

Young children, however, dislike frequent finger pricks and may prefer urine tests but many older children and adolescents find them more convenient and preferable to urine tests. A combination of urine tests and random finger prick blood tests, done at a different time each day are helpful in building up a blood glucose profile of the individual child, provided of course that any major changes in activity or lifestyle from day-to-day are also recorded; these are so variable in children and significantly alter the blood sugar levels.

All children should keep a diary recording daily insulin dosage and times of urine and blood glucose tests, ketones, and comments on activity, illness and infections and hypoglycaemic attacks.

If urine testing is not available, then control has to be assessed by watching for appearance of symptoms of hyperglycaemia — polyuria, especially at night, thirst, a feeling of tiredness, poor weight gain, or the smell of ketones in the breath.

Other indicators of control

Measurement of glycosylated HbAlC gives a good indication of how well control has been over the previous 2—3 months and reflects the average levels of blood glucose in that period. Well-controlled diabetics are about 2 per cent above the normal level of 6—8 per cent.

Maintenance of normal growth and development. Poor control may result in growth failure, although the extremes of the Mauriac syndrome — stunted growth, hepatomegaly and delayed puberty — should rarely be seen today. Excessive weight gain, especially in adolescents and girls, is an indication to reduce both calorie intake and insulin.

Is good control important? Paediatricians seldom see the long-term complications of diabetes but have an important role in their prevention. Present evidence suggests that good control is important, and that the incidence of microvascular complications is lower in patients who maintain a blood glucose below 200 mg/100 ml and avoid frequent high surges.

Specific problems

Hypoglycaemia

A mild hypoglycaemic attack should be induced in all newly diagnosed diabetics so that both child and parents recognize the early symptoms, which although variable, tend to be the same for each child.

Symptoms include feeling faint, sweaty, cold, confused or unable to concentrate, tachycardia, headache and hunger. Parents notice a change in mood and irritability or inappropriate and bizarre behaviour. Unconsciousness or coma may occur with or without a convulsion.

The usual causes are a delayed or missed meal, excessive exercise or games at school without taking extra carbohydrate, or excessive insulin, usually a mistaken overdose.

Management

All diabetic children should carry glucose tablets,

sugar or sweet biscuits at all times. When symptoms first appear, immediately take several glucose tablets. If the child is drowsy or cannot eat, give a sweet drink with added sugar. If unconscious, give 25 or 50 per cent dextrose intravenously or glucagon 0.5–1.0 mg intramuscularly. After regaining consciousness, give milk drinks and biscuits unless the next meal is due.

Attacks during the day can be avoided by reducing the morning dose of insulin or taking extra carbohydrate before periods of excessive activity — games, football, swimming etc. Nocturnal hypoglycaemia can be avoided by reducing the evening dose of insulin and giving an adequate evening snack before bed. The Somogyi phenomenon is a reactive hyperglycaemia, with glycosuria and ketonuria following unrecognized, or transient or nocturnal hypoglycaemic episodes. The usual cause is too high a dose of insulin and can be avoided by reducing the dose.

Hyperglycaemia, intercurrent illness and vomiting

1. Any intercurrent illness will increase insulin requirements, upset control, and reduce appetite and food intake.
2. *Never* reduce or omit insulin if the child is ill, vomiting or not taking food. More — not less — insulin may be required.
3. Give the usual daily dose of insulin if the blood sugar is normal, and additional soluble insulin if it is high, even if the child is not eating.
4. Give the daily carbohydrate allowance as frequent, small snacks, and encourage the child to drink milk, Coca-Cola/Pepsi-Cola or other carbohydrate-containing drinks.
5. Admit to hospital if vomiting is persistent, or signs of dehydration or ketoacidosis develop.

Emotional problems

These can be minimized by continuous support and careful education of both child and parents, promoting a responsible and balanced attitude to diabetes and removing much of the fear of the disease from the family, so that it interferes as little as possible with normal life and activities. Cultural attitudes and beliefs, however, make it very difficult for some families to accept this. Much depends on the initial attitude of the doctor and his enthusiasm as to how the family will respond. The child should be helped to take some responsibility

for his own care from an early age, consistent with his ability. Avoid imposing impossibly strict regimes of control; it is often necessary to compromise and do what is realistic with the family.

Emotional problems and some rebellion are common among adolescents who question why they have been inflicted with this life-long disease and have to put up with its treatment; they resent the dietary restrictions, doing urine tests and parental oversight. They also worry about the long-term complications. Careful handling and open discussion with a sympathetic doctor is essential to restore their confidence.

Disorders of the thyroid gland

Physiology

Thyroxine (T_4) is the main hormone of the thyroid gland which regulates tissue metabolism. Secretion is controlled through a feed-back servo mechanism. Thyrotrophin-releasing hormone (TRH) is secreted from the median eminence of the hypothalamus into the hypophyseal portal circulation. This regulates the secretion of thyroid-stimulating hormone (TSH) from the anterior pituitary, and which, in turn, stimulates the thyroid gland to produce both thyroxine (T_4) and tri-iodothyronine (T_3). These hormones regulate their own secretion by a negative feed-back on the anterior pituitary (T_4) and hypothalamus (T_3). (Figure 16.1)

Biosynthesis of thyroid hormones

Plasma iodide is trapped in the thyroid gland

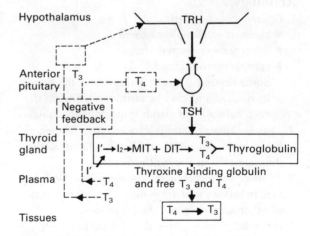

Figure 16.1 Production and control of thyroid hormones

and the uptake is regulated by thyroid stimulating hormones. Thyroid iodide is then organified to thyroid iodine which combines with tyrosine to produce thyroid hormones. These are stored within the gland as thyroglobulin until released into the circulation by proteases. There, both T_4 and T_3 combine with carrier proteins called thyroid binding globulin and thyroid binding pre-albumen. These bound forms of T_4 and T_3 provide a circulating reserve of thyroid hormone, although only the free forms are metabolically active. Free T_3 is the main active hormone and is five times more potent than T_4; it is less strongly bound to protein. Eighty per cent of T_3 is derived from the peripheral de-iodination of T_4 which serves as a reservoir for T_3.

Thyroid function in the fetus and neonate

The thyroid gland has developed and is active by 12 weeks of fetal life, and immunoreactive TSH can be detected in the pituitary. The fetus is dependent on its own intact pituitary–thyroid axis for production of thyroid hormone, since maternal thyroid hormones do not cross the placenta – unlike maternal antithyroid drugs and maternal antithyroid antibodies which readily cross and may damage the fetal thyroid. Within a few hours of birth there is a sharp rise in TSH levels, thought to be due to the stress of birth, and lasts for up to several weeks before gradually returning to normal values. A similar rise in T_3 and T_4 occurs to levels which would be compatible with hyperthyroidism in adults, returning to normal more slowly than TSH.

Congenital hypothyroidism

Aetiology

1. *Defects in embryogenesis*:
   - agenesis or complete absence.
   - dysgenesis or partial absence.
   - ectopic thyroid gland.
     Some thyroid tissue remains along the line of its descent and may be visible as a lingual thyroid. All aberrant glands function inadequately.
2. *Defective hormone synthesis*. Five enzyme deficiencies have been described, each associated with a different step in the synthesis of T_4.
3. *Pituitary and hypothalamic hypothyroidism*. Both are rare in infancy and are associated with deficiency of other anterior pituitary hormones.
4. *Antenatal goitrogens*. Iodide and carbimazole ingested by the mother can cross the placenta and block the synthesis of thyroid hormone by the fetal gland. Maternal iodine deficiency will similarly prevent adequate production of hormone by the gland.

Effects

As well as its general effects on metabolism, thyroxine is crucial for normal growth, development and maturation of the brain and other organs in fetal life and early childhood. Complete absence results in cretinism with symptoms apparent within a few weeks of birth. Early and prompt treatment may reverse some of the adverse effects but there appears to be a critical period in brain development after which treatment may not be fully effective. In general, the earlier treatment is started (within 6 weeks of birth) the more favourable is the outcome, with normal or near normal intelligence, while late treatment is associated with a poor outcome. Follow-up studies, however, show considerable overlap with some early diagnosed and treated cases showing significant learning difficulties at school, and a small number mental retardation, while occasionally late diagnosed cases do well.

Screening for congenital hypothyroidism has been practised on a nationwide scale in many Western European countries, Canada, USA and Japan in the past 10 years using a TSH assay on dried blood spots on filter paper, and is combined with screening for phenylketonuria and other inborn errors about the seventh day of life. TSH is preferred to a T_3 or T_4 assay because there is little overlap between normal and hypothyroid values, with few false positives so repeat tests are seldom necessary. It does not, however, exclude the rare pituitary and hypothalamic causes. The European studies have shown an incidence of congenital hypothyroidism of about 1 in 3500 births – about twice as high as that obtained from retrospective surveys. It is twice as common in girls. In USA it is uncommon in blacks. A small number of infants with hypothyroidism may be missed because of a delayed rise in TSH to the hypothyroid range, or mild disease, or errors in the screening of samples and reporting or follow-up, or due to loss of specimens.

Clinical presentation

The infant appears normal at birth, but prolonged neonatal jaundice, poor feeding and poor muscle tone are common. A considerable number are post mature. Additional and later features are lethargy, poor feeding and poor weight gain, constipation, low pitched hoarse cry, sparse coarse hair and dry skin, protruding tongue and coarse heavy featured facial appearance (Figure 16.2). The anterior fontanelle is often large and an umbilical hernia present. Individually, any of these features may be found in many normal babies, but together they indicate hypothyroidism. In the severe cretin, these features appear within 4–8 weeks but milder degrees may be much more difficult to diagnose and appear less dramatically in later infancy and childhood with poor growth and slow development as the main features.

Diagnosis

Consider hypothyroidism in any child whose development is slow. Serum thyroxine is low, although in the early weeks of life in normal infants it is higher than at any other time in life. Serum TSH is high except in rare cases of pituitary failure when it is low. Bone age is retarded. A thyroid scan is

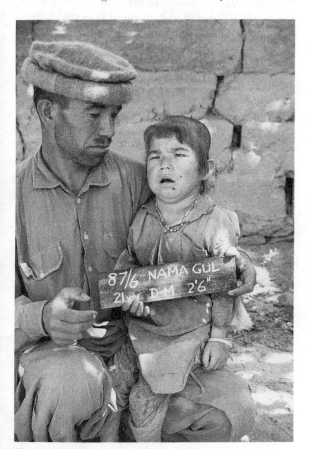

Figure 16.2 Cretin showing typical appearance

seldom necessary, except to identify a large ectopic gland.

Treatment

L-Thyroxine sodium is the treatment of choice. The starting dose in infancy is 25 μg once daily increasing after a few weeks to 50 μg. In late infancy and early childhood the usual daily requirement is 100 μg. Further increments are necessary as the child becomes older, the final adult dose being 200 to 300 μg daily. The adequacy of the dose can be ascertained by monitoring linear growth, clinical signs and TSH levels. Following treatment, TSH levels slowly fall to normal. If treatment is inadequate, serum TSH will rise again. Overdosage of thyroxine produces irritability, weight loss and premature closure of cranial sutures (craniostenosis) which may itself cause developmental delay. T_4 levels should be maintained in the upper half of the normal range. Parents must be aware of the need for regular daily treatment and that it must be continued for life.

Prognosis

The prognosis for linear growth and skeletal maturation is good. Intellectual progress, as indicated above, depends very much on the age at which treatment is started, and if delayed beyond age of 3 months the chances of eventually attaining normal intelligence are poor. It is quite likely that some of the damage in severe hypothyroidism is antenatal since maternal thyroid hormone does not cross the placenta.

Acquired hypothyroidism – juvenile myxoedema

Aetiology

1. Autoimmune thyroiditis (chronic lymphocytic thyroiditis; Hashimoto's thyroiditis). This is much the commonest cause.
2. Rarer causes are:
   - late onset of defects in embryogenesis or hormone synthesis (strictly speaking these are 'congenital')
   - infiltration of the gland in storage and other disorders
   - secondary to pituitary lesions and TSH deficiency, or hypothalamic lesions and TRH deficiency

- iodine deficiency (see below: endemic goitre)

Autoimmune thyroiditis

This is the most important cause of acquired hypothyroidism in childhood. Girls are much more commonly affected than boys, and there is often a strong family history of thyroid and other autoimmune disorders.

Clinical features

The onset is usually insidious as autoimmune thyroiditis increasingly damages the gland, (though a small number go on to develop autoimmune thyrotoxicosis). Diagnosis is often delayed unless an obvious goitre (sometimes tender) develops. The most important sign is a slowing of growth. Bone age is significantly retarded and dental development delayed. Changes in personality — often considered by parents as a good sign — are common as the child becomes more placid, quieter and better tempered. School performance and mental ability, however, remain good, and may delay the diagnosis.

Other features which gradually appear include increasing constipation, intolerance to cold, the hair becomes coarse, dry and brittle, and the skin cold and dry. Children are seldom obese, and often appear rather muscular, though there may be some facial puffiness. There is an association between hypothyroidism and a slipped femoral capital epiphysis. An unusual and paradoxical finding in some children is precocious sexual development. In girls there is breast development, hypertrophy of the labia minora, galactorrhoea (which may mimic a pituitary tumour) and cystic ovarian enlargement. In boys testicular enlargement occurs without a corresponding development of pubic hair.

Diagnosis

A low T_4 and raised TSH levels are diagnostic. If hypopituitarism or a hypothalamic cause is suspected, TSH levels may be normal or low, and a TRH stimulation test will be helpful. Many cases will have significant titres of antithyroglobulin and antimicrosomal antibodies. A thyroid scan is seldom necessary.

Bone age will be retarded and may show epiphyseal dysgenesis. This is the stippling defect present in the epiphyses and indicates the date of onset of the hypothyroidism, e.g. stippling of the upper femoral epiphysis would indicate that the child was hypothyroid at 9 months of age. Anthropometric measurements, if available, will show a reduction in growth velocity.

Associated conditions

There is an increased incidence of hypothyroidism in a number of other disorders and evidence of these should be sought:

- insulin dependent diabetes mellitus — 5 per cent have hypothyroidism
- other autoimmune disorders — including the polyglandular syndromes (Addison's disease, pernicious anaemia, mucocutaneous candidiasis, pheochromocytoma)
- non-endocrine autoimmune disorders — e.g. immune complex nephritis and thrombocytopoenia
- Down's syndrome
- congenital rubella
- slipped femoral capital epiphysis

Treatment

This is simple replacement with L-thyroxine once daily for life, in a dosage of between 100 and 300 µg daily (see treatment of congenital hypothyroidism, above). Therapy is monitored by the fall in TSH and maintenance of T_4 within the upper half of the normal range, as well as by the clinical response especially increase in linear growth and bone maturation.

In cases of long-standing or severe disease, treatment is started with low doses and gradually increased over several weeks to full replacement dosage. As well as a reversal of the clinical features, other side effects of treatment may include emotional and behavioural disturbances, muscle pains, transient mild hair loss, slipped femoral capital epiphysis (due to increased activity) and pseudotumour cerebri.

Prognosis

This is good. Catch-up growth is good with adequate treatment, skeletal maturation is normal and intellect is not impaired.

Goitre

A goitre is an enlarged easily visible thyroid gland. The thyroid is enlarged if the lateral lobe is larger than the terminal phalanx of the child's thumb. Swellings may be diffuse or asymmetrical with single or multiple nodules. Diffuse swellings suggest:

1. autoimmune thyroiditis, with hypo- or hyper-thyroidism, or simple colloid goitres
2. compensatory enlargement due to congenital enzyme defects or ingestion of goitrogens, either natural substances or drugs (e.g. iodides, sulphonamides and para-amino salicylic acid)
3. endemic goitre

Most diffusely enlarged thyroids are due to autoimmune thyroiditis, and present evidence suggests that most non-specific goitres and adolescent goitres are part of a wider spectrum of autoimmune thyroiditis.

Nodular goitres

These require examination to exclude malignancy. Thyroid carcinoma, although uncommon, occurs at any age and metastasizes early to lower cervical lymph nodes. The gland is particularly sensitive to X-irradiation. There was a high incidence of thyroid carcinoma about 30 years ago when it was fashionable to give X-ray treatment to the face and neck for such benign conditions as enlarged tonsils and adenoids, ringworm and other skin disorders.

Painful goitres

Suppurative thyroiditis is acute in onset and causes severe neck pain. Less severe chronic pain and tenderness are sometimes associated with chronic autoimmune (lymphocytic) thyroiditis.

Endemic goitre

Endemic goitre has been recognized from ancient times and is recorded in Hindu writings 4000 years ago, although only recently has been recognized to be due to environmental iodine deficiency and an inadequate intake in the diet.

It exists in many parts of the world, especially mountainous areas and places far away from the sea. A wide belt of endemic goitre exists from Pakistan in the West, across the Himalayas, Nepal, Northern India and across into Bangladesh, Burma and Thailand to Vietnam and Malaysia. Sporadic pockets are found elsewhere in India and throughout SE Asia; New Guinea; the Middle East; Central Africa and the Congo basin (Zaire); across the Andes in South America, and the Alps in Europe.

In endemic areas there is a high incidence of deaf-mutism, mental deficiency and other neurological and developmental disorders, as well as growth failure and dwarfism. The predominant clinical features vary somewhat in different parts of the world, thus in New Guinea hypothyroidism is relatively uncommon, while neurological disorders are common; in Nepal, where goitre is superendemic, nearly one-third of the population have features of hypothyroidism. When over 50 per cent of the population have a goitre, the incidence of deaf-mutism and mental retardation rises rapidly affecting up to 4 per cent of the population in some villages. Prevalence rates are highest, as expected, in the groups most vulnerable to physiological stresses — school children, especially around puberty, and pregnant and lactating mothers, so there is a high female/male ratio. Endemic goitre and cretinism are not confined to man in these areas; similar changes can be seen in goats and other domestic animals.

Control

This is one of the easiest and cheapest of diseases to control. The aim of management is to ensure a regular supply of iodine in physiological amounts. On a national scale the easiest and most practical method is to fortify common salt with potassium iodide or iodate — 10 mg of potassium iodide added to 1 kg salt will provide the daily requirement of 10 µg iodide in 10 g salt. It is easy, cheap and has proved very effective and does not require the use of scarce and costly resources of the health services. Other methods which have been tried include the addition of iodide to water supplies or bread, and the injection of iodized oil once every few years (4 ml oil containing 2.15 g iodine). Additional iodine can be supplied in the form of iodized sweets or tablets for children and pregnant women.

Thyrotoxicosis (Graves' disease)

The basic defect is an autonomous overproduction of T_3 and T_4 by a diffusely enlarged hyperplastic gland, which is no longer under pituitary control. Thyrotoxicosis is now considered to be part of the spectrum of autoimmune thyroiditis, and high levels of circulatory antithyroglobulin and antimicrosomal antibodies may be found. It is however, much less common than hypothyroidism in childhood. Girls are five times more frequently affected than boys and there is a high familial incidence of both thyroid and other autoimmune disorders.

Rare causes of thyrotoxicosis include a functioning thyroid adenoma or carcinoma; a TSH secreting pituitary adenoma and excessive ingestion of thyroid hormones or iodine.

Clinical features

The onset is generally more gradual than in adults, and diagnosis often delayed because large goitres and eye signs, such prominent features in adults, are not common. Early symptoms are often attributed to psychological causes — irritability, nervousness, restlessness, emotional outbursts and an inability to concentrate. Progress at school is poor and a deterioration in handwriting is especially noticeable. Later, more classical symptoms appear with increased appetite, weight loss, heat intolerance, excessive sweating, tiredness and muscle weakness. Examination shows a persistent tachycardia, full peripheral pulses, systolic hypertension, and exophthalmos, eyelid retraction and stare. Hands are warm, moist and tremulous. An audible bruit may be heard over the diffusely enlarged gland.

Diagnosis

Is based on the clinical features and finding of a raised T_4 and T_3 and low TSH with no response to TRH stimulation. Thyroid antibodies are frequently raised. Bone age is generally advanced.

Treatment

Medical

Medical treatment is preferred in children using either carbimazole or propylthiouracil for 2 to 3 years until disease activity subsides, the thyroid ceases its autonomous secretion and again comes under pituitary control.

Carbimazole 10 mg three times a day initially, is the most commonly used drug, reducing the dose after 3 to 4 weeks as determined by the clinical state. Excess carbimazole will cause a goitre. About 50 per cent of children will relapse if treatment is less than 2 years. A variable number will relapse after 2 to 3 years treatment and therapy may be required for up to 6 years. Side effects of carbimazole include skin rashes, agranulocytosis and aplastic anaemia (with little warning from the peripheral white cell count), a systemic lupus-like syndrome and hepatitis.

- Thyroxine may be used concurrently to prevent an increase in size of the gland.

- Propranolol, 10 mg three times a day, may be used initially to block the systemic effects of thyrotoxicosis.
- Propylthiouracil. Start with 100−300 mg a day initially and reduce after 3−4 weeks, depending on the clinical state, to about half or one-third of the starting dose. Side effects are similar to those of carbimazole.

Surgery

Subtotal thyroidectomy, carried out by an experienced thyroid surgeon, is effective when medical management has failed or the patient is unable to tolerate drugs. Surgery carries the same risks as in adults, and about 50 per cent may be expected to become hypothyroid after operation.

Radiotherapy

Radioisotopes are seldom used in children unless all other forms of treatment are contra-indicated, because of the risk of inducing thyroid cancer.

Neonatal thyrotoxicosis

This occurs in the infants of mothers who have thyrotoxicosis or who have had the condition irrespective of their present state. It is due to high titres of thyroid stimulating immunoglobulins (usually IgG) crossing the placenta; it is important to realize that these persist long after the mother has become euthyroid or after thyroidectomy.

A persistently high fetal heart rate — above 160 per minute — suggests fetal thyrotoxicosis.

Affected babies are often born prematurely and of low birth weight. A goitre is present in about half, though not always easy to detect. Typical symptoms and signs of hyperthyroidism develop within a few days of birth, though occasionally appear as late as 2 weeks. Babies are restless, irritable, and hungry; weight gain is poor with feeding problems and diarrhoea. There is tachycardia and a wide pulse pressure; congestive heart failure may develop. Exophthalmos is common. Hyperpyrexia is an additional feature. Although the condition is self-limiting, it carries a significant mortality if untreated and symptoms may occasionally persist for over 6 months. Treatment is with carbimazole 1−2 mg/kg/day in three divided doses and if necessary propranolol 2 mg/kg/day in three divided doses.

Possible long-term effects in some infants include craniosynostosis with subsequent developmental impairment, and hyperactivity. Intellectual development may be impaired in a few.

Congenital adrenal hyperplasia (adrenogenital syndrome)

Congenital adrenal hyperplasia (CAH) is the commonest adrenal disorder of childhood with an incidence of between 1 in 5000 and 1 in 25 000 births. It is an autosomal recessively inherited disorder in which there is an absence of one of the essential enzymes involved in adrenal steroid biosynthesis. The great majority of cases are due to deficiency of the enzyme 21-hydroxylase which blocks the production of cortisol, while smaller number are due to a deficiency of 11-hydroxylase, blocking the production of mineralocorticoids. Deficiency of other enzymes is rare. A simplified scheme of steroid synthesis is shown in Figure 16.3.

The principal effects of CAH are:

1. Excessive production of ACTH, due to interruption of the pituitary—adrenal feedback mechanism.
2. Adrenal hyperplasia, due to excessive stimulation by ACTH.
3. Excessive production of androgens due to increased stimulation at steps above the enzyme block causing virilization of female infants *in utero* and ambiguous genitalia at birth (Figure 16.4). Minor degrees of virilization cause enlargement of the clitoris, more severe forms result in rugosity of the labia, or fusion of the labia with a scrotal appearance, and a penile urethra. The internal genitalia are normal.

21-hydroxylase deficiency

This is now known to exist in at least three and possibly four distinct clinical forms.

Figure 16.3 *Simplified pathway of adrenal steroid synthesis*

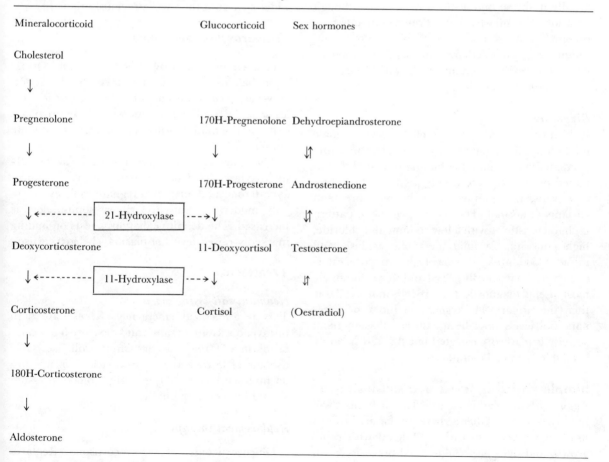

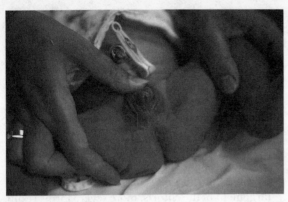

Figure 16.4 Congenital adrenal hyperplasia showing ambiguous genitalia in a girl (Reproduced courtesy of Dr A.W. Ferguson)

Classical salt-losing form

About two-thirds of all cases are salt losers. Girls are readily identified at birth because of virilization. Boys generally remain unrecognized, unless there is a known family history, until they present with an acute salt-losing adrenal crisis usually in the second or third week of life, though occasionally somewhat later. Pre-term infants may present within a few days of birth. Prodromal symptoms include lethargy and feeding problems which progress to vomiting, dehydration, circulatory collapse and death.

Diagnosis

A history of sudden death of a previous male infant in similar circumstances may alert an astute paediatrician, as may the finding of a slightly enlarged penis and more deeply pigmented scrotum and penis, though these may be no more than variants of normal. The serum electrolyte pattern is characteristic — with a low sodium and chloride, high potassium, a mild metabolic acidosis and raised blood urea. Plasma 17-hydroxyprogesterone levels are markedly raised and this is the single most useful diagnostic test. If it is not available then the urinary 11-oxygenation index or pregnanetriol levels may be measured. Plasma renin activity is markedly elevated but this test is rarely available to most laboratories.

Simple virilizing form: non salt-losing

Again, girls are readily identified at birth. Boys will not be recognized (unless there is a family history) until they present in early childhood with rapid growth and signs of pseudo-sexual precocity — an enlarged penis and pubic hair, but the testes remain infantile in size, indicative of a peripheral virilizing effect. The bone age is advanced. Diagnosis is as above, the differential diagnosis is from a virilizing adrenal tumour.

Late onset and 'cryptic' forms

These present in later childhood or adolescence with virilization, menstrual disturbances and endocrine symptoms suggestive of 21-hydroxylase deficiency. Girls show only mild clitoral enlargement and slight fusion of the labia minora, but none of the typical signs of *in utero* virilization. Boys or young men may exhibit few signs other than mild biochemical disturbances, oligospermia and subfertility; other signs of excessive androgen secretion such as hirsutism may be difficult to evaluate in men. Recently, family studies among clinically normal relatives of 'classical' cases have revealed biochemical and endocrine abnormalities compatible with a mild deficiency of 21-hydroxylase — so-called 'cryptic' cases indicating that the disorder has a far wider spectrum than was previously thought.

11-hydroxylase deficiency

This is characterized by hypertension and virilization. Salt loss is not a feature. Hypertension is not, however, seen in all patients, the reasons for this are not yet understood. As with 21-hydroxylase deficiency, a milder form may not present until late childhood.

The diagnostic tests are the same as for 21-hydroxylase deficiency though plasma 17-hydroxygesterone and urinary pregnanetriol levels are only moderately raised. Urinary sodium loss is increased. The definitive diagnosis rests on finding markedly raised levels of plasma 11-deoxycortisol.

Treatment

Neonatal salt-losing crisis.

This is a medical emergency. Resuscitate with intravenous isotonic saline and dextrose 5 per cent, or plasma if there is circulatory collapse. Give a bolus of intravenous hydrocortisone 50 mg and 9α-fludrocortisone 100 µg orally. Blood pressure should be monitored daily.

Replacement therapy

1. Glucocorticoids: use hydrocortisone. Replace-

ment doses are 5 mg twice or three times daily in infancy $(20\,mg/m^2/day)$, though perhaps twice daily dosage ensures better compliance with treatment. High doses of glucocorticoids will cause growth suppression especially during early infancy and childhood, at the same time advancing bone age. Temporary increases may be required at times of stress − e.g. acute intercurrent infections − and repeated admissions to hospital may be necessary in early life depending on parental ability to cope.

2. Mineralocorticoids: use 9α-fludrocortisone, 100 μg daily in infancy and 200 μg daily in older children. It is important to maintain adequate treatment with mineralocorticoids throughout childhood even though the need for salt may appear to diminish, as these reduce the requirements for glucocorticoids and so, in the long-term, ensure that linear growth is not suppressed.

3. Salt losers will need additional salt, 2−3 g daily should be added, in divided doses, to feeds.

Surgery
Surgical correction of virilized girls should be carried out between 6 and 12 months of age and includes clitorectomy and vaginoplasty. Several operations may be necessary to achieve a normal introitus. Affected girls are entirely normal females and can have children, so it is extremely important that they are given the correct sex as soon as possible after birth, and well before the child becomes aware of her sex, by the age of 18 months. Nothing is more tragic than to assign the wrong sex to these children.

Monitoring treatment
Unfortunately, no single biochemical test exists with which to monitor control and progress, and so a combination of both anthropometric and biochemical means are used. These include growth velocity and skeletal age and clinical evidence of excessive steroid administration. Measurement of 17-hydroxyprogesterone is currently the best biochemical test. Serum electrolytes and urinary pregnanetriol or 17-oxosteroids are not particularly sensitive. Plasma renin activity is closely related to salt status, and may prove a more useful means in the future of assessing adequacy of control.

The aims of treatment are to provide adequate replacement therapy, to suppress excess androgen production and to allow normal growth in childhood and pubertal development. Adequately treated children should enter puberty at the normal time. Delay in the menarche in girls suggests inadequate treatment with raised androgen (testosterone) levels. A change of treatment to dexamethasone, with a longer duration of activity is often helpful, in a dosage of 0.25 to 0.75 mg daily, and is probably the treatment of choice in adults.

Genetics of CAH

Recently, interest in the genetics of CAH has been stimulated following the discovery that the gene for 21-hydroxylase lies very close to the HLA-B locus on chromosome 6 and shows some linkage with it, the incidence of BW47 being increased in both salt-losing and simple virilizing forms. Conversely, the haplotype HLA-B8:DR3, strongly associated with autoimmune disorders, appears to have a negative association with 21-hydroxylase deficiency.

Biochemical tests have not proved sensitive enough to distinguish normals from heterozygote carriers, but using HLA genotyping, it is now possible through family studies on parents and siblings to identify which siblings are carriers and which are normal.

Prenatal diagnosis of affected infants is now readily possible by finding raised 17-hydroxyprogesterone levels in amniotic fluid between 14 and 20 weeks. The use of DNA probes in the future raises the possibility not only of prenatal diagnosis in the first trimester, but also of prenatal treatment to suppress virilization of affected females by giving dexamethasone to the mother.

The small child

The small child is a common problem presented to paediatricians. Parents are much more likely to worry about a child who is small than one who is tall. The great majority of small children will be normal, thus, by definition 10 per cent of children will be on or below the tenth percentile in height for their age. Children on the third percentile are two standard deviations (−2 s.d.) below the mean; more than 80 per cent below the third percentile will be normal with either familial short stature or constitutional growth delay, and less than 20 per cent will have a pathological cause. The majority of children who are −3 s.d. or more below the mean height for their age, however, are likely to have a pathological cause for their small size.

Familial short stature

This may be assumed if the child's projected final height falls within 10 cm of the average height percentile of the mother and father. Growth is parallel to the third percentile, the bone age and clinical findings are normal.

Constitutional growth delay

The child is at the lower end of the normal range of timing of skeletal and pubertal development. Growth is normal during infancy but slows down in early childhood, and entry into puberty and the adolescent growth spurt are delayed for up to 2 years (after 14 years in girls and 16 years in boys) although catch-up does occur and the final adult height and sexual development are normal. During childhood bone age corresponds more to height age rather than chronological age. There is often a family history.

The following scheme represents one approach to the assessment and investigation of the small child.

1. After careful and accurate measurement, the height and weight are plotted on a percentile chart appropriate for the child's sex and, if standards exist, for the race or community to which the child belongs. This will show whether the child is indeed small or not.
2. The heights of both parents must be measured, and other siblings if available, so that the family pattern can be ascertained.
3. The mid-parental height can then be plotted on the chart at age 19 years. In the case of boys, the final height should lie between the father's height and the mother's height plus 12.5 cm; for the girls the final height should lie between the mother's height and father's height minus 12.5 cm.
4. Record the birth weight and gestation of the child. These will indicate whether the child was 'small for dates' or showed evidence of intrauterine growth retardation, and has remained small ever since − prenatal short stature. Unfortunately this important piece of information is frequently not available.

5. Further assessment of growth in height and height velocity (increase in height (cm) per year) will be necessary to show whether the child is growing steadily along the same percentile or falling away. This can only be made at intervals of at least 4 to 6 months, and preferably over at least a 1 year period since any errors in measurements over shorter periods of time will be too large to make reliable assessments. Seasonal variations in growth must also be taken into account.
6. A full and detailed medical history is essential, including maternal health and illness during pregnancy; birth history, a feeding history, and previous illnesses as well as a family history. Records from an infant welfare clinic, if available, are helpful.
7. A careful physical examination follows, and both this and the history should be directed towards identifying stigmata suggestive of or typical of specific disorders. Dysmorphic features may suggest a syndrome or chromosomal abnormality; abnormal body proportions may suggest a bone dysplasia, while children with growth hormone deficiency and congenital adrenal hyperplasia tend to be small and rather fat.

The following specific disorders need to be considered:

1. *Intrauterine growth retardation.* Although the aetiology in many remains unknown, there is an association with congenital infections and malformations, dysmorphic syndromes and chromosomal abnormalities. Twins and survivors of multiple pregnancy frequently suffer from intrauterine growth retardation.
2. *Dysmorphic syndromes,* with abnormal facies and other physical features are generally associated with proportional short stature. Their recognition is aided by reference to one of the standard texts.*
3. *Chromosomal abnormalities.* Most of the major abnormalities compatible with survival are readily identified, but many of the minor autosomal disorders, with partial deletions or translocations are often accompanied by delayed growth throughout childhood, short stature, some developmental delay and a variety of dysmorphic features. Turner's syndrome must be considered in all small girls, even though

* e.g. Smith, D. W. (1982). *Recognizable Patterns of Human Malformation.* 3rd edn, W B Saunders, Philadelphia.

they may be otherwise physically normal, and without any stigmata. The incidence is about 1 in 60 girls who are below the third percentile in height.

4. *Disproportionate small stature.* The most likely cause is one of the many forms of bone dysplasia. These can be broadly divided into two groups, with either short-limbed, or short-trunk dwarfism. Diagnosis is based on clinical and radiological findings. Metabolic forms of rickets — vitamin D resistant and renal — also show some shortening of the lower limbs.

5. *Malnutrition.* This remains, worldwide, the commonest cause of growth failure and is seen in its extreme form as marasmus. The diagnosis is not usually difficult.

6. *Gastrointestinal disease.* Coeliac disease is the commonest cause, and is often surprisingly silent and symptomless. Chronic infections and infestations, including giardiasis must be considered. Cystic fibrosis is being diagnosed more frequently in the Middle East and may need to be excluded if there is a history suggestive of malabsorption and recurrent chest infections. Crohn's disease is an occasional cause of growth failure in older children, and should be considered if there are unexplained gastrointestinal symptoms.

7. *Congenital heart disease* is readily diagnosed. Growth impairment is related to the severity of the cardiac lesion and is greatest in cyanotic heart disease. Surgical correction of the cardiac lesion is generally followed by a growth spurt.

8. *Chronic respiratory disease* is readily identified; severe asthma, cystic fibrosis and occasionally severe bronchiectasis are the usual causes. Children with chronic asthma severe enough to require continuous treatment with oral steroids will almost certainly show growth failure and alternative forms of therapy, e.g., inhaled corticosteroids (beclomethasone or budesonide) or sodium cromoglycate should be tried. As a last resort, alternate day oral steroids may be given, as growth suppression is much less on this regime.

9. *Severe chronic anaemia.* Children suffering from one of the severe congenital haemolytic anaemias e.g., thalassaemia major or sickle cell anaemia or one of its variants, invariably show poor growth and also delayed onset of puberty. High transfusion regimes in thalassaemia improve growth rates.

10. *Chronic renal disease.* Growth failure is a constant feature of chronic renal failure, usually due to severe congenital anomalies, and renal tubular disorders. The diagnosis, however, may not be readily apparent.

11. *Endocrine disorders.* Most endocrine disorders are associated with a disturbance of growth, including hypothyroidism, poorly controlled diabetes mellitus and Cushing's syndrome. Probably the commonest cause is prolonged or excessive corticosteroid therapy.

Hypopituitarism and growth hormone deficiency

Growth hormone deficiency may be due to diseases affecting either the pituitary or hypothalamus, including tumours such as a craniopharyngioma or adenoma, infections, trauma and a number of rarer genetic syndromes. Deficiency may be isolated or part of panhypopituitarism. Recently, many cases of growth hormone deficiency previously attributed to idiopathic hypopituitarism have been shown to be the result of hypothalamic rather than pituitary failure since these patients show a significant rise in plasma growth hormone levels when given an injection of growth hormone releasing hormone (GHRH).

Children with idiopathic hypopituitarism are a normal size at birth but growth begins to slow down during infancy and continues throughout early childhood, dropping eventually to well below the third percentile; they often appear well-nourished or even fat in relation to their small stature and have a characteristic 'baby' face. Boys may have an underdeveloped penis and scrotum. Lesser degrees of growth hormone deficiency may be more difficult to recognize but all will show a steady failure of growth. A skull X-ray is essential to exclude signs of a craniopharyngioma — an enlarged pituitary fossa, erosion of the clinoid processes or suprasellar calcification. It may also reveal a small or 'empty' pituitary fossa consistent with idiopathic hypopituitarism. A confirmatory CT scan should be done if facilities are available.

Probably the largest and most important group of children with growth hormone deficiency and growth failure now are those who have received cranial irradiation as part of the treatment of leukaemia. The most vulnerable groups appear to be children under the age of 3 years and those who have relapsed or received more than one course of irradiation. The hypothalamus seems to be much more sensitive to damage than the pituitary. The effects may become evident within a year of treatment although the full effects may not be seen until several years later when up to 70 per cent of children will show evidence of growth hormone deficiency and growth failure.

Emotional deprivation

Severe emotional deprivation is a well recognized cause of growth failure, the father is often violent, bad-tempered or alcoholic, the mother depressed. The child fails to thrive physically and emotionally, is neglected, abused and withdrawn. Older children show behaviour problems and regression at school. Although the condition may strongly be suspected from the history, it is essentially a diagnosis made by excluding all other pathological causes. Endocrine studies are, however, difficult to interpret because some degree of hypopituitarism develops in all severely emotionally deprived children, probably due to hypothalamic suppression by the higher centres. Growth hormone, thyroid and other endocrine functions return to normal during recovery.

Points to note are:

1. All chronic diseases will interfere with normal growth in children.
2. If there are no clues in either history of physical findings to suggest a cause, then the following should be considered at any age:
   - coeliac disease
   - hypothyroidism
   - Turner's syndrome − all small girls
   - growth hormone deficiency

In late childhood consider also Crohn's disease and hypogonadism.

Investigations

The aim is to screen for and eliminate as many pathological causes as possible. It is emphasized again that certain disorders, in particular coeliac disease, Turner's syndrome and Crohn's disease may be quite symptomless.

General
- full blood count and blood film
- urinalysis, microscopy and culture
- plasma electrolytes, calcium, phosphorus, alkaline phosphatase − to exclude renal disease, renal tubular acidosis and metabolic rickets
- liver function tests and α-1-antitrypsin
- serum iron and red cell folate
- X-ray wrist and (L) hand − for bone age/skeletal maturity − bone age is normal in dysmorphic syndromes and skeletal dysplasia but retarded in chronic diseases

Specific
- skeletal survey − spine, long bones and skull, antero-posterior and lateral views − for bone dysplasias and pituitary fossa
- jejunal biopsy − to exclude coeliac disease
- barium meal and follow-through to small bowel − to exclude Crohn's disease
- ultrasound of renal tract
- chromosomes − karyotype − to exclude Turner's syndrome
- sweat test − if symptoms suggest cystic fibrosis

Endocrine
- thyroid function tests − TSH and T_4
- plasma cortisol levels − midnight and 9.00 a.m.
- growth hormone tests
- computerized tomography of skull/pituitary and other areas, e.g., abdomen, as indicated

Tests of growth hormone secretion

Growth hormone is secreted in pulses over 24 hour period, under normal physiological conditions, with peaks and troughs of hormone levels. A single random estimation is therefore of little or no value in deciding whether a child is secreting sufficient hormone for normal growth. Unfortunately, as yet, there is no single satisfactory test of growth hormone secretion. A number of physiological or pharmacological stimuli can be used to measure hormone release but the insulin test remains the standard with which others are compared.

Peak levels of between 15 and 20 mU/l or above are regarded as evidence of normal secretion; peak levels below 7 mU/l indicate severe growth hormone deficiency, and peak levels between 7 and 15 mU/l are suggestive of partial growth hormone deficiency.

Insulin test

Insulin induced hypoglycaemia stimulates growth hormone secretion. There is a danger, however, that the test may induce severe hypoglycaemia if the child is known or suspected to have hypopituitarism, and a separate intravenous cannula should be inserted so that 50 per cent glucose can be given immediately if severe hypoglycaemia develops.

The test should be performed after an overnight fast. Soluble insulin 0.1 units/kg is given intravenously and samples for glucose and growth hormone taken at 0, 15, 30, 45, 60, 90, 120 and 150 minutes. Cortisol, TSH and other hormone levels can also be estimated. A fall in blood sugar to below 40 mg/dl (2.2 mmol/l) or between 50 and 60 per cent of the fasting value within 20–30 minutes produces satisfactory hypoglycaemia.

Glucagon

After an overnight fast give glucagon 100 μg/kg i.m. (maximum dose 1 mg). Blood samples are taken at 0, 30, 60, 90, 120, 150, 180 and 240 minutes, since peak response may be delayed. Capillary samples may however be taken. Cortisol levels can be measured at the same time.

Clonidine

Clonidine is given orally 4 μg/kg and blood samples taken at 0, 30, 60, 90, 120 and 150 minutes. The test is safer and simpler than the insulin test but may be accompanied by hypotension and drowsiness.

Exercise and sleep

These are physiological stimuli that can be used. Exercise must be vigorous and sustained for about 10 minutes on a bicycle ergometer or treadmill. A single blood sample only is required 30 minutes from the start of the exercise. It is not, however, a suitable test for very young children. Growth hormone secretion is increased during deep sleep. A cannula is inserted before the child goes to sleep. A single sample may be taken 1 hour after the onset of deep sleep, or several samples at intervals from 30 to 120 minutes. It can be usefully combined with midnight cortisol levels.

Sex steroid priming

Pre-pubertal children, with a bone age of over 10 years, who are small but otherwise normal, often have a refractory response to growth hormone stimulation making interpretation of results difficult. Secretion can be 'primed' or increased by giving sex hormones before performing the test. Girls are given ethinyl oestradiol 100 μg orally daily for 3 days before the test; boys are given testosterone 100 mg (as esters) intramuscularly 3 days before the test.

Growth hormone releasing hormone (GHRH)

Synthetic analogues of this hormone are now available making it possible to determine whether the pituitary or hypothalamus is primarily at fault. GHRH 1.5 μ/kg is given intravenously after an overnight fast and blood collected at 0, 15, 30, 45, 60, 90, 120 and 150 minutes. Satisfactory peak growth hormone levels suggest that the lesion lies in the hypothalamus and not the pituitary.

Further reading

Barnes, N.D. (1984). Clinical aspects of acquired thyroid disease in childhood. In: *Paediatric Endocrinology in Clinical Practice* (Ed. A. Aynsley-Green), MTP Press, Lancaster, 55–71.

Drucker, S. and New, M.I. (1987). Disorders of adrenal steroidogenesis. *Pediatric Clinics of North America*, **34** (4), 1055–1066.

Editorial (1987). Congenital adrenal hyperplasia. *Lancet*, **ii**, 663.

Fisher, D.A. (1987). Effectiveness of newborn screening programs for congenital hypothyroidism: prevalence of missed cases. *Pediatric Clinics of North America*, **34** (4), 881–890.

Fisher, D.A., Pandian, M.R. and Carlton, E. (1987). Autoimmune thyroid disease – An expanding spectrum. *Pediatric Clinics of North America*, **34** (4), 907–918.

Grant, D.B. (1984). Congenital hypothyroidism: pathogenesis, screening and prognosis. In: *Paediatric Endocrinology in Clinical Practice* (Ed. A. Aynsley-Green), MTP Press, Lancaster, 45–54.

Hughes, I.A. (1984). Medical and psychological management of congenital adrenal hyperplasia. In: *Paediatric Endocrinology in Clinical Practice* (Ed. A. Aynsley-Green), MTP Press, Lancaster, 83–115.

Mahoney, C.P. (1987). Differential diagnosis of goitre. *Pediatric Clinics of North America*, **34** (4), 907–918.

Ramalingaswami, V. (1973). Endemic goitre in South-East Asia. *Annals of Internal Medicine* **78** (2), 277–283.

17

Parasites

A parasite by definition is a living organism that can only feed off another living organism (the host) in order to survive. The host may be man or animal. Some parasites will attach themselves to man if the normal animal host is not available while others may need two or three hosts to complete their life cycle.

Parasites may attach themselves by the skin, directly to the intestinal tract or to the intestinal tract via the skin and lungs.

Those that parasitize non-invasively through the skin alone are comparatively harmless, although their bites may subsequently become infected. However, some of these may be parasitized themselves (for example, the *Anopheles* mosquito by the malaria parasite *Plasmodium*) and pass their 'guest' on to the new host.

Parasitic infestation should be considered in the following five clinical syndromes among children:

1. unexplained anaemia
2. unexplained fever
3. chronic diarrhoea and ill health
4. asthma
5. skin rashes

Table 17.1 on pages 240–1 gives a summary of anti-parasitic drugs.

Worms

Ascaris

General
Ascaris lumbricoides (the large roundworm) occurs widely throughout the world, mainly among children. One in four of the world's population are thought to be infested. They live off the contents of the small intestine, are cream coloured, and up to 40 cm long.

Life cycle (Figure 17.1)
The female is fertilized in the small intestine and

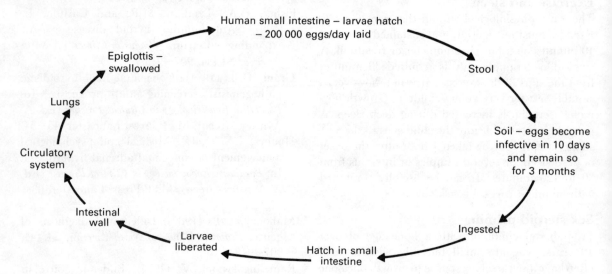

Figure 17.1 Diagram of the life history of the *Ascaris lumbricoides* in man — the dog roundworm (*Toxocara canis*) and the cat roundworm (*Toxocara catis*) have similar cycles in the dog and cat

produces as many as 200 000 eggs per day, which are passed in the faeces. The eggs remain viable in the soil for 10 days and are killed by sunlight. If ingested, the egg hatches in the small intestine.

The hatched larva migrates through the intestinal wall via the blood stream into the lungs. It then penetrates the alveolar wall and is transported by ciliary action up to the epiglottis and is then swallowed to reach its ultimate destination in the small intestine where it develops into the male or female adult worm.

Clinical picture

The migrating larvae damage the lung, may produce a verminous pneumonia, or, because they are antigenic, asthma. In the author's experience in Central Africa, worm infestation was one of the commonest causes of childhood asthma.

The effects of the adult worm depend entirely on the worm load. This may be very low, and little harm is caused, apart from the shock to the parent or child when one is passed out of the rectum.

In heavy infestations general toxaemia also occurs as well as malabsorption with resulting malnutrition.

Diagnosis is by finding the worm (not difficult) in the faeces. In cases of asthma, the faeces should be scanned for eggs. This is also not difficult as they are numerous.

Management

Levamisole is now the drug of choice. The dose is 2.5 mg/kg in a single dose. If this is not available, then piperazine hydrate 75 mg/kg given on two successive days gives a 90 per cent cure rate and is cheap. When surgical treatment is needed it must be carried out in conjunction with medical treatment. A bolus of worms may cause intestinal obstruction when surgical treatment will be needed.

Prevention

The infestation is contracted by children ingesting soil which is contaminated with faeces. Control is, therefore, by improved hygiene and sanitation and more important periodic mass treatment of children in an affected area.

Hookworm

General

Infestation of hookworm (*Ankylostoma duodenale* and *Necator americanus*) may result in worms remaining in the gut for many months or years, and should always be kept in mind in diagnosis of severe anaemia.

The worm is only 1 cm long but has a mouth, teeth and oesophagus. The mouth is attached to the gut mucosa by suction and the teeth penetrate the mucosa and blood is then sucked into the worm.

Life cycle (Figure 17.2)

The eggs are laid by the adult female in the gut and pass out with the faeces. Within 24 hours in warm,

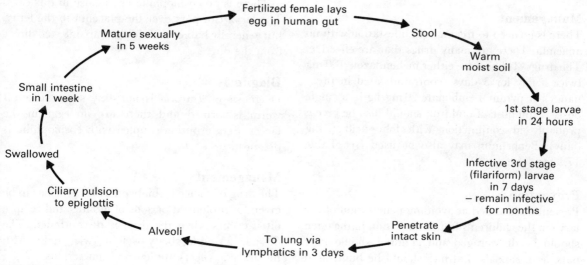

Figure 17.2 The life cycle of the hookworm.

moist soil the egg hatches into a larva which is non-invasive.

Within 7 days this develops into the invasive filariform larva which remains viable in the soil for several months. This generally invades by penetrating the skin of the foot, but very occasionally may be ingested.

After penetration the larva reaches the lung via the blood stream by the third day and its progress from there to the small intestine is identical to *Ascaris lumbricoides* and occurs within 7 days. The larva develops into the adult worm by 5 weeks.

Clinical picture

The problem the worm causes to the human depends on its progress.

1. Site of invasion: intensive irritation which may become secondarily affected.
2. Migration of the larva through the lungs: this does not cause the pneumonia of ascariasis but may cause mild asthma.
3. Adult worm in the gut: symptoms are due to severe iron deficiency anaemia as the worm ingests blood for its iron content. This is known as hookworm anaemia (HA) and is the major hazard of the infestation.

Diagnosis

The characteristic eggs may be found in a fresh stool or rectal smear but an experienced laboratory would be desirable for diagnosis. Eosinophilia is common.

Management

There is no need to treat a light infestation with no anaemia. There are many drugs that are effective. The drugs of choice are either mebendazole 100 mg twice a day for 3 days (contraindicated in pregnancy) or pyrantel embonate 20 mg/kg in a single dose. A full dose of oral iron should also be given, probably in conjunction with folic acid (5 mg daily). Bephenium may also be used (see Table 17.1 for dosage).

Prevention

Prevention is aimed at avoiding penetration of the larva in the children's feet. Defaecation in the open should be discouraged and children should play outside in sandals. Latrines should be built, used and kept clean. These apparently simple procedures are very difficult to attain in most rural areas where the disease is endemic.

Toxocara canis

General

This is a roundworm infection common in dogs all over the world. The human is not a compatible host but may become infested when the eggs are ingested from the fur or tongue of the domestic animal.

A similar infestation occurs in cats (*Toxocara catis*) but, although some authorities insist to the contrary, there is very little clinical evidence that this form of the worm affects humans.

Life cycle

The cycle in the dog is similar to that of ascariasis in man.

Clinical

Man is a strange host to the *Toxocara*, and after hatching from the eggs in the small intestine, the larva 'gets lost' and migrates in most of the tissues. This is particularly so in the skin where an irritating migrating eruption is common and the condition is known as visceral larva migrans (VLM).

The infestation may take another form involving the eye only. Instead of wandering all over the body, the larva makes straight for the retina where it settles, producing a granuloma which may resemble a retinoblastoma, but most certainly will cause blindness.

There is no eosinophilia or malaise in this case. The larva can pass over the placenta to the fetus, but generally babies and children are infested direct from the dog.

Diagnosis

Diagnosis of *Toxocara* is not easy since no adult worm is formed and there are no eggs in the faeces. Skin eruption coupled with eosinophilia is diagnostic.

Management

The drug of choice is thiabendazole. This has to be given for prolonged periods of months and relapse often occurs when the drug is discontinued. The dose is 25 mg/kg body weight twice daily with meals. Side-effects are few and not serious.

The patient's condition should be carefully

monitored during treatment. As the ocular form of the disease is a result of inflammatory reaction to the larva, short courses of steroids may help, but these should be given under supervision of an ophthalmologist.

Prevention

The disease occurs most commonly in children as a result of ingestion of eggs from dogs' faeces. This is caused when the child is licked by the dog or kisses its fur, as dogs clean their fur with the tongue. Health education and regular worming of dogs and puppies is therefore essential.

Strongyloides stercoralis

General

This worm inhabits the small bowel and normally causes few problems. However, in the case of severe malnutrition hyperinfection occurs resulting in:

- severe acute and chronic diarrhoea simulating coeliac disease,
- Gram-negative septicaemia,
- asthma-like symptoms (due to mass migration of larvae — see below), and
- encephalitis.

Life cycle (Figure 17.3)

Non-infectious larvae are excreted in the faeces of infected man. In warm moist soil the larvae develop into male and female worms which mate and produce filariform larvae which are infective to man. They penetrate the skin, generally the foot. They are carried to the lungs via the blood stream, and penetrate the alveoli. Here they are coughed up and swallowed, ending up in the mucosa of the small intestine. In this environment they undergo the same cycle as in the warm moist soil. New larvae (non-infective) produced by the recently developed male and female worms are then excreted in the faeces and the cycle is repeated.

Anus infection may occur if the filariform (infective) larvae are produced in the bowel. These will re-enter man via the perianal region, migrate through the tissues to the lungs and return to the small bowel. This state may repeat for years.

Clinical picture

There may be no symptoms. However, in auto-infection the filariform larvae may cause intense perianal irritation, skin rashes and even a snake-like wheal in the skin itself. These rashes and wheals tend to occur on the trunk of the body.

Apart from the hyperinfection symptoms already mentioned, the only other symptom in uncomplicated *Strongyloides* infection are mild abdominal discomfort and occasional diarrhoea.

Diagnosis

This is confirmed by examination of the stool for mobile larvae. Occasionally jejunal biopsy is necessary.

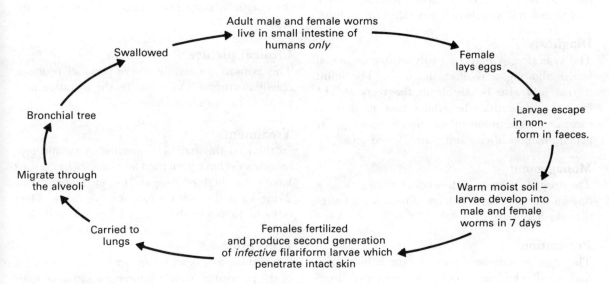

Figure 17.3 The life cycle of the *Strongyloides stercoralis*

Management

Thiabendazole is the drug of choice and the dosage is 25 mg/kg twice per day for 3 days.

Prevention

As for hookworm disease.

Whipworms

General

Whipworms (Trichuris) occur in humid climates in developing countries. They may be as long as 5 cm and the habitat of the adult worm is in the mucosa of the large bowel. It is not blood-sucking but lives off the intestinal faeces. Because of the life cycle it is commonest in children.

Life cycle

The adult female produces a large number of eggs per day and these are passed out in the faeces. The eggs mature in warm, moist soil in about 2 weeks. When the soil is ingested by children, the eggs produce larvae in the colon which develop into adult worms in 3 months.

Clinical picture

There may be no symptoms at all and so no treatment is required. However, there may be severe bloody diarrhoea (but without fever as in amoebic dysentery and bacillary dysentery).

Rectal prolapse may be a feature (when the adult worms may actually be seen on the rectal mucosa). As a result of the bloody diarrhoea there may be anaemia and there is generally eosinophilia.

Diagnosis

The typical eggs may be easily visible on rectal smear allowing a positive diagnosis. The adult worms may also be visible in the rectum. The length of time that the adults take to develop means that symptoms of the disease may appear general months after visiting an infested area.

Management

The drug of choice is mebendazole 100 mg twice a day for 3 days. This may have to be repeated after 3 weeks have passed.

Prevention

The eggs can only be ingested by the habit of pica and small children should be prevented from sampling soil.

Threadworms

General

The threadworm (*Enterobius vermicularis*) has an international distribution and is extremely common. They seldom grow larger than 1-2 cm and resemble threads of cotton. Like whipworms, they reside in the colon.

Life cycle

The gravid female migrates from the caecum to the rectum and lays its eggs around the anus and perineum at night. After disgorging the eggs the female disintegrates. The eggs mature rapidly in 6 hours. Reinfection occurs by one of four ways:

1. transfer of the eggs from anus to mouth via fingernails
2. by contact of fingers with other contaminated areas such as toilet seats, towels, and flannels
3. inhalation and swallowing of eggs in dust-laden atmosphere
4. reinfestation − the larvae hatch on the perineum and migrate to the colon via the anus.

In the first three the mature ova hatch in the duodenum and migrate to the colon, where the mature worm develops. The whole process takes about 6 weeks.

The female worms may be seen by the child's mother, emerging from the anus. Alternatively, sticky tape may be stuck to the perianal area early in the morning and removed in 30 minutes, to give the diagnosis since many eggs will adhere to the tape.

Clinical picture

This is most commonly severe perianal pruritus, chiefly nocturnal. Occasionally, the irritation may result in nocturnal enuresis.

Treatment

In the past this has been unsatisfactory and piperazine salts have been tried for years. Better results have been obtained from the use of thiabendazole 25 mg/kg a day with meals for one week. Over 60 kg body weight the dose is 1.5 gm twice daily.

Prevention

General hygiene is important with regular washing of the perineum. Small children should have nails cut short and wear cotton gloves at night. It is generally necessary to treat the whole family, as some children may be asymptomatic.

Flat worms

General

Tapeworms are segmented worms classified as cestodes (flatworms). They can vary in size from as long as 30 feet (*Taenia saginata*, the beef tapeworm) to as short as 20 to 45 mm (*Hymenolepis nana*, the dwarf tapeworm).

Man usually becomes infected through the ingestion of the larval form encysted in uncooked meat or through contamination of food and water by the eggs.

Tapeworms are cosmopolitan and can be contracted throughout the world. With the notable exceptions of two potentially serious conditions, cysticercosis and hydatid disease, cestode infections cause few clinical problems, but when a patient is informed that he is acting as host to such an unwanted guest, he becomes understandably alarmed.

Life cycle (Figure 17.4)

Taenia saginata, the beef tapeworm, has adopted man as the only definitive host. Man usually contracts the tapeworm by eating uncooked 'measly' beef.

Taenia solium, the pork tapeworm, has man as the only definitive host. Man acquires *T. solium* infection by eating uncooked 'measly' pork and the larval cysticerci, dormant in the meat, hatch in man's intestine to develop into the adult worms. After the *T. solium* larvae hatch from the eggs they migrate into the tissues and there encyst causing cysticercosis.

Man may also ingest the eggs from food or water contaminated by human faeces or, in certain circumstances, by regurgitating the eggs from the adult worm in his intestine.

This type of re-infestation comes about when a segment full of eggs, the proglottid, becomes detached from the adult worm, disintegrating and so liberating its load of eggs. Detachment of the proglottid may occur if a patient vomits severely or is given inappropriate treatment.

Clinical picture

Any tissue may be involved but the serious symptoms arise from invasion of the central nervous system. Epilepsy is the commonest symptom but hydrocephalus, occular involvement and nodules in muscle and skin are also found.

Diagnosis

Initially there are usually few symptoms and the diagnosis may be made several years after tissue invasion. If nodules are visible or palpable, tissue biopsy will reveal the cyst. The cysts frequently

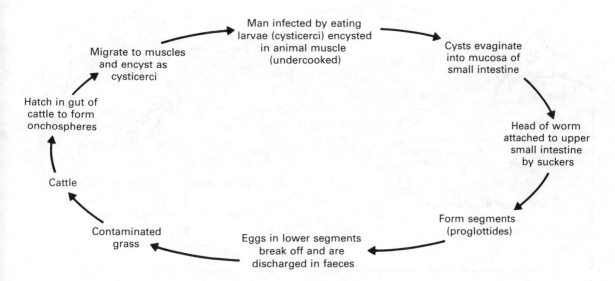

Figure 17.4 The life cycle of the *Taenia saginata* and *Taenia solium*

calcify over a variable time and may be revealed on X-ray. The CT scan has now a part to play in revealing intracerebral pathology.

Management
Niclosamide is generally considered the drug of choice for the treatment of all tapeworm infections and has superceded other drugs. The adult dose in *T. saginata* infection is two grams before breakfast in two divided doses, one hour apart. Unfortunately there is no treatment for cysticercosis.

Prevention
Thorough cooking of meat will kill the larvae and render meat safe to eat. Freezing meat for over three weeks will kill larvae but ordinary refrigeration does not.

Fish worms

General
Diphyllobothrium latum, the fish tapeworm, is acquired by man through eating raw or uncooked fish.

Life cycle (Figure 17.5)
This is complex, in that there are two intermediate hosts; the first is a freshwater crustacean of the *Cyclops* species and the second is a freshwater fish. Man ingests uncooked fish and the encysted larva in the fish's muscle develops into the adult worm. This may grow up to 5 or 10 metres. Kippering or smoking of fish does not render the flesh safe for eating.

Clinical picture
Infection with *D. latum* may cause a megaloblastic anaemia through the tapeworm either competing for or blocking the absorption of vitamin B_{12} but despite its great length, it usually causes few symptoms.

Treatment
Niclosamide 2 g on the first day followed by 1 daily for 6 days.

Prevention
Health education in particular to persuade people from eating raw fish. The parasite is destroyed by cooking.

Dwarf tapeworm

Life cycle
Hymenoleptis nana, often called the dwarf tapeworm because it only measures 25–45 mm, is a common parasite in North Africa, southern Europe and many tropical countries. Infection is spread from man to man. In some areas 5 to 10 per cent of children may be infected.

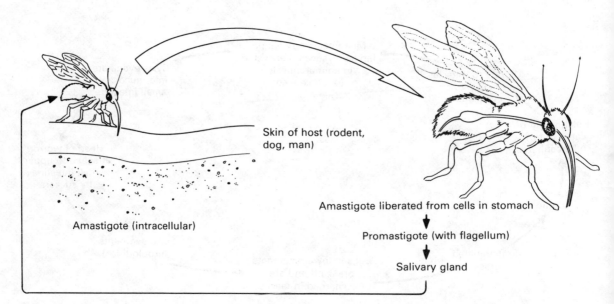

Skin of host (rodent, dog, man)

Amastigote (intracellular)

Amastigote liberated from cells in stomach

Promastigote (with flagellum)

Salivary gland

Figure 17.5 The life history of visceral leishmaniass

Clinical picture

Largely asymptomatic, although heavy infestations may cause diarrhoea.

Management

Niclosamide is the drug of choice but treatment may not be necessary.

Dog tapeworm

General

The dog tapeworm *(Echinococcus granulosus)* causes hydatid disease in man.

Life cycle (Figure 17.6)

Infected dogs have 3−6 mm adult tapeworms in their small intestine. Eggs are liberated in the faeces and contaminate the grass. The herbivore, generally the sheep, is the intermediate host. When the eggs are ingested they are liberated in the gut and enter the circulation, where they settle in the capillaries in various viscera. Thus the hydatid cysts is formed. Dogs become infected by eating tissues containing the cyst. Man is infected in the same way as herbivores and develop hydatid disease.

Clinical picture

The dog catches the adult worm by eating the offal of sheep, cattle, pigs or camels which act as an intermediate host for the larval cysts.

Hydatid disease is not uncommon in shepherds and those herding animals. Man contracts hydatid disease from swallowing the eggs from unwashed hands after petting dogs or from eating vegetables polluted by dog or wild carnivore faeces. The larvae hatch in the bowel and are then transported by the blood to any tissues or organs.

The most common sites are liver, lungs, kidney and abdominal viscera since they act as filters with their rich blood supply.

The symptoms of hydatid disease may present in two ways; either as those from mechanical pressure due to a space occupying mass or a cyst may leak or rupture causing an acute hypersensitivity reaction since the cyst fluid is very allergic. Often, however, the patient may be asymptomatic.

Diagnosis

This can be made only if the disease is kept constantly in mind. Often the diagnosis is made at operation for a mass previously suspected of being malignant.

X-rays, ultrasound and CT scans can be used to localize cysts. In the past the intradermal Casoni injection of hydatid antigen was used for diagnosis, but this has been superceded by specific serological tests, or which complement fixation, haemaglutination and enzyme immunoabsorbent assay (ELISA) are the most common.

Treatment

There is no effective and safe medical treatment for

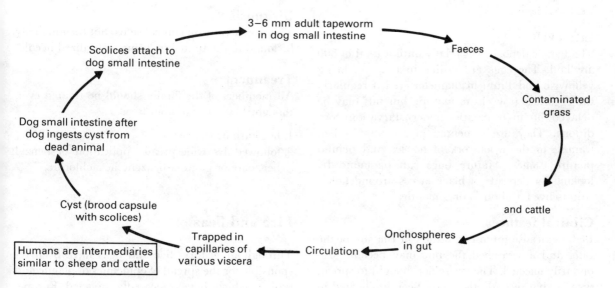

Figure 17.6 The life cycle of the dog tapeworm *(Echinococcus granulosus)*

established hydatid disease, although albendazole has had some limited success (see Table 17.1 for dosage). However, where cysts are found surgical removal is the only real treatment. Extreme care must be taken to remove cysts intact.

With the introduction of niclosamide, tapeworm infections have become much more straightforward to treat. Only cycticercosis and hydatid disease present real problems.

Prevention
Health education in hyperendemic areas. Children should be discouraged from being licked by dogs or kissing them. Vegetables such as watercress should be thoroughly washed in a mild antiseptic solution. Sheep carcases should be burned or buried and not left for dog consumption.

Parasites causing skin irritation

Bedbugs

General
Bedbugs exist all over the world, and although there are 70 different species, only two are parasitic to man: the *Cimex lectularius* (usually in temperate climates) and the *Cimex hemipterus* which lives in the tropics.

They live off human blood like mosquitoes. Also like the mosquito, they are nocturnal in their feeding habits. They can resist starvation well and go for weeks without a feed.

Life cycle
The female deposits eggs daily until a total of 500 are laid. The eggs are visible to the eye, being yellowish and 1 mm in diameter. If fed regularly the eggs take 6 weeks to mature, but this may be delayed up to 6 months under starvation conditions. They are cemented in crevices in bed frames, in the woodwork of houses and behind picture frames. Mature bugs can be found by looking for deposits of black faeces around holes. Adults live for about 5 or 6 months.

Clinical features
Bedbugs cause intense irritation at the site of the bite, and if scratched the bite may become secondarily infected. They were not thought to spread disease, but recently they have been implicated in the spread of the hepatitis B virus.

Treatment and control
The bugs are extremely sensitive to heat and fumigation of a room and its contents with sulphur dioxide for 6 hours is highly effective and safe.

Scabies

Scabies is a common skin condition which occurs world-wide and is caused by the mite *Sarcoptes scabiei*. It affects all social classes.

Life cycle
The gravid female burrows into the stratum corneum of the skin and forms tunnels in which to lay her eggs. The female lives for a month and lays about four eggs. These hatch into larvae in about 4 days. These migrate to the surface and change into eight-legged nymphs which become adult in 10 days. They may infest another person or re-infest the same one.

Clinical picture
The commonest sites of infestation are the hands, feet, buttocks, elbows and axillae. While they are feeding the skin becomes irritated and a sensitivity rash follows causing intense irritation. The burrows may become secondarily infected with bacteria, particularly the group A haemolytic streptococcus. Acute glomerular nephritis may follow.

Nocturnal itching is common and a diagnostic sign.

Diagnosis
This is generally on clinical signs, but the mite may be found in the tunnel by using a sterilized needle.

Treatment
All members of the family should be treated even though they are symptom free:

1. hot bath or shower,
2. followed by widespread application of benzyl benzoate or gamma-benzene hexachloride.

Lice and fleas

Throughout history, lice and fleas have been responsible for the spread of epidemics of plague and typhus which have repeatedly ravaged Europe. That this does not happen today is due mainly to a high standard of living and hygiene, but where there is poverty or social disintegration through war these diseases often reappear.

Lice and fleas are spread by close contact between humans or animals. Children are particularly at risk from infestations. They tend to be more sociable than adults and congregate at school and play. Children are liable to share their clothes, towels and hair brushes without reflecting on personal hygiene. They also have a natural reluctance to bathe and hair wash regularly.

Lice

Lice are obliged to live on or in close proximity to their hosts and are therefore termed obligate ectoparasites. They soon die if separated from their host. Lice are also very host-specific and it is uncommon to find one species of louse parasitizing more than a single host species.

Three types of louse regularly infest man: *Pediculus corporis*, the body louse; *Pediculus capitis*, the head louse; and *Pthirus pubis*, the pubic or crab louse. As their names suggest, each tends to restrict itself to a certain area of the body although occasionally transfer elsewhere can occur.

Body lice

Life cycle
Pediculus corporis is the largest of the three. It lives in body hair and underclothes. The female prefers to lay her eggs in clothing fibres next to the body. However, in hirsute people she will lay her eggs in the shaft of the hairs. The adult female louse lives for about a month and lays four to five eggs daily. The nymphs hatch after 8 days at normal surface body temperature (30−32°C). They then undergo three successive moults in the next 2−3 weeks becoming adults. During this time they need to take blood meals from their host between three and five times a day.

Clinical picture
Pediculus corporis is the vector of epidemic louse-born typhus. During World War I thousands of troops and their attending physicians died of the disease. Typhus is a disease of poverty and social disintegration. It is more likely to occur in winter and spring months.

Although rare in Europe, typhus still occurs in poor temperate climates and in tropical countries of high altitude such as Ethiopia, Afghanistan and the Himalayas, Indonesia, China and the Phillipines.

Typhus is caused by *Ricketsia prowazekii* which reproduces in the epithelial cells of the louse gut. When the irritating bite is scratched the infected faeces of the louse are rubbed into the abrasion so transmitting the disease.

Lice have also been responsible for another ricketsial disease, trench fever, so termed because of its association with the squalor of the trenches in the 1914−18 war and on the Eastern front in 1943.

P. corporis can transmit relapsing fever through the innoculation of the spirochaete *Borrelia recurrentis*. It is a disease, like typhus, of poverty and overcrowding. Relapsing fever is endemic in Ethiopia and parts of Asia. Besides transmitting serious diseases, *P. corporis* has an extremely irritating bite. Scratching the lesion frequently leads to super-infection. Children are liable to develop impetigo as a complication.

Head lice
Pediculus capitis, the hair louse, is not usually a vector of serious disease. It is more of a nuisance and is common in children of nursery and school age. The life cycle of *P. capitis* is similar to *P. corporis* except that the female always cements her eggs to the base of the hairshaft. The eggs are called 'nits'.

Pubic lice
Pthirus pubis, the pubic or crab louse, is usually transmitted by sexual or other close personal contact. It does not transmit any serious disease but the bites are irritating and leave a characteristic blue spot. *Pthirus pubis* possesses large crab-like claws on the second and third pairs of legs by means of which it attaches to hairs. It cannot survive more than 24 hours away from man and only attaches its eggs to hair.

Treatment
The treatment of all louse infestations consists of two parts. The first is to kill all the adult lice and destroy the eggs on the body. The second part is to make sure that lice and their eggs are eradicated from clothing.

In the past, benzyl benzoate and gamma benzene hexachloride were effective treatments. The irritating nature of benzyl benzoate and resistance to gamma benzene hexachloride however have meant that carbaryl and malathion are now preferred drugs.

Carbaryl can be applied as a lotion to the body or as a shampoo to the scalp. The lotion must be allowed to dry naturally on the body and then after 12 hours the hair should be combed thoroughly to remove nits before rinsing. The shampoo should be allowed to remain for 5 minutes before combing and washing.

This treatment may be repeated after a week. Malathion is also available as a lotion and a shampoo preparation. The lotion should be applied to the body for 5 minutes, then rinsed off, and the body hair combed to remove dead lice and nits. The shampoo should be applied to dry hair, allowed to dry and washed off after 12 hours.

In children, where the infestation may be heavy, a second application is often necessary. Hair should be cut short, especially at the back of the head and neck, and nits removed with a fine comb.

Prevention

Clothes should be boiled for 20−30 minutes to destroy the adult lice and their firmly attached eggs. Ironing into the folds and pleats of garments will also help in eradication.

Fleas

General

There are over 2000 different species of flea but only one is specific to man, *Pulex irritans*. However, it is not uncommon for man to be troubled and bitten by animal fleas when he lives in close contact with domestic or wild animals. Fleas can jump 2−3 m by means of powerfully developed hind legs.

Life cycle

The flea is a temporary obligate parasite and both the male and female flea need blood for completion of their life cycle. Unlike lice, fleas can survive for weeks away from their hosts if conditions are favourable.

The female flea lays 10 to 25 eggs per day and is indiscriminate where she lets them fall. The eggs, however, are sticky so that they attach themselves to fur, feathers, hair or in the nest of the specific host. Depending on temperature, the eggs hatch within 2 or 3 days, liberating a larva.

The larva feeds on detritus and after 2 weeks weaves a cocoon within which the flea pupa will develop. The pupa will not hatch into the adult unless conditions are favourable.

Clinical picture

Fleas cause local irritation from their bites but can also transmit disease. Plague is transmitted to man under conditions of overcrowding and poor hygiene by the black rat flea, *Xenopsylla cheopis*.

Xenopsylla cheopis can also transmit murine typhus to man. It is transmitted from the rat. Man can also occasionally become infested with the dog and cat tapeworm, *Dipylidium caninum*, by swallowing the flea *Ctenocephalides canis*.

Children are more likely to be infected than adults and usually the infestation causes few symptoms.

Treatment

The bite of fleas can be extremely irritating and hypersensitivity to the flea bite may develop. Antihistamines will aleviate symptoms and the application of crotamiton ointment is soothing. Monosulfiram soap or a 25 per cent solution may be applied to the body after dilution in two to three parts water.

Clothes may also be rinsed in the solution before washing. This will kill any fleas on the body or garments.

Prevention

To eradicate fleas from pets and the house, animals should be dusted with a non-toxic flea powder, or made to wear an impregnated flea collar. The carpets, which commonly harbour fleas, should be thoroughly vacuumed and cleaned.

Amoebiasis

Amoebiasis is caused by the parasite *Entamoeba histolytica*. It is a disease of poor environmental hygiene rather than of the tropics. The amoebae live in the colon off gut bacteria. The amoebae are only harmful to the gut mucosa and become invasive in 20 per cent of those people infested.

Life cycle

Outside the protection of the host the amoebae become encysted and dormant. They are excreted in the stools of people who do not have amoebic dysentery (carriers). The cysts contaminate food and water and are ingested. They pass into the colon where the cyst goes and the amoeba appears. The amoebae in most cases (80 per cent) live on the surface of the colon mucosa. As they move to the left colon where the faeces are more formed they stop feeding and encyst, eventually passing out in the stool as cysts. Occasionally in children who have acute diarrhoea and there is 'intestinal hurry', live amoebae are passed out in the diarrhoea stools. This does not mean that the diarrhoea was caused by the amoebae.

In a small number of cases the amoebae become invasive. They destroy the gut mucosa forming shallow ulcers and eat the capillary red cells rather than the gut bacteria. This results in amoebic dysentery. Occasionally the amoebae then enter the portal blood system and end up in the right lobe of the liver. They live off the liver cells and form liver abscesses. Small abscesses may then enter the systemic blood system and end up in the brain. The liver abscess itself may grow so big that it ruptures into the pleural cavity or pericardium.

Clinical picture

The majority of children infested may have no symptoms at all. Amoebic dysentery resulting from amoebic ulcers in the colon may be of acute onset in children (but of very slow onset in adults) with bloody diarrhoea.

Fluid loss is not as great as in viral and bacterial diarrhoea and rehydration may not be necessary, but generally amoebic dysentery co-exists with acute viral diarrhoea which often results in severe dehydration.

It is only after the dehydration of the viral diarrhoea is corrected that the amoebic dysentery becomes evident. Untreated amoebic dysentery is generally self-limiting and lasts for about 6 weeks. However it may then recur. The colon can be severly ulcerated. A diagnosis of ulcerative colitis in childhood should not be made in the tropics until amoebiasis has been excluded.

Liver abscess is not common in childhood but must be suspected when a child has fever with a large and tender liver. Jaundice is not common but when present the condition may resemble viral hepatitis. Rupture of the abscess will result in severe toxaemia, and there may be lung symptoms.

In the Middle East amoebic liver abscess must be differentiated from hydatid disease of the lung and liver, which is more common.

Diagnosis

A fresh, warm stool only should be examined for the amoebae or cysts. Stales tools are of little value. The amoebae or cysts can be seen under microscope.

Ninety per cent of all cases of amoebic dysentery have antibodies in the serum but this is a more specialized investigation not readily available.

Amoebic liver abscesses have to be diagnosed by aspiration. The pus is pink and contains cysts and amoebae. This again is a specialized procedure.

Treatment

Amoebic dysentery
Combination of: metronidazole 400 mg orally three times a day for 5 days
and: emetine hydrochloride 65 mg daily by injection for 5 days

Amoebic liver abscess
Combination of: metronidazole 400 mg three times a day for 5 days
and: diloxanide furoate 0.2 g three times a day for 10 days.

If diloxanide furoate is not available the dose of metronidazole should be doubled.

In the past a combination of emetine hydrochloride and chloroquine was used but this is more toxic to the child than the above.

The abscess may have to be aspirated.

Giardiasis

General

Giardiasis is caused by the parasite *Giardia lamblia* which is a flagellate protozoon (mobile parasite with a tail) which lives on the mucosa of the small bowel (jejunum) and encysts when it falls off the mucosa and passes down the bowel.

As with the *Entamoeba histolytica*, *Giardia lamblia* may infest a large percentage of the world's population.

Life cycle

Outside the protection of the small intestine the parasite encysts and may exist for some months in warm, moist conditions of the soil. Once ingested in contaminated food and water the cyst dissolves and the parasite lives on the mucosa of the small bowel. Like *Entamoeba histolytica* they multiply by fission.

If they fall off the gut mucosa they are passed down the gut, encyst, and pass out in the faeces.

The parasites do not damage the small gut as far as is known, but in heavy infestations it is thought that they interfere with enzyme activity and so prevent the breakdown and absorption of carbohydrates and fats.

Clinical picture

Most children infested with *Giardia lamblia* do not develop giardiasis but heavy infestations can produce a coeliac syndrome with steatorrhoea and failure to thrive.

Minor manifestations result in vague abdominal pains or chronic diarrhoea.

Management

The drug of choice is metronidazole 200 mg three times a day for 5 days. If this is not available, mepacrine can be used 50 mg three times a day for 5 days.

Schistosomiasis (bilharzia)

Schistosomiasis is caused by blood worms or flukes infesting humans. The parasites require an intermediary host in the form of a fresh water snail.

Three types affect man.

1. *Schistosoma haematobium* affecting man in Africa and Arabia and causing urinary schistosomiasis.
2. *Schistosoma mansoni* affecting man in Africa and occasionally Arabia, and causes bowel schistosomiasis.
3. *Schistosoma japonicum* affecting man in the Far East and causing bowel schistosomiasis.

Each *Schistosoma* has its own particular snail for an intermediary host.

Life cycle (Figure 17.7)

There are male and female schistosomata that carry out a sexual cycle in the human. The eggs of the female are laid in small venules and migrate into a hollow viscus. In the case of *S. haematobium* this is the urinary tract and the eggs are passed out in the urine. In the case of *S. mansoni* and *S. japonicum* this is the gut and the eggs are voided in the faeces.

The eggs hatch out in fresh water to form little 'worms' (miracidia) which either die or penetrate the shells of suitable snails. Here they divide asexually (the asexual cycle) and are eventually

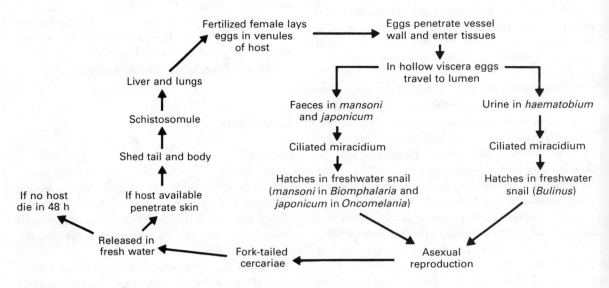

Figure 17.7 The life history of *Schistosoma haematobium* and *Schistosoma mansoni*

passed out into the water as cercariae (small mobile 'worms'). These penetrate the human skin and find their way to the liver via the lungs where they become male and female and pass into the mesenteric veins in the case of *S. mansoni* and *S. japonicum* and the bladder plexus of the veins in the case of *S. haemotobium*. Here fresh eggs are fertilized and the cycle restarted.

Clinical picture

In children in endemic areas the initial symptoms of skin rash (site of penetration) fever and loss of weight do not occur because of intrauterine immunity.

The main problem is due to tissue response to eggs that are not released. This results in granulomatous lesions which may resemble papilloma (bilharziomata).

Schistosoma haematobium

The bilharziomata arise in the bladder and commonly cause haematuria. This in itself is not harmful and it may be the commonest cause of haematuria in Central Africa. However, obstruction to the ureters may occur with resulting hydronephrosis. At first this is reversible with treatment but in long-standing cases it is irreversible. In these cases also the bladder may be the site of urinary stone formation or may shrink due to calcification. If the child reaches adulthood he may develop carcinoma of the bladder. In long-standing cases the eggs may metastasize into the lungs resulting in pulmonary hypertension. Cases have also been reported of bilharziomata in the meninges.

Schistosoma mansoni and japonicum

Most patients may be symptomless, but long-standing cases may lead to hepatosplenomegaly as a result of portal hypertension due to obstruction of the portal veins. Iron deficiency anaemia may also occur. Occasionally bilharzioma grow so large in the gut that they resemble papilloma resulting in melaena and diarrhoea. In adults malignant changes occur.

It is important to remember in Africa that combined infestations (*S. haematobium* and *S. mansoni*) frequently occur.

Diagnosis

As adult worms are not easily available, the eggs should be looked for. This is probably best carried out by the nearest laboratory but the following points are important and will help in finding the eggs.

Schistosoma haematobium

Urine
As most eggs are voided at midday, specimens should be collected at this time and the urine should be sedimented by centrifuge.

Rectal biopsy
This is not difficult as *Schistosoma haematobium* is trapped in the rectal mucosa. The mucosa is 'stripped' with the aid of forceps and placed under a coverslip on a slide. It is examined under low-powered microscope.

Schistosoma mansoni and japonicum

Stools
This should be carried out using a concentration technique by the local laboratory. Rectal smear alone is not sensitive enough.

Rectal biopsy
As above.

Immunodiagnostic tests
Immunodiagnostic tests using patients' serum are also available.

Treatment.

Many drugs are available, but unfortunately most may be toxic to the patient. The best combination of drugs for *S. haematobium* is given as a single dose:

metriphonate 12.5 mg/kg
+
niridazole 25 mg/kg

This combination is effective for *S. mansoni* and *S. japonicum*, but less so than *S. haematobium*.

Praziquantel (single oral dose 40 mg/kg) is effective against all strains but is expensive.

Stibocaptate 6 mg/kg twice per week until five doses have been given. Effective against all strains, but can be dangerous to the host.

Test of cure

Do not examine for worms under 3 months after end of treatment as worms may still be excreted up to then.

Prevention

Control of the disease can only be brought about by destroying the intermediate host, the snail. Children should be prevented from paddling or swimming in static water which is known to be inhabited by the snail.

Leishmaniasis

Leishmaniasis is a parasitic infection common to the countries bordering on the Mediterranean, as well as the Indian subcontinent. It occurs in two forms, visceral leishmaniasis and cutaneous leishmaniasis (Baghdad boil). Cutaneous leishmaniasis is rare in children and only visceral leishmaniasis will be dealt with here.

Aetiology

Parasitic infection caused by the protozoan *Leishmania donovani*.

Table 17.1 *Antiparasitic drugs*

Parasite	Drugs	Dosage	Major side effects
Protozoa			
Amoebiasis	Metronidazole	50 mg/kg/day orally every 8 h for 7 days	Gastrointestinal upset, metallic taste, mutagenic effect. Contra-indicated in blood dyscrasias, active CNS disease and hepatic dysfunction.
Giardiasis	Metronidazole	10–15 mg/kg/day orally every 8 h for 10 days	As above. Contra-indicated in blood dyscrasias and CNS disease.
	Tinidazole	10–15 mg/kg/day every 8 h orally for 5–7 days	
Leishmaniasis	Sodium stibogluconate	10 mg/kg/day i.m., i.v. (max. 600 mg). For Indian disease for 6–10 days For African disease up to 30 days	Nausea, vomiting, urticaria, bradycardia.
Worms			
Ascariasis	Levamisole	2.5 mg/kg orally single dose	Gastric irritation.
	Mebendazole	100 mg twice a day orally for 3 days	Contra-indicated in children under 2 years.
	Piperazine	15 mg/kg/day orally for 2 days	Contra-indicated in epilepsy. Large doses cause vomiting, blurred vision, muscle weakness.
	Pyrantel pamoate	11 mg/kg/orally single dose	
Hookworm	Bephenium	<23 kg: 5.0 g/day >23 kg: 10.0 g/day in 2 divided doses, may repeat for 3 days	Withhold food for 2 hours after medication; may cause nausea, vomiting, diarrhoea.
	Pyrantel	11 mg/kg orally single dose	
	Mebendazole	100 mg twice a day orally for 3 days	
Hydatid	Albendazole	10–14 mg/kg/day for several months	

Table 17.1 *Antiparasitic drugs (continued)*

Parasite	Drugs	Dosage	Major side effects
Tapeworm	Niclosamide	After overnight fasting 1.0 g (2 tabs) chewed at 1 hour interval, purge 2 hours after last dose. Half dose for children under 6 years	Gastrointestinal discomfort.
Tapeworm	Praziquantel	50 mg/kg single dose	
Strongyloides	Thiabendazole	25 mg/kg dose orally twice daily for 3–14 days	Caution in hepatic disorders; gastric irritant; may cause dizziness.
Toxocara	Thiabendazole Mebendazole	25 mg/kg/dose orally twice daily for extended period 100 mg twice daily orally	
Enterobius	Mebendazole Pyrantel	100 mg twice daily for 3 days 11 mg/kg orally single dose	Mild gastrointestinal discomfort. Transient SGOT elevation; caution in pre-existing liver disease.
Flukes			
Schistosoma All species	Praziquantel Niridazole	40 mg/kg orally single dose 25 mg/kg orally three times a day for 5–10 days	Minor gastrointestinal disturbance. Neuropsychiatric symptoms.
S. haematobium	Metriphonate	10 mg/kg/dose for 3 days every 2 weeks	
S. mansoni	Oxamniquine	15 mg/kg/dose orally 12-hourly for 2–3 doses	Vertigo
Filaria	Diethyl carbamazine	6 mg/kg/day three times a day orally for 7 days	Headache, malaise, nausea, vomiting.

Reservoir

The amastigote occurs in rodents, dogs and man and is intracellular (Leishman–Donovani body).

Life cycle

The vector is the female sandfly. The fly takes the amastigote in a blood meal. In the vector's stomach, the amastigotes are liberated from the cells, multiply by fusion, develop flagella and become promastigotes. The promastigotes migrate from the gut to the mouth and are injected at the next meal.

Infection in man can also occur from blood transfusion and very rarely from person to person.

Incubation period

Two weeks to 3 years.

Course of disease

If not contained locally by macrophages, lymphocytes and plasma cells, there is widespread dissemination in the reticulo-endothelial system, resulting in intermittent fever, sometimes with a 'double peak' in 24 hours. Pyrexial phases are later interspersed with apyrexial phases.

There is generalized enlargement of all parts of the reticulo-endothelial system but the spleen is the most significant. Later there is hepatosplenomegaly.

In late stages the spleen becomes very large and tender. There is also cachexia, normochromic and normocytic anaemia, with recurrent respiratory infections.

Diagnosis

There is a leucopenia, hyperglobulinaemia and thrombocytopenia.

1. Direct diagnosis by splenic puncture is the most accurate. Leishman and Donovan bodies (intracellular evidence of the parasite) are diagnostic.
   It is less easy to detect the parasitized cell in bone marrow and blood cultures.
2. Indirect diagnosis. Antibodies by immunofluorescent antibody and ELIZA tests.
3. 'Field test'. Formal gel test. One millilitre of serum is shaken up with one drop of 40 per cent formaldehyde. This test is positive if the serum gels in 30 minutes.

Differential diagnosis

aleukaemic leukaemia
typhoid
brucellosis
histoplasmosis
AIDS

Treatment

1. Supportive, improving nutrition with blood transfusion and correction of bacterial infection.
2. Drug therapy. Pentavalent organoantimony drugs. Sodium stibogluconate 0.1 ml/kg i.v. or i.m. daily up to a total dose of 6 ml in a day for 2 weeks.
3. Aromatic diamidine drugs. Hydroxy-stilbamadine isethionate 3−4 mg/kg/day for 10 days. Total of three courses separated by 7 days rest period.
4. Amphotericin-B has been used but is very toxic.
5. Sodium stibogluconate is probably the drug of choice.

Malaria

This is the commonest and most serious of the diseases acquired in the tropics. It is caused by a parasite known as *Plasmodium*. Part of its life cycle occurs a certain female mosquito, the anopheline.

When the infected mosquito feeds on human blood at night it injects the infecting agent of the plasmodium parasite, the sporozoite, into the human bloodstream. The sporozoite then completes its life cycle in the human. Malaria may also be acquired by man through infected blood transfusions.

There are four different *Plasmodium* species causing four different types of malaria.

1. *Plasmodium falciparum* (malignant tertian malaria)
2. *Plasmodium vivax* (tertian malaria)
3. *Plasmodium ovale* (tertian malaria)
4. *Plasmodium malariae* (quartan malaria)

Life cycle

The malaria parasite has two cycles. A sexual cycle occurs in the infected mosquito. The union of a male and female gametocyte in the mosquito produces sporocytes which migrate to the salivary glands of the mosquito and are injected into the human (see Figure 17.8).

The sporozoites undergo an asexual cycle in the human.

On entering the human the sporozoites leave the blood and enter the liver cells and here divide asexually to produce a structure full of little 'eggs' known as merozoites. This structure is known as schizont. When this is mature it ruptures out of the liver cell and thousands of merozoites enter the blood stream where many invade red cells. Here they form a second schizont. When this is mature it is full of fresh merozoites which rupture out of the red cell, destroying it, and the merozoites invade more red cells, and so it goes on.

1. In the case of *P. vivax* and *P. ovale* merozoites can re-invade liver cells and so relapses may occur in these infections even though the parasite has been cleared from the blood stream by drugs. Merozoites of *P. falciparum* and *P. malariae* cannot do this and so relapses do not occur when the parasite is cleared from the peripheral blood.
2. In the case of *P. vivax*, *P. ovale* and *P. malariae* schizonts are commonly seen in the peripheral

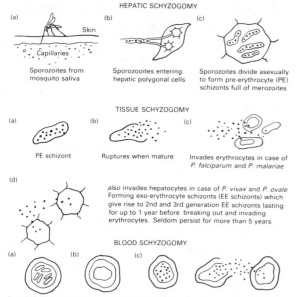

HEPATIC SCHYZOGOMY

(a) Skin
Capillaries
Sporozoites from mosquito saliva

(b) Sporozooites entering hepatic polygonal cells

(c) Sporozoites divide asexually to form pre-erythrocyte (PE) schizonts full of merozoites

TISSUE SCHYZOGOMY

(a) PE schizont

(b) Ruptures when mature

(c) Invades erythrocytes in case of P. falciparum and P. malariae

(d) also invades hepatocytes in case of P. vivax and P. ovale Forming exo-erythrocyte schizonts (EE schizonts) which give rise to 2nd and 3rd generation EE schizonts lasting for up to 1 year before breaking out and invading erythrocytes. Seldom persist for more than 5 years

BLOOD SCHYZOGOMY

(a)   (b)   (c)

(a and b) All *Plasmodium* multiply asexually to produce *trophozoites*. The trophozoites then divide asexually producing *merozoites*. (c) The cell is now fully parasitized. (d) The cell ruptures and releases the merozoites which invade other erythrocytes. (e) Some do not invade erythrocytes but change into sexual forms called gametocytes.

SEXUAL CYCLE

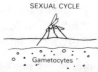

Gametocytes

At an evening feed mosquitoes suck gametocytes into the stomach. Gametocytes mate to form *ookinetes*. The ookinete forms an oocyst after migrating through stomach wall The oocyst ruptures releasing many thousands of sporozoites which migrate to the salivary gland.

Figure 17.8 The life histories of the four different types of malaria parasites, *Plasmodium falciparum*, *P. vivax*, *P. ovale* and *P. malariae*

blood. This is not so, however, in the case of *P. falciparum* as schizonts are generally formed in capillaries. Heavy peripheral parasitaemia in *P. falciparum* indicates a severe infection.
3. Some merozoites do not form schizonts in the peripheral blood but instead form male and female gametocytes. If these are ingested by a blood sucking mosquito they start up the sexual cycle in the mosquito.

Clinical picture

1. *Fever* occurs every time the merozoites rupture out of the red cells. In the case of *P. vivax* and *P. ovale* this occurs every 3 days (tertian) and in the case of *P. malariae* every 4 days (quartan). *P. falciparum* does not have this pattern and fever may occur daily. *P. falciparum* produces the most

serious form of malaria and is sometimes known as 'malignant tertian'.
Hyperpyrexia is common in *P. falciparum* malaria.
2. *Anaemia*. This is a haemolytic anaemia and is most severe in *P. falciparum* infection.
3. *Jaundice*. This is generally mild and occurs in all types. It may be severe in some cases of *P. falciparum* infection, when there has been liver cell damage.
4. *Splenomegaly*. This is common in all types and the spleen may become very large. In areas where malaria is endemic most children will have enlarged spleens due to malaria infections.
5. *Cerebral malaria*. This is an encephalitis that is sometimes difficult to diagnose in children and is generally a result of heavy *P. falciparum* infection. However, many children with first *P. falciparum* infection may present with hyperpyrexia, fits and unconsciousness without actual brain damage.
6. *Nephrotic syndrome*. This is generally a severe type of nephrosis occurring in children and associated with *P. malaria*. It is thought to be due to an immunological process affecting the glomerular basement membrane.
7. *Acute diarrhoea*. This is common in children and is associated with malaria.
8. *Recurrent malaria*. When a child is infected by the parasite he may die (particularly in the case of *P. falciparum*) or he may recover without treatment. In this case he builds up antibodies to the common parasite in his area. Re-infection in the case of *P. falciparum* may occur but tends to get less severe with each attack. The result of this is that the child becomes immune by the time he reaches late childhood. As in measles, transplacental protection may be given by the mother. In the case of *P. vivax* and *P. ovale*, infections are less severe and recurrent fevers may occur, but tend to be due to the re-invasion of the liver cells during the primary infection (not possible in the case of *P. falciparum* and *P. malariae*).
These attacks tend to die out after 3 or 4 years.
9. *Immunosuppressant effects* of an attack of malaria. All forms of malaria depress the immune system of the child. The white cell count is low and the child is more susceptible to some forms of cancer (Burkitt's lymphoma) and hepatitis B infections. All this adds to the problems of a severely malnourished child and an attack of malaria can precipitate kwashiorkor.

Diagnosis

This is achieved by examining a stained dried blood film for the parasites.

A single negative film does not mean that the child has not got malaria, and in endemic areas most healthy children have a mild parasitaemia (parasites in the blood). Diagnosis is made by combining physical signs mentioned before with the blood film.

Treatment

General

1. Hyperpyrexia. It is important to *reduce the high fever* quickly with salicylates and wrapping the child in a tepid wet towel. Do not use a fan. This actually prevents the child from losing heat.
2. *Correct dehydration* due to pyrexia and diarrhoea by nasogastric or parenteral fluid.
3. *Control febrile convulsions* by intramuscular paraldehyde 0.1 ml/kg, or intravenous diazepam 250 µg/kg.
4. The anaemia may be severe enough to require *blood transfusion*. 15–20 ml/kg should be given slowly.

Chemotherapy

Most drugs are used to remove the schizonts from the peripheral blood. Chloroquine and quinine are the best drugs to achieve this. They are effective for all types of malaria, but in the case of *P. vivax* and *P. ovale* relapses will occur unless drugs effective against the schizonts in the liver cells are given as well. The drug of choice here is primaquine.

Recently in some areas of the world the parasite is becoming resistant to chloroquine. In these cases quinine may be effective. Failing this pyrimethamine + sulfadoxine (Fansidar[TM]) is the drug treatment of choice. Dosages for the various drugs are given below.

Chloroquine

This is safest given by mouth. One tablet is 150 mg base

Under 1 year	½ tablet daily for 5 days.
1–5 years	1 tablet daily for 5 days.
5–12 years	2 tablets daily for 5 days.

In seriously ill children the drug may be given i.m. 6 mg/kg/day for 3 days.

For safety this is given in divided dose separated by 2 hours, i.e. 3 mg/kg followed in 2 hours by 3 mg/kg. However, this treatment should be reserved for unconscious children and change should be made to oral treatment as soon as possible.

Quinine

This is safest given by mouth.

Under 1 year	100 mg daily for 5 days.
1–5 years	300 mg daily for 5 days.
5–10 years	600 mg daily for 5 days.
Over 10 years	1000 mg daily for 5 days.

Each day the dose should be given in divided doses so that it can be given three times per day.

In serious cases it may be given intravenously at 10 mg/kg to be repeated in 8 hours. Change to oral as soon as possible.

Pyrimethamine + sulfadoxine (Fansidar [TM])

Under 5 years	½ tablet daily for 5 days
5–10 years	1 tablet daily for 5 days
Over 10 years	2 tablets on first day — 1 tablet daily for 5 days

Each tablet contains 500 mg sulphadoxine and 25 mg pyrimethamine.

Primaquine

This drug should not be given to children with G-6-PD deficiency. The tablets consist of primaquine diphosphate 26.5 mg containing 15 mg of primaquine base. Dosage is expressed as a weight of the base.

Under 5 years	7.5 mg of base daily for 10 days
Over 5 years	15 mg of base daily for 10 days

Cerebral malaria

Although the diagnosis of cerebral malaria is not always easy to confirm, all unconscious or 'fitting' children with *P. falciparum* parasitaemia should be suspect and treated as such.

1. Institute intravenous therapy with 1/5 isotonic saline and 5 per cent glucose.
2. Control fits with paraldehyde or diazepam.
3. Start at once with intravenous quinine with a dose of 100 mg if under 5 years of age, and 200 mg if over 5 years. This should be repeated in 8 hours.

Table 17.2 *Malaria chemoprophylaxis*

In chloroquine sensitive areas

Chloroquine

0−1 year	50 mg	weekly
1−5 years	100 mg	weekly
6−10 years	200 mg	weekly
Adults	300 mg	weekly

Pyrimethamine

0−1 year	12 mg	weekly (½ tablet)
1−5 years	12 mg	weekly (½ tablet)
6−10 years	25 mg	weekly (1 tablet)
Adults	50 mg	weekly (1 tablet)

In chloroquine resistant areas

Pyrimethamine + sulfadoxine (Fansidar)

0−1 year	¼ tablet	weekly
1−5 years	½ tablet	weekly
5−10 years	1 tablet	weekly
Adults	1 tablet	weekly

   1 tablet contains 25 mg pyrimethamine and 500 mg sulphadoxine

Pyrimethamine + dapsone (Maloprim™)

0−1 year	2.5 ml	twice weekly
1−5 years	5 ml	twice weekly
5−10 years	10 ml	twice weekly
Adults	1 tablet	twice weekly

   5 ml syrup contains 3 mg pyrimethamine + 25 mg dapsone
   1 tablet contains 12.5 mg pyrimethamine + 100 mg dapsone

N.B. Prophylaxis should be started before leaving a non-malarial area and continued for one month on return.

4. When the child becomes conscious revert to oral chloroquine in doses stated.

Intravenous chloroquine and intramuscular chloroquine may be given if quinine is not available but it must be stressed that this mode of administration of chloroquine is dangerous and sudden deaths have frequently been reported. Oral chloroquine is safe.

Malaria prophylaxis

The mosquito feeds at night so accommodation in malaria-infested areas should have windows and doors screened to prevent the mosquito entering. Mosquito nets should also be used over beds at night. At sundown long-sleeved shirts and trousers should be worn, and insect repellent applied to the exposed areas.

Chemoprophylaxis is summarized in Table 17.2.

18

Skin Disorders

Disorders of the skin are some of the most common everyday clinical problems in paediatrics, yet they are among the most neglected. Some of the more common problems are discussed here.

Pigmentary conditions

Mongolian blue spot

This is a hyperpigmented bluish-black area over the sacrum, buttocks and lower back resembling a bruise. It is present at birth and gradually fades during the first year or two of life in the majority of children although it persists in a few to adult life. It has no clinical significance.

Hypopigmentation

Vitiligo

The aetiology is unknown although in some instances there may be a familial predisposition. There is a loss of pigmentation and melanocytes in patches over different parts of the body (Figure 18.1). These are not present at birth, but appear gradually during childhood and are often progressive. The lesions vary in size and may cause major cosmetic and psychological problems when present on the face and other exposed parts of the body. Spontaneous remissions are uncommon but do occur. There is no satisfactory treatment although some cosmetic ointments do help. It is estimated that 1 per cent of the world's population is affected, involving all races.

Postinflammatory

This is seen in hyperpigmented children after recovery from burns or severe infections involving whole skin thickness. Full healing occurs but there is a total loss of melanocytes and the area remains depigmented. As in vitiligo, this can be very disfigur-

ing, and there is no effective treatment although cosmetic ointments may help.

Albinism

This is not a common condition but probably occurs more frequently in blacks. It is present at birth and is due to a failure of melanocytes to produce melanin. It is inherited as a recessive disorder. There is often parental consanguinity. The eyes are pink or pale blue due to a lack of pigment in the iris. The hair is white and the skin is

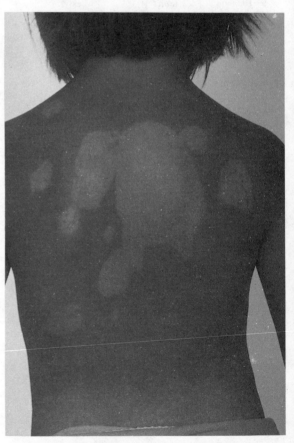

Figure 18.1 The well-marked areas of depigmentation in vitiligo (Gower Medical Publishing Ltd)

pink; there may also be a deficiency of sweat glands. Affected children show marked photophobia and nystagmus, and there may be some degree of mental retardation. The condition is extremely distressing; there is a marked sensitivity to sunlight or exposed skin, resulting in a high incidence of skin cancer. There is no treatment. Affected children should be protected, as far as is practical, from the sun and wear dark glasses.

Naevi

Naevi may be divided into involuting (those that disappear) and non-involuting (those that do not).

Involuting naevi

Erythema nuchae
These are present at birth over the occiput at the junction of the hairline and neck; less often also over the eyelids, forehead and upper lip. They are quite benign and disappear within a few months. No treatment is required though parents may need reassurance.

Cavernous and mixed capillary–cavernous haemangioma
These vascular naevi are often referred to as 'strawberry naevi' (Figures 18.2 and 18.3). Although the vascular elements are present at birth, they are often not visible, or are seen as small insignificant marks on the skin, and occur on any part of the body. There is no sex or genetic predisposition. One or more naevi appear within a few weeks of birth and there follows a proliferative phase of rapid growth which continues until about 6 or 7 months of age, by which time the naevus may have reached a very large size. Depending on its position, it may become traumatized or infected. As it begins to involute the centre becomes white due to local thrombosis. The natural history is one of spontaneous regression and so parents must be dissuaded from seeking surgical treatment in infancy, when the naevus is at its largest, because the end result is likely to be much less disfiguring when it is left alone.

Non-involuting naevi

There is only one of major importance and this is

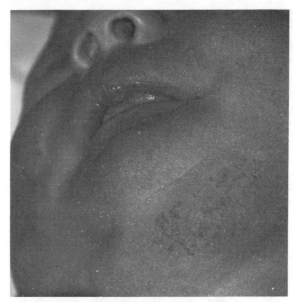

Figure 18.2 A deep cavernous haemangioma

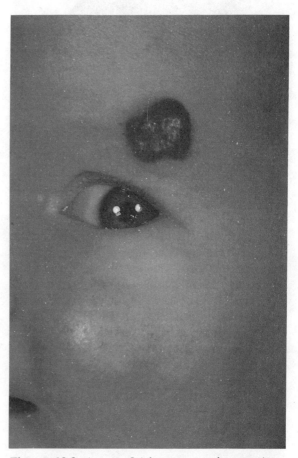

Figure 18.3 A superficial cavernous haemangioma (strawberry naevus) (Gower Medical Publishing Ltd)

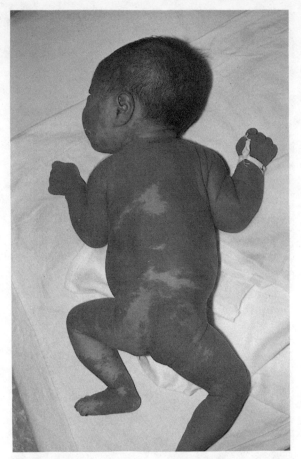

Figure 18.4 A superficial haemangioma (port-wine stain)

due to congenital abnormalities of the skin capillaries. The naevi may occur on any part of the body as a red stain in the skin. A common site, unfortunately, is on the face, where it is referred to as a 'port wine stain' (Figure 18.4). If it is above the palpebral fissure on the face, it may be part of the Sturge–Weber syndrome, in which there is a similar vascular malformation involving the meninges and choroid plexus on the same side of the head. Congenital glaucoma may also occur in the eye on the same side as the vascular lesions. There is no treatment.

Bacterial skin infections

Impetigo

Impetigo is the commonest skin infection, due mainly to group A β-haemolytic streptococci or

Staphylococcus pyogenes. It is highly contagious and spreads rapidly causing epidemics in schools, nurseries or other institutions where children are in close contact. The intact skin normally provides a very efficient barrier against infection, but any break in the skin, however small, is a portal of entry for surface colonizing bacteria. Thus impetigo may follow abrasions, cuts, trauma, or insect bites. Predisposing factors include poor hygiene and social conditions, and a warm humid climate or environment, as well as other skin disorders such as scabies, pediculosis, dermatitis, eczema or herpes simplex.

Classical impetigo is a primary infection with group A β-haemolytic streptococci most often involving the face, neck and hands (Figure 18.5). Initially small pustules are produced which rupture forming a superficial erosion from which infected serum oozes and dries forming the characteristic golden yellow crusts. Regional lymphadenitis may develop. Secondary staphylococcal infection from skin commensals is common. Streptococci which

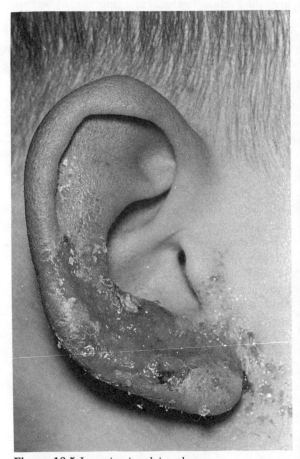

Figure 18.5 Impetigo involving the ear

infect the skin are a different type from those which cause pharyngitis; the reasons for this are not known. Some strains which cause impetigo are also nephritogenic and are associated with acute glomerulonephritis, but acute rheumatic fever does not follow impetigo.

Treatment

As impetigo is highly infectious, affected children should be kept from school. At home, all children in the family should be inspected and treated, or the infection will persist. Local treatment consists of removing infected crusts by washing with saline or cetrimide with chlorhexidine. Topical antibiotics are seldom necessary but dilute potassium permanganate or 1 per cent aqueous gentian violet may be applied to the lesions. A course of penicillin (or erythromycin in penicillin hypersensitive individuals) must also be given. Other antibiotics are rarely required.

Bullous impetigo

This is due to infection with *Staphylococcus aureus*. The bullae are usually larger than the small vesicles of streptococcal impetigo, and thin-walled, filled with a clear fluid, bursting quickly to produce a crust around the edges, the base drying quickly. Spread tends to be more localized unless it follows varicella or multiple insect bites. Local treatment is the same as for classical impetigo but systemic treatment is with erythromycin, fucidic acid or flucloxacillin since the majority of staphylococci are penicillin resistant.

Dactylitis

Dactylitis refers to superficial blisters filled with pus and surrounded by an area of erythema at the tip of a finger or thumb. The majority are due to group A β haemolytic streptococci. Treatment may require incision and drainage of the pus followed by local treatment and systemic penicillin.

Paronychia

This is a localized form of cellulitis around the nail and nail bed. Treatment is as for dactylitis although antistaphylococcal antibiotics may be required. In children who constantly suck their fingers or thumb, infection with *Candida* may cause a chronic paronychia.

Erysipelas

Erysipelas is a distinctive form of superficial cellulitis due to group A β-haemolytic streptococci. It spreads rapidly, the skin becoming swollen, shiny and hot with a distinct edge. Superficial bullae may develop due to local tissue oedema. There is a marked systemic disturbance with fever, rigors and chills, and toxaemia. Affected children should be treated in hospital with systemic penicillin as septicaemia is a common complication.

Cellulitis

Cellulitis is an inflammation of the skin due to infection with a variety of organisms which include *Staphylococcus aureus*, some types of streptococci, *Haemophilus influenzae* type b and pneumococci. The edge is indistinct, unlike erysipelas, the skin hot, indurated and tender with lymphangitis and involvement of regional lymph nodes. Cellulitis overlying osteomyelitis is usually due to *Staphylococcus aureus*. Facial and periorbital cellulitis are serious conditions and there may be spread of infection into the ethmoid sinuses, the orbit and central nervous system. A blood culture should always be taken before starting treatment with systemic antibiotics. Orbital cellulitis, with signs of proptosis and ophthalmoplegia requires surgical treatment in addition to antibiotics.

Folliculitis and furunculosis

Folliculitis refers to a superficial infection of the hair follicle. A furuncle is a deeper infection in the hair follicle; lesions are indurated and inflamed, and often multiple, especially on the scalp and buttocks. A boil is a furuncle in which necrosis has developed in the centre with suppuration. The infecting organism is generally *Staphylococcus aureus*. Local treatment, combined with good hygiene is usually sufficient.

Other staphylococcal skin infections

Several less common skin infections are recognized, occurring either as isolated cases or in epidemics due to localized infections with specific strains or phage types of *Staphylococcus aureus* which produce specific exotoxins. Evidence from epidemics suggests that the infecting organism is generally non-invasive and that several types of skin infection may be caused by one epidemic strain. Local and systemic anti-staphylococcal treatment is necessary to eradicate the organism.

Staphylococcal scalded skin syndrome (SSSS); Ritter's disease

This affects mainly young children. The onset is sudden with fever, irritability and a generalized scarlet fever-like rash starting over the face and neck, axillae and groins and rapidly involving the whole body. The rash may fade on pressure and is often tender to touch. Within 24 to 48 hours superficial bullae appear, containing clear fluid and over the next few days large areas of skin exfoliate exposing a raw moist area which quickly dries. Healing takes place without scarring within a week to 10 days. Mucous membranes are not usually involved. In spite of the apparent severity of the disease, systemic symptoms are often surprisingly mild, complications few and mortality low.

The syndrome is caused by infection with specific phage types of *Staphylococcus aureus* producing an exfoliative exotoxin ('exfoliatin') which induces splitting of the skin within the epidermis at the level of the stratum granulosum.

Toxic shock syndrome (TSS)

The onset is sudden with fever, a diffuse macular scarlet fever-like rash, hypotension and shock, and a wide spectrum of systemic symptoms, ranging from a mild illness to one with an occasional fatal outcome. Symptoms include diarrhoea and vomiting at the onset of the illness; myalgia; disturbances of hepatic and renal function; thrombocytopoenia and disseminated intravascular coagulation and central nervous system involvement with confusion, disorientation and changes in consciousness but without focal neurological signs. Mucous membrane changes range from mild erythema — conjunctival injection, a strawberry tongue and vaginal hyperaemia — to severe erosions. Desquamation of the rash occurs 1 to 2 weeks later and is especially marked over the hands and feet. The hair and nails may also be shed some weeks later.

The toxic shock syndrome is thought to be the result of a localized infection with a strain of *Staphylococcus* producing a specific exotoxin which splits

the skin at the base of the epidermis, not within the epidermis as in the SSSS. Blood cultures are seldom positive. Recently cases have been reported in association with the use of some types of tampons during menstruation.

Staphylococcal scarlet fever

In this condition a generalized scarlatiniform rash develops resembling that produced by streptococci, but it does not exfoliate and is accompanied by few systemic symptoms.

Toxic epidermal necrolysis (TEN)

Histologically, this differs from the SSSS in that the skin splits below the basal layer of the epidermis, with detachment from the underlying dermis. The basal layer of the epidermis may show inflammatory changes and some necrosis. The condition is uncommon in children and is almost identical histologically to drug induced TEN in adults. Systemic disturbance is marked, with fever and malaise, and there may be extensive involvement of mucous membranes.

Napkin dermatitis; nappy rash: ammoniacal dermatitis

Inflammation of the skin in the napkin area, perineum, thighs and lower abdomen may vary from a mild erythema to severe excoriation with ulceration and blistering, though sparing areas within skin-folds. Contributory factors to irritation and inflammation include soap, detergents and chemicals used in washing napkins; ammonia produced by the breakdown of urea in urine by urea-splitting skin bacteria, and secondary bacterial infection with skin organisms and candida.

Prevention consists of changing wet nappies immediately and never allowing a baby to lie in a wet nappy; avoiding the use of plastic pants, and boiling nappies, after which they should be thoroughly rinsed to remove all traces of soap and detergent.

Treatment

1. It is essential to keep the skin dry and avoid contact with urine. Apply zinc and castor oil cream, or water repellent cream such as dimethicone 1 per cent in cetrimide, or similar proprietary preparation.

2. Keep the inflamed area exposed to dry the skin — warm sunlight or a lamp at a safe distance.
3. Apply nystatin cream or miconazole nitrate 2 per cent cream or clotrimazole 1 per cent cream.
4. Do not use topical antibiotics.
5. Topical steroids, e.g. hydrocortisone 1 per cent should never be applied until infection has been controlled, usually 2 or 3 days after starting treatment with nystatin.

Seborrhoea of the scalp: seborrhoeic dermatitis

This results from an accumulation of normal secretions of the sebaceous glands into greasy crust on the scalp of young infants. It is often associated with a dry scaly seborrhoeic rash on the face and behind the ears which spreads to involve the chest, back and abdominal wall, the skin being inflamed and red. Secondary infection with skin bacteria and candida is common.

Treatment

After gently shampooing the scalp, apply arachis oil or olive oil and allow it to soak into the squames. Shampoo again and repeat the process every 12 or 24 hours. Clean the face with boiled water and apply baby oil. An alternative treatment is to apply 2 per cent sulphur—salicylic acid ointment to the scalp after shampooing.

Fungal infections

Candida albicans (thrush: moniliasis)

Candida (Monilia) is a normal commensal inhabiting the skin, mouth, intestinal tract and vagina, but can readily become pathogenic. Oral thrush is common in infants and young children producing white patches over the buccal mucosa, palate and tongue, which though normally benign, may be painful and interfere with feeding. In debilitated, malnourished and immunosuppressed children it can spread throughout the whole of the intestinal tract and appear at the anus. The fungus multiplies readily on areas of warm moist skin such as the groin, where it may complicate nappy rash

(Figure 18.6), and fingers where it may cause paronychia in thumb suckers. Secondary monilial infection may also complicate stomatitis of measles or herpes, seborrhoeic dermatitis, eczema and psoriasis. Systemic candidiasis may develop after prolonged steroid or antibiotic therapy and in immunosuppressed patients.

Treatment

Oral thrush readily responds to a course of nystatin suspension, 100 000 units 6 hourly. If the response is slow, topical application of 1 per cent aqueous gentian violet, though messy, is very effective. Poor hygiene and dirty feeding bottles will cause persistent or recurrent infections and failure of treatment; in breast fed babies maternal thrush on the nipples must be excluded, and treated with nystatin cream. Other effective though more expensive topical applications are miconazole, clotrimazole and amphotericin B.

Ringworm (tinea)

This is the name given to an infection of the skin and hair by three types of fungi — *Microsporum, Trichophyton* and *Epidermophyton*. Man is the primary host to several species of each of these three types, infection with other species is secondary and acquired from infected animals, the usual primary hosts being dogs, cats, cattle, sheep, goats and rodents.

Tinea capitis

Tinea capitis is an infection of the hair and scalp, usually with a *Microsporum* or *Trichophyton* species, and is probably the commonest fungal infection in

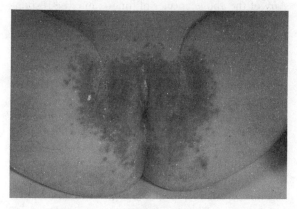

Figure 18.6 *Candida* (thrush) involving the nappy area. (Gower Medical Publishing Ltd.)

251

children. Infecting fungal hyphae grow into the roots of the hair and, depending on the species then grow either along the surface of the hair shaft or invade the shaft and grow inside. The damaged hair becomes fragile and breaks off leaving circular patches of hair loss or alopoecia.

Tinea capitis is infectious and readily transmitted amongst children in close contact with each other in schools and nurseries; articles that are shared or in communal use such as brushes and combs in hair-dressers, hats, towels, etc are sources of infection.

Diagnosis is made by microscopic examination of skin and hair scrapings, and culture of infected hairs. These are readily obtained as they are fragile and easily broken off near the scalp. Some species fluoresce under Wood's (ultra-violet) light.

Treatment

All infected hair must be removed or shaved off. Affected children should be kept away from school and all contacts carefully examined and treated if infected. To be effective, a systemic antibiotic must be used to penetrate the hair root, topical treatment alone is not adequate. Griseofulvin is given orally, two or three times a day after meals in a dose of 10 mg/kg/day for 6 to 8 weeks and continued for 2 weeks after clinical cure. Potential side effects are hepatotoxicity and phototoxicity. Selenium sulphide, applied topically, is sporicidal and a twice-weekly shampoo with a 2.5 per cent suspension, when combined with griseofulvin, is very effective in rapidly making hair non-infectious. Clotrimazole 1 per cent or miconazole 2 per cent cream may also be applied to the scalp.

Tinea corporis

Any of the above species of fungus may be responsible for infection of the skin of the face and body (Figure 18.7). Typically there may be one or many circular, ring-like patches of erythematous, dry scaly skin, of varying size occurring on any part of the body. The lesions are often slightly itchy and have a discrete edge which may be papular. Pustules suggest secondary bacterial infection. Excessive heat and humidity are aggravating factors especially if there is widespread infection. Domestic animals, including sheep and goats may be a source of continuing infection.

Tinea cruris is a localized form of tinea corporis involving the groins and inner aspects of the upper thighs. It is circumscribed, scaly erythematous and

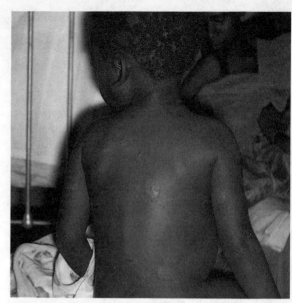

Figure 18.7 Ringworm of scalp and trunk in an African child

slightly itchy and is always bilateral. Diagnosis is made by microscopic examination of skin scrapings and culture.

Treatment

Topical treatment is almost always effective and griseofulvin is rarely required. Suitable preparations include:

- clotrimazole 1 per cent or miconazole 2 per cent or econazole nitrate 1 per cent cream applied two or three times daily
- benzoic acid compound ointment (Whitfield's ointment)
- undecenoic acid or zinc undecenoate ointment and powder
- magenta (Castellani's) paint
- tolnaftate 1 per cent cream

Tinea pedis: athlete's foot

Tinea pedis is a fungal infection of the skin on the soles of the feet and between the toes. The soles of the feet are dry, scaly and itchy; between the toes the skin is often scaly, inflamed and macerated, and there may be secondary bacterial infection. Communal sources of infection include swimming pools, changing rooms and gymnasia where children walk about in bare feet. Tinea of the hands involving palms and fingers is much less common.

Diagnosis and treatment is the same as for tinea

corporis. The feet must be kept dry and if possible sandals and woollen socks worn, and changed frequently, they should be boiled when washed. Nylon socks and rubber-soled shoes should not be worn as they make the feet sweat. Zinc undecenoate powder may be sprinkled in the socks.

Tinea versicolor: pityriasis versicolor

This is an infection of the superficial layer of the epithelium caused by the yeast *Malassezia furfur*. It produces sharply circumscribed small hyper- or hypopigmented finely scaling lesions which are widespread over the trunk and more proximal parts of the limbs (Figure 18.8). There is little erythema or inflammation. The lesions may sometimes be mistaken for vitiligo in dark-skinned persons though is generally obvious and confirmed by examination of skin scrapings. As with other fungal skin infections, the disorder is aggravated by hot moist conditions and excessive sweating.

Treatment

Topical applications of Whitfield's ointment, 1 per cent clotrimazole or 2 per cent miconazole cream and selenium sulphide suspension are effective and should be continued for about a week after the rash has cleared. Clothing should be boiled and changed frequently.

Viral infections of the skin

Warts

Warts are the commonest viral infection of the skin in children, and are caused by several different strains of the human papilloma virus. Warts vary

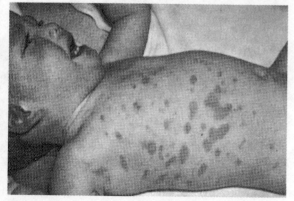

Figure 18.8 Tinea versicolor

considerably in size, shape and distribution but are all benign, despite the anxiety caused to parents.

The common wart: verrucae vulgaris

These are usually found on the hands and fingers, less often elsewhere on the limbs. Plantar warts are common in older children and acquired in the same way as tinea pedis. The pressure of walking presses the wart into the sole of the foot, and as it grows becomes painful.

Treatment

The multiplicity of treatments available reflects some of the difficulty in eradicating them. Left alone, many will eventually disappear over a 1 to 2-year period.

The following are effective treatments:

- application of a 40 per cent salicylic acid plaster after removing the superficial thickened skin with a scalpel or pumice stone, and changed every 2 to 3 days
- paint with 25 or 50 per cent podophyllin in collodion, cover with an occlusive dressing
- a mixture of lactic acid 16.7 per cent and salicylic acid 16.7 per cent in collodion (Salactol™)
- curettage under local anaesthesia
- freezing with carbon dioxide snow or liquid nitrogen

Flat warts: plane warts

These are small flat-topped warts, often multiple, and found especially on the hands and face. There is a tendency to develop over sites of minor trauma. They are resistant to local treatment and are best left alone, since most forms of treatment will damage and scar the more delicate skin of the face, and, given time will disappear spontaneously.

Anogenital warts are fleshy, moist and some times vascular warts found anywhere on the perineum and also mucosal surfaces. Infection is usually transmitted from the hands of parents, though occasionally syphilitic condylomata lata have to be considered in the differential diagnosis. Applications of podophyllin 25 per cent in paraffin left on for several hours before washing are effective, as is diathermy.

Molluscum contagiosum

The lesions are small round papules mainly found

on the face and upper part of the body, smooth and with a central umbilication. There is no surrounding erythema. Like warts, they are contagious and spread rapidly amongst close contacts, and can also be transmitted by sexual contact.

Treatment

The contents of the central core can be removed by expressing with fine forceps, sharp needle or curette. Alternatively, the lesions can be painted with podophyllim.

Herpes simplex

The typical lesions of herpes are painful groups of vesicles with an erythematous base; these quickly rupture, exposing the base which then crusts over and may become secondarily infected (Figure 18.9). They heal without scarring. Although primary herpes is often a stomatitis in young children, it may also present as a kerato-conjunctivitis or vulvo-vaginitis, or on the hands or trunk. Constitutional disturbance, with fever, malaise and regional lymphadenopathy is common. Kaposi's varicelliform eruption is a generalized secondary herpetic infection of atopic eczematous lesions. After a primary infection, a carrier state develops and persists for life. The virus may remain quiescent or be reactivated with colds, upper respiratory and other infections and may be particularly troublesome in some children as recurrent cold sores.

Treatment is mainly symptomatic. Careful attention to oral hygiene and fluid intake is important in stomatitis. Idoxuridine in an 0.1 per cent solution or acyclovir 5 per cent ointment can be applied to oral lesions four times a day. Topical applications of a local anaesthetic may help to relieve pain.

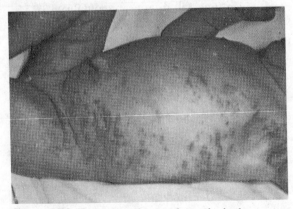

Figure 18.9 Herpes simplex involving the body

Acyclovir ointment or an ointment of 5 per cent idoxuridine in dimethyl sulphoxide can be applied to skin lesions four times a day. They must be kept well away from the eyes. Acyclovir suspension, 200 mg five times a day may shorten the infection if treatment is started early. Antibiotics may be needed to control secondary infection. Topical or systemic steroids must never be used. Recurrent cold sores respond to treatment with acyclovir ointment if treatment is started immediately the sores reappear.

Herpes is highly infectious and infected children should be isolated, special precautions being taken to avoid contact with immunosuppressed and eczematous children.

Eczema

The terms eczema and dermatitis have the same meaning. Eczema is an inflammatory reaction of the skin characterized in the acute form by erythema, oedema, vesiculation and exudation, and in the chronic state by hyperkeratosis and lichenification. Intense itching may accompany both.

Exogenous causes include many irritants and allergens which may be chemical, infective or due to medicaments, e.g:

- napkin dermatitis
- contact dermatitis — metals, especially nickel and chromium
  − chemicals in plastics (epoxy resins and adhesives), rubber (shoes and 'trainers') and dyes (hair dyes, clothing)
- preservatives — cosmetics, foods
- wool alcohols — lanolin, cosmetics, creams
- medicaments — neomycin; benzocaine; preservatives in creams and other topical applications

Seborrhoeic dermatitis (see page 251) and atopic eczema are the commonest endogenous causes of eczema in childhood.

Atopic eczema

This is a part of the atopic triad of asthma, eczema and hay fever/allergic rhinitis syndrome. There is often a strong family history. The aetiology is unknown but genetic factors suggest an autosomal dominant condition requiring specific environmental stimuli for full expression. Breast feeding and the total avoidance of cow's milk and its products in the first 6 months of life may modify the severity of the disease in some cases, in others avoidance of protein-containing foods such as eggs, fish and wheat may help. The role of food allergy in eczema is still extremely controversial. Atopic patients have a variety of immunological abnormalities including raised IgE antibody levels against a diverse range of allergens including house dust mites, pollens, foods and animals. Skin tests are generally unhelpful, however, in atopic eczema. A role for environmental factors is suggested by the increased incidence of atopic disorders in West Indian and Asian children born and living in Britain compared with children living in their home countries.

Atopic eczema usually presents from about 3 months of age, and involves the face, forearms and trunk with erythematous dry patches of skin appearing followed by papules and vesicles. Itching may cause affected infants to rub their cheeks against the cot sheets. Other sites involved are the creases behind the ears, flexures of the knees, elbows and wrists. The differential diagnosis in infancy is from seborrhoeic dermatitis which presents earlier, involves the face, trunk, and flexures of the groins and axillae and is less irritating.

In older children a mixture of acute and chronic lesions may be present with lichenification and thickening of the skin of the hands and feet and flexures of the elbows, knees, wrists and ankles, as well as patches of varying size over the trunk. Severe itching results in scratching and further excoriation and bleeding and secondary infection from commensal skin organisms, staphylococci, *Candida* and occasionally herpes. Regional lymph nodes are frequently enlarged.

Pityriasis alba refers to the scaly, dry, slightly depigmented patches of mild eczema commonly found on the face and cheeks of children. The differential diagnosis is from vitiligo which has sharp edges, and pityriasis versicolor.

Atopic eczema is subject to periods of quiescence and acute exacerbations. The cause of these is not always clear but may be associated with periods of stress, infections or exposure to known (or unrecognized) allergens. In some atopic children eczema often improves around the age of 2 or 3 years, though only to be replaced by asthma. Fortunately the majority of children will improve as they get older, and in many eczema will have completely regressed as they reach adolescence.

Management

This can be difficult and tedious for parents. The aim is to keep the eczema quiescent, promptly treat acute exacerbations and prevent scratching.

Basic management and maintenance

1. Avoid known aggravating factors:
   - keep dust down to a minimum,
   - use pillows and bedding made of synthetic fibres rather than feathers,
   - use cotton clothing, rather than clothes made from wool or synthetic fibres,
   - keep contact with animals to a minimum
2. Encourage breast feeding throughout infancy; avoid cow's milk, all dairy products and eggs. Goat's milk is less allergenic than cow's milk, and may be tried, but many children are still allergic to it.
3. Never use commercial soaps, they are highly alkaline and irritant. Use an emollient oil or emulsifying ointment, both as a soap substitute and in the bath. Aqueous cream or similar preparation can be used regularly during the day. The liberal use of emollients will reduce, to some extent, the need for steroids. A useful preparation is urea 10 per cent in hydrocortisone 1 per cent cream.
4. Use hydrocortisone 1 per cent — the least potent steroid — for maintenance treatment. Avoid using any steroids on the face; if one is necessary then use hydrocortisone 0.5 per cent sparingly. More potent steroids will cause atrophy of the skin and telangiectasia.
5. Thickened lichenified areas of chronic eczema can be improved by the use of a steroid under an occlusive dressing at night, e.g. on the hands, feet or limbs. Alternatively, preparations containing 2−5 per cent tar and 1−2 per cent ichthyol in zinc paste are particularly helpful, especially under an occlusive dressing, which also helps to prevent scratching.
6. Sleeplessness due to scratching can be helped by trimeprazine syrup 2−3 mg/kg at night.

Management of acute exacerbation

1. All skin lesions, even if not obviously septic, will be heavily colonized or infected by a mixture of skin organisms, staphylococci, and possibly

streptococci. A five-day course of erythromycin or co-trimoxazole should always be given.

2. Used judiciously, short courses of a more potent steroid will quickly control an acute exacerbation, though very potent steroids should be avoided if possible.

3. Topical antibiotics are combined with many steroid preparations, they may be helpful in short courses but excessive use may sensitize the skin (especially neomycin) and result in the development of antibiotic resistant organisms.

4. Sedation with trimeprazine by day as well as at night may be required to prevent scratching. Clemastine (0.5–1.0 mg) is an alternative sedative.

Note: Systemic steroids should never be used in the treatment of acute or chronic eczema.

Keloid formation

This can be a significant problem for patients with highly pigmented skins (Figure 18.10). Keloid is due to the overgrowth of collagen at the site of an injury or burn. It resembles an overgrowth of scar tissue, and can be very disfiguring. Treatment is unsatisfactory, since surgical removal will stimulate the recurrence of an even larger keloid. Local infiltration of hydrocortisone repeatedly over a period of several months has met with some success with one of the authors. Local X-ray treatment must never be used because of the risk of malignant change.

Further reading

Hansen, R.C. (1983). Staphylococcal scalded skin, toxic shock, kawasaki disease. *Pediatric Clinics of North America*, **30** (3), 533.

Morley, W.M. (1984). Diseases of the skin. In: *Textbook of Paediatrics* (Eds J.O. Forfar and G.C. Arneil) 3rd Edn, Churchill Livingstone, Edinburgh, 1630.

Stein, D.H. (1983). Superficial fungal infections. *Pediatric Clinics of North America*, **30** (3), 545.

Tunnessen, W.W. (1983). Cutaneous infections. *Pediatric Clinics of North America*, **30** (3), 515.

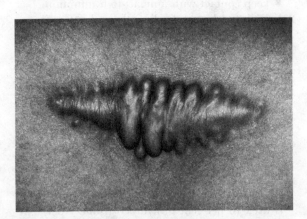

Figure 18.10 Keloid formation in the scar of a wound. (Gower Medical Publishing Ltd)

19

Eye Disorders

The eye is subject to a large variety of diseases and some of the common ones in childhood are described below. The structure of the eye is shown in Figure 19.1.

Diseases of the eyelid

The corneal reflex protects the eye when dirt or a foreign body touches the cornea or sclera. The muscles of the eyelid are innervated by the fifth and seventh cranial nerves and if damaged result in loss of the reflex, contamination of the eye by dirt and dust and infection of the sclera and cornea.

Styes

A 'stye' is an infection of the eyelash follicle. It is not usually serious and responds to local bathing with warm saline.

Meibomian cyst

A Meibomian cyst is caused by inflammation of a Meibomian gland situated on the inside of the eyelid. Treatment is the same as for a stye but an antibiotic ointment may also be used, three times a day for 5 days. Tetracycline is the antibiotic of choice.

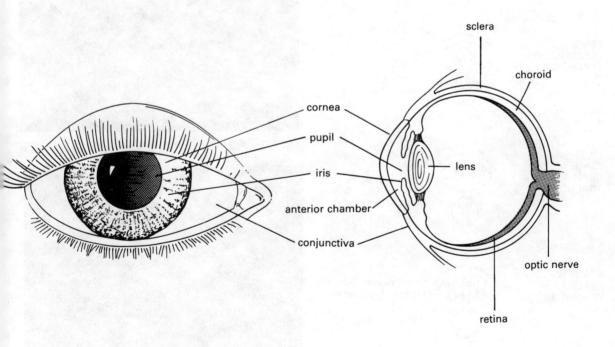

Figure 19.1 The structure of the eye

Trachoma

This is the most serious disease of the eyelid as the inflammation and resultant scarring spreads on to the cornea. It is an infectious disease caused by *Chlamydia*, an obligate intracellular organism, and is spread by flies. The disease is common throughout the Mediterranean and North Africa, the Middle East, Asia, and tropical Africa. The four stages of the disease are shown in Figure 19.2. In stage II the pannus (infiltration) may spread over the whole of the cornea resulting in blindness.

There is no lasting immunity and repeated infections may cause progressive damage to the cornea. Repeated scarring of the lid results in it being turned inwards (entropion) and the eyelashes then cause further irritation and scarring of the cornea. The causative agent may be demonstrated in Giemsa stained conjunctival scrapings. Early diagnosis is important, but the infection responds well

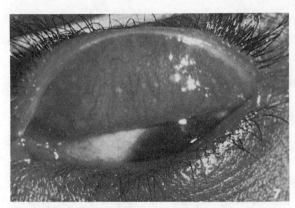

Figure 19.3 Early trachoma

NORMAL
lid (tarsal surface) — vertical tarsal vessels clearly visible

cornea — sometimes crescent but no infiltration or pannus

STAGE I DEVELOPING TRACHOMA — hyperaemia hiding tarsal vessels
— early infiltration and pannus progressus

STAGE II ESTABLISHED TRACHOMA — follicles
— infiltration, pannus and limbal follicles

STAGE III HEALING TRACHOMA — fine linear scars
— pannus regressus

STAGE IV HEALED TRACHOMA — tarsal vessels again visible plus scarring
— Herbert's pits

Figure 19.2 The development of trachoma

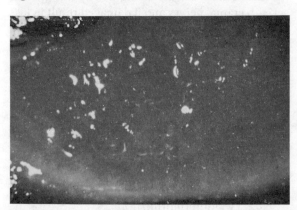

Figure 19.4 Advanced trachoma

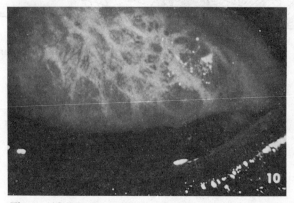

Figure 19.5 Late trachoma

258

to tetracycline eye ointment 1 per cent instilled into the eye three times a day for a month. A further course may be given after an interval of 15–20 days. Secondary bacterial infection is common and may result in permanent damage to the eye. Entropion requires surgical treatment. (See Figures 19.3, 19.4 and 19.5.)

Chalazia

This is a painless mass in the eyelid caused by blockage of a Meibomian gland (Figure 19.6). If infected, it should be treated as for a 'stye', and removed by surgical excision afterwards.

Blepharitis

This is a chronic inflammation of the eyelid margins involving the eyelashes and is usually due to *Staphylococcus aureus* (Figure 19.7). There may be a purulent discharge. It is often associated with dandruff. The lid margin should be cleaned with warm cotton wool saline soaks, followed by the application of tetracycline eye ointment for at least 7 days.

Diseases of the conjunctiva

Conjunctivitis is usually bilateral. The eyes are inflamed and often painful, with a purulent and often profuse discharge (Figure 19.8). Milder forms result in a 'sticky eye' especially noticeable on waking. In allergic conjunctivitis there is intense irritation, and then the eye may be secondarily infected.

Conjunctivitis is classified as follows:

- bacterial
- viral
- chemical
- allergic

Bacterial conjunctivitis

The commonest infecting organism is *Staphyloccus aureus*, but any common bacterial pathogen may be involved. It responds well to either chloramphenicol 1 per cent or tetracycline 1 per cent eye ointment four times a day for up to 5 days after washing the eye gently with cooled boiled water or sterile saline. Steroid eye preparations must never be used in the treatment of bacterial conjunctivitis.

Viral conjunctivitis

Trachoma (see above) is the commonest cause. Conjunctivitis is a feature of measles but if the eye becomes secondarily infected in malnourished

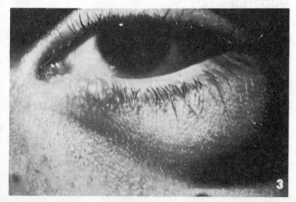

Figure 19.6 A chalazian

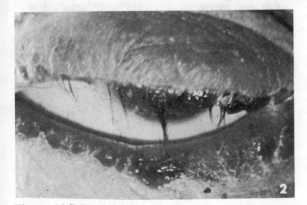

Figure 19.7 Blepharitis

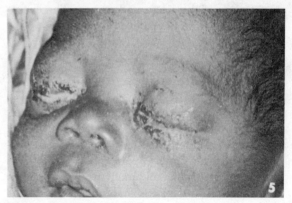

Figure 19.8 Purulent conjunctivitis

children, keratomalacia and loss of vision may develop especially if vitamin A deficiency is present. Secondary infection with herpes simplex virus may result in a staphyloma and perforation of the eye. Treatment is as for bacterial conjunctivitis, with the addition of vitamin A by mouth.

Chemical conjunctivitis

A wide range of household and industrial chemicals may cause accidental damage to the eye and permanent blindness. An iatrogenic chemical conjunctivitis results from the overzealous or prolonged use of local treatment − drops or ointment − in the eye. Cobra venom and cantharides (powder made from the blister beetle) are other poisons occasionally causing conjunctivitis.

Treatment
The eye must be immediately and thoroughly washed and irrigated with isotonic saline or cooled boiled water and continued several times a day over the next 24−48 hours. Secondary infection requires systemic antibiotic treatment. Cobra venom causes severe pain and local anaesthetic drops may be necessary.

Allergic conjunctivitis

Simple, mild irritation responds to antihistamine (antistine privine) eye drops or hydrocortisone eye drops or ointment. Spring catarrh is an extremely irritating but benign condition affecting children of school age. Spontaneous improvement may be expected in older children. Diagnosis is made from the observation of raised conjunctival tissue around the junction of the sclera and cornea. The excess tissue may have to be removed by scraping.

Diseases of the cornea

The general term for disease causing inflammation of the cornea is keratitis. Whatever the cause, keratitis is characterized by an increased production of tears, intense pain, photophobia and blurred vision. Unlike conjunctivitis, inflammation is not marked. Keratitis may be classified as follows:

Vitamin A deficiency

The cornea loses its lustre and tone but inflammation, unless due to secondary bacterial infection, is minimal. The cornea softens and may perforate with protrusion of the iris, which then becomes stuck to the back of the cornea. As healing takes place, white scarring of the cornea occurs with loss of vision. This is accelerated if the child has an attack of measles, when the causal organism is probably the herpes simplex virus. It occurs only in malnourished children and is known as keratomalacia.

Treatment
In the early stages vitamin A 100 000 units should be given daily for 6 days using atropine 1 per cent and tetracycline eye ointment daily for the same period. If corneal scarring is recent and extensive this may have to be treated by corneal grafting. If there is some vision present the eye should be left alone.

Bacterial ulcers

These are secondary and follow trauma to the eye (Figure 19.9). Pus may be produced in the anterior chamber of the eye (hypopyon). Corneal ulceration and perforation may result if the condition is untreated.

Treatment
Vigorous treatment with tetracycline or chloramphenicol eye ointment four times a day and atropine 1 per cent eye ointment may be necessary for up to 5 or 6 days.

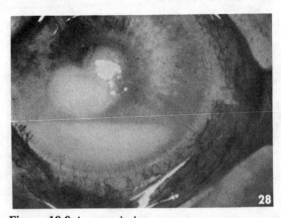

Figure 19.9 A corneal ulcer

The eye lesions in leprosy are a keratitis or iridocyclitis, and occur more often in Asia than in Africa. Damage to the facial nerve may result in inability to close the eyes, causing a chronic conjunctivitis and keratitis and, ultimately, blindness.

Viral ulcers

These are usually due to infection by herpes simplex but sometimes chickenpox may involve the cornea.

Treatment
Acylovir ophthalmic ointment should be instilled 4-hourly in the eyes, and continued for at least 3 days after healing is complete. Alternatively idoxuridine eye ointment is instilled 4-hourly. Atropine 1 per cent eye ointment should also be instilled up to four times a day to reduce blepharospasm. Prolonged treatment may be needed and scarring may occur. Topical steroids must never be used.

Diseases of the lens

Cataract is the term given to a lens which is opaque or no longer transparent. Cataracts in infancy and childhood may be either congenital or acquired.

Congenital cataracts

These usually result from intra-uterine viral infections such as rubella. They are readily detected as the whole of the centre of the cornea of one or both eyes appears opaque. The infant is blind and may develop nystagmus. Treatment is surgical removal of the cataract, though the results are often disappointing.

Cataract in later childhood

Commoner causes include:

● trauma
● complication of long-term steroid therapy
● metabolic diseases such as poorly controlled diabetes mellitus and very rarely, galactosaemia

Treatment
All cases will need surgery at the appropriate time. Vision may temporarily be improved by instilling 10 per cent phenylephrine drops daily. Vitamin D

deficiency in early infancy may produce bilateral cataracts.

Iridocyclitis

Inflammation of the iris may frequently extend into the anterior vitreous. It is a common complication of juvenile rheumatoid arthritis especially in the early onset pauci-articular type in girls. There is a strong correlation with the presence of antinuclear antibodies. Iridocyclitis may precede joint symptoms. All children with rheumatoid arthritis should have a slit-lamp examination, since early recognition and treatment is essential to preserve vision.

Systemic bowel disease — ulcerative colitis and Crohn's disease — may also be complicated by an iridocyclitis.

Diseases of the retina

1. *Congenital toxoplasmosis* produces a characteristic chorio-retinitis followed by scarring, and is a common cause of loss of vision, though usually only one eye is involved. Diagnosis is made on the typical fundal findings and a positive toxoplasma dye test. It may be the only manifestation of congenital toxoplasmosis. Treatment is with sulphonamides and pyrimethamine or clindamycin for 3 to 4 weeks.
2. Infestation with *Toxocara canis* may produce a systemic illness with visceral larva margins, but sometimes the only manifestation in children may be ocular disease. The larvae produce either a pre-retinal or subretinal granuloma. Diagnosis is made on the fundal findings and a positive enzyme-linked immunosorbent (ELISA) antibody test. Many cases settle without treatment but a short course of systemic steroids for 3—4 weeks may help.
3. *Vitamin A deficiency* — see above.
4. *Retinitis pigmentosa* is a sex-linked condition characterized by night blindness, peripheral visual field contraction and a pigmentary retinopathy. Loss of vision is progressive as retinal cells degenerate. There is no effective treatment.
5. A *pigmentary retinopathy* is also a feature of a number of rare syndromes.
6. *Retrolental fibroplasia* is a disorder due to oxygen toxicity in the premature infant. Excessive

administration of oxygen is followed by the proliferation of new blood vessels growing towards the periphery of the retina and into the vitreous. Haemorrhages from these vessels are followed by the development of fibrous tissue, and loss of vision. Detachment of the retina may occur. Prevention depends on careful monitoring of arterial oxygen levels in preterm infants, and keeping this within normal physiological limits. There is no effective treatment.

7. *Sickle cell retinopathy* is seen especially in the HbSC disease, and less often in sickle cell anaemia. The retinopathy results from localized thromboses due to sickling within the peripheral retinal arterioles. Abnormal vascular shunts develop with new blood vessel formation, and vitreous haemorrhages may also occur.

Onchocerciasis: river blindness

This is a major cause of blindness in tropical Africa, Central America and the Yemen. Its health, economic and social consequences make it a major endemic disease of such importance that WHO, in conjunction with other agencies, has established a large onchocerciasis control programme.

The causative agent is a filaria worm, *Onchocerca volvulus*. Adult filariae may live up to 10–15 years in humans, either in a free form in the skin or encysted form (nodules or onchocercomas). The adult female produces microfilariae which live from 18–30 months in the skin, passing through the eye and other tissues. Transmission is via the blackfly (buffalognat, *Simulium*) which is both vector and intermediate host in whom further development of microfilariae takes place. The blackflies are found especially near rivers and irrigated areas where their larvae develop. The risk of eye lesions and blindness is related to the frequency of blackfly bites, proximity of housing to a river and duration of exposure.

The clinical syndromes in onchocerciasis are:

1. cutaneous syndromes with intense itching, depigmentation and atrophy of the skin or lymphoedema and thickening of the skin
2. presence of nodules of varying size in the skin

3. ocular syndrome – this is due to the presence of living or dead microfilariae in various parts of the eye, night blindness is the earliest symptom followed by progressive loss of vision, lesions seen include:
   - punctate keratitis followed by sclerosing keratitis
   - iridocyclitis and sequelae
   - chorioretinitis
   - optic nerve neuritis and optic atrophy.

Diagnosis requires ophthalmoscopy and slit-lamp examination, and cutaneous biopsies to demonstrate microfilariae.

Treatment
The drug of choice is diethylcarbamazine. Control of the vector is by mass campaigns aimed at eradication of simulium larvae from breeding grounds using DDT or biodegradable organophosphorus compounds.

Tumours of the eye

The following tumours may involve the eye or orbit:
- retinoblastoma (Figure 19.10)
- rhabdomyosarcoma
- optic nerve glioma
- Burkitt's and other lymphomas
- secondary deposits from a neuroblastoma or leukaemia
- benign haemangiomas and dermoid cysts

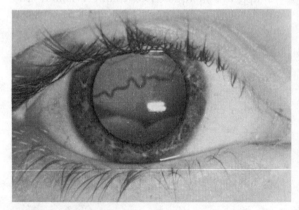

Figure 19.10 A retinoblastoma

20

Accidents, Injuries and Child Abuse

Accidents and injuries

Accidental injury in childhood has been classed as the most important epidemic in the Western world. Unfortunately, with the introduction of the motor car, greater sophistication in medical therapy (pills, medicines) and household cleaning materials and the necessity for both parents to go out to work, leaving the child in the care of a less responsible person (elder brother or sister), accidental injury is rapidly becoming a major problem in developing countries.

Incidence

It is difficult to estimate the incidence of accidents of all types in developing countries but in England and Wales in 1987 accidents of all types and violence accounted for 30 per cent of all deaths between the ages of 1 and 14 years (34 per cent for boys and 25 per cent for girls). Under the age of 1 year it was only 3 per cent. These figures compare with some of those assessed in developing countries. In Libya, as in many other countries, road accidents have become so common that they are the major cause of death in all under the age of 25 years.

Factors involved in the cause of accidents

There are three main factors:

1. The age and mentality of the child is most important. The younger the child, the more care it needs but a mentally retarded child, such as one suffering from Down's syndrome, aged 6 or 7 years is just as vulnerable as a 2-year old toddler of normal intelligence. Intelligence and limb co-ordination are very important factors and children should be carefully protected until they can look after themselves.
2. The causative agent. These are many and are

mentioned below when dealing with specific problems. Many accidents can be prevented with a little care in the home and toddlers should never be allowed to play near main roads.
3. The environment. This is very important and will help to determine the exact circumstances in which the accident took place.

Accident prevention

In any country this can be best be carried out by education through the media. Television and radio are excellent media for this and many accidents in the home can be prevented in this way. The media can also stress the importance of never leaving toddlers in the care of other children. Long-term medical therapy with the aid of tablets or liquids should always be avoided when home conditions are poor and parental intelligence low. However, if tablets are given, the media publicity can show how they can be safely stored.

It is important for every country to be able to obtain as much information as possible on the incidence of different types of accident, as this varies from country to country. It is then possible to plan a national policy for accident prevention. This can best be carried out by an accident committee formed at government level.

Poisons

Most children in rural areas and 'shanty' towns in developing countries generally live in one-roomed houses, and play out of doors. In these houses there are generally no cupboards or shelves. For this reason never give parents or children long-term medication in the form of tablets or medicine. Antibiotics should be given by injection.

It is generally not advisable to give long-term therapy for epilepsy (sedatives), rheumatism (salicylates) and anaemia (iron tablets or medicine).

If medicine is demanded by parents, as is very common, then a stock of coloured sugar and water should be kept for this purpose. If these guidelines are carried out, some of the accidental poisoning mentioned below could be avoided.

Products such as kerosine, caustic soda, bleach and cleaning materials etc, are always kept in the house and poisoning from these products may be unavoidable, particularly if they are kept in soft drink bottles.

General measures

If the child is fully conscious, remove the poison by emptying the stomach. Syrup of ipecachuana, 15 ml given with a drink, will induce vomiting within 20–30 minutes and may be repeated if necessary.

Gastric lavage is unpleasant and should be reserved for iron-containing medicines, or when a large quantity of drugs has been taken.

Contra-indications to both methods are:

- following the ingestion of kerosine or some other oily substance
- following the ingestion of corrosives

In these cases no attempt should be made to empty the stomach.

Children should be kept under observation for at least 24 hours after ingestion, even though the child is symptom free and the case appears to be mild. However, if the child is unconscious and the facilities are available, he should be intubated with a cuffed endotracheal tube, while gastric lavage is being carried out. This procedure protects the lung from aspiration of any stomach contents during the process of gastric lavage.

If the child is unconscious, then further management is as for the unconscious child (see page 195).

Kerosine

Kerosine poisoning may damage the respiratory system and the central nervous system.

- Respiratory system – The main danger is a lipid (chemical) pneumonia, from inhalation or aspiration.
- Central nervous system – Coma and death from CNS depression after absorption may occur. The fatal dose is 1 ml/kg. CNS depression is probably due to hypoxia from the lipid pneumonia.

Treatment

1. Do not give emetics or gastric lavage as this will cause lipid inhalation.
2. Give corn oil or milk by mouth. This delays absorption and allows kerosine to be excreted by the bowel. Small doses of purgative may help excretion.
3. Give antibiotics in full doses for 7 days.

N.B. Always admit mild cases for at least 48 hours and X-ray the chest if this is possible before discharge from hospital to exclude lipid pneumonia (Figure 20.1)

Household corrosives

These cause burns to the mouth and throat but if sufficient is swallowed there may also be scarring to and perforation of the oesophagus.

Treatment

1. Avoid gastric lavage and emetics, as these may lead to perforation.
2. Alkalis are of little value as the damage is due to acute burns.
3. Surgery with emergency gastrostomy may be the only hope in some cases.
4. In severe cases scarring results in stricture of the oesophagus (Figure 20.2) Dexamethasone may inhibit some scarring and stricture formation.

Bleaches

These are mild corrosives, and may cause gastritis but little burning or scarring. However the chlorine that will be released in most cases may cause pulmonary or laryngeal oedema.

Treatment

1. Oral fluids should be given in copious amounts.
2. If large quantities have been swallowed gastric lavage should be carried out using isotonic saline. This should be followed by 30 ml of antacid such as aluminium hydroxide gel.

Salicylates (including aspirin and oil of wintergreen)

The main problem is a metabolic acidosis occurring about 4 hours after taking the overdose, resulting in deep rapid respirations. This may lead to irritability, coma and death. Purpura may also develop as a result of hypoprothrombinaemia and reduction

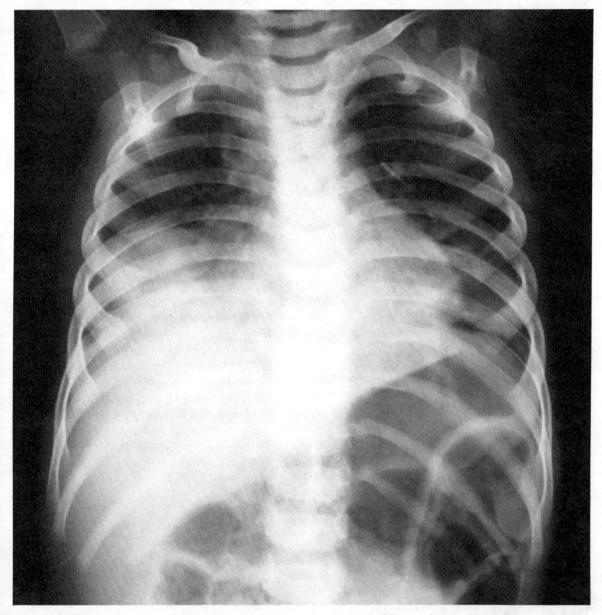

Figure 20.1 Chest X-ray showing chemical pneumonitis at the right base following kerosene ingestion

in vitamin K levels. Electrolyte disturbances together with alterations in blood sugar levels (increase or decrease) may develop. If salicylate levels can be estimated, levels below 40 mg/100 ml 4 hours after ingestion are seldom harmful, whereas levels over 100 mg/100 ml are lethal.

Treatment

1. Gastric lavage with 1 per cent sodium bicarbon-

ate should be carried out even when the history of ingestion is over 4 hours.
2. Set up an intravenous drip with isotonic saline and 5 per cent glucose at the rate of 150 ml/kg/ 24 hours.
3. If acidotic, and plasma bicarbonate cannot be estimated, assume severe acidosis of less than 10 mmol/1 of bicarbonate. Use the formula 'body weight in kg × 8 × 0.3'. This gives the amount of sodium bicarbonate in mmol needed to make

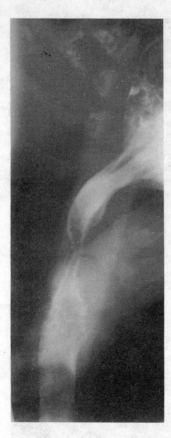

Figure 20.2 Barium swallow showing oesophageal stricture following ingestion of caustic soda

the urine alkaline (an alkaline diuresis will increase the excretion of salicylates). One ml of 8.4 per cent sodium bicarbonate = one mmol of bicarbonate. Give the sodium bicarbonate in the drip chamber and not as a single intravenous bolus.

4. Give vitamin K 5 mg intramuscularly.
5. In severe cases peritoneal dialysis or exchange transfusion may be necessary.

Iron

Overdose with oral iron leads to gastric erosion, severe abdominal pain, haemorrhage and shock. There may also be severe liver damage and renal failure. As little as 1 g of ferrous sulphate may be fatal in a young child. A serum iron level of 500 µg/dl (90 µmol/l) is indicative of severe iron poisoning.

Treatment

1. Gastric lavage with 1 per cent sodium bicarbonate, or desferrioxamine 2 g/litre.
2. Specific therapy is with desferrioxamine which chelates iron. Immediately after lavage leave 2 to 5 g desferrioxamine in 50 ml water in the stomach. Desferrioxamine colours the urine orange.
3. Give intravenous desferrioxamine 15 mg/kg infused over an hour, repeat every 4 hours until a maximum of 80 mg/kg has been given over 24 hours. Too rapid an infusion may cause hypotension or anaphylaxis.
4. If it is impossible to give an intravenous infusion, intramuscular desferrioxamine 1 g every 4 hours can be given. Injections are painful.

Burns and scalds

A child with severe burns (Figure 20.3) or scalds should be managed as follows:

1. Weigh the child.
2. Try to estimate the percentage area of skin that has been burned or scalded (see Figure 20.4).
3. If the child has inhaled smoke or toxic fumes, is anoxic or the face is involved with burns to the respiratory tract, then humidified oxygen should be given together with methyl prednisolone (2−3 mg/kg per dose). N.B. If this is combined with diuretics in severe burns it may cause severe potassium loss.
4. Sedation. Potent analgesia may be required to relieve pain and shock. The following are suggested:

   Morphine or
   diamorphine   0.1 mg/kg
   Papaveretum up to 1 year 0.2 mg/kg
                1 year   2.0 mg/kg
                7 years   5.0 mg/kg
                14 years   10−15 mg/kg
   Pethidine   1 m/kg

5. Gently remove all clothing over the affected area.
6. (a) If more than 10 per cent body surface is involved, intravenous therapy is essential to prevent the onset of shock from fluid losses, irrespective of the depth of the injury. This therapy may have to be continued for up to 72 hours to compensate for fluid loss and restore blood volume.
   (b) Give plasma, frozen plasma, plasma protein fraction, dextran or gelatin (Haemaccel™) in preference to isotonic saline. However, isotonic saline or blood may have to be given if the other fluids are not available.

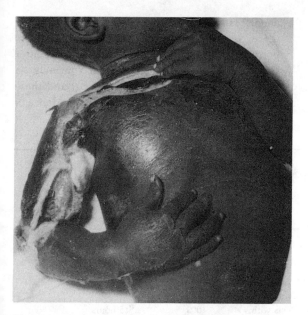

Figure 20.3 Extensive burns following a fall on to an open fire

Estimation of burned area

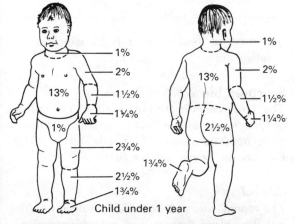

Child under 1 year

Percentages which change most with growth

Age in years	< 1	1	5	10
	% of total surface area			
Half of head	9½	8½	6½	5½
Half of thigh	2¾	3¼	4	4½
Half of leg	2½	2½	2¾	3

Figure 20.4 Estimation of burned area

(c) Transfuse a volume of plasma equivalent to the child's total plasma volume (40 mg/kg) for every 15 per cent burnt skin area. Give half the calculated volume in the first 8 hours. The remaining half should be given over the next 16 hours to keep the haemato-crit normal and a urinary output of 1 ml/kg/hr. Serial haematocrit samples can be taken using capillary blood. Serial estimations are a useful guide to monitoring fluid balance.

(d) Limit oral fluid intake of water to about three-quarters of normal fluid intake to prevent excessive dilution of extracellular fluid resulting in hyponatraemia.

(e) Whole blood is seldom needed in the shock stage but may be required later. If burns exceed 40 per cent of the body surface, transfuse between 20 and 40 per cent of the child's blood volume. (N.B. blood volume in infancy is 80 ml/kg).

7. Watch for renal failure. If the burns are more than 15−20 per cent of the body surface, monitor the urinary output hourly by inserting an indwelling catheter. However it is important to keep it in for as short a period as possible because of the risk of urinary tract infection, as well as urinary stone formation.

8. Give tetanus toxoid if the child has been actively immunized. If not, give human antitetanus globulin ('humotet').

9. Appropriate antibiotic therapy should give protection against staphylococci and β-haemolytic streptococci. The antibiotics of choice are penicillin, erythromycin or flucloxacillin.

10. Nurse all burnt children on sterile towels with the burns exposed until they have dried. Protection with a mosquito net may be necessary to keep off flies as well as mosquitoes.

11. Irrigate all chemical burns, especially those involving the eyes and mucous membranes thoroughly with water.

Injuries caused by wild animals

These generally happen in the rural areas but snake bites occur anywhere. Wild animals attack man for three reasons:

- to kill for food
- to defend itself or its young
- to warn off interlopers

Snake bites

There are three types of poisonous snake (snakes with fangs):

- the elapids (land snakes, including cobras, with small fixed fangs)

- sea snakes (also have small fixed fangs, but common only in Asian sea water
- vipers (long erectile fangs, triangular heads and short, fat bodies)

The main clinical features of the three types of snake bite are shown in the following table:

Table 20.1 *Clinical features of snake bites*

Snake	% No poisoning	Effects of poisoning Local	Systemic	% Mortality	Average death time
Elapids	50%	Slow swelling, followed by necrosis	Neurotoxic Palsies Respiratory Paresis	10%	5−20 hours
Seasnakes	80%	None	Myotoxic effects with moving paresis	10%	15 hours
Vipers	30%	Rapid swelling Occasionally necrosis	Bleeding diathesis and shock	1−15%	2 days

Diagnosis

The type of snake bite is very important and diagnosis can be made from the local lesion. Viperine poisoning is the only type usually accompanied by shock. The other two types progress rapidly, within 2 to 3 hours, to respiratory failure.

Management

1. A child can die from shock, and calm reassurance is the most important first line of treatment.
2. If antivenom is not available, tetanus toxoid may be given for reassurance.
3. Tourniquets may have been applied and these should be released.
4. Hourly blood pressure and pulse rates.
5. Urinary input and output charts.
6. Cleansing of area of necrosis.
   - Local site should be left alone, as should blisters and swellings.
   - Necrosis, however, should be excised.

Specific treatment

1. Blood transfusion helps in viperine shock.
2. Steroids may be helpful systematically.
3. Antivenom. Polyspecific antivenom, if given correctly, is the most important therapeutic agent. However, it should not be given until there is clear clinical evidence of systemic poisoning. This may be hours or even days after the bite. It should not be given routinely as severe immediate reactions may occur and these are very often fatal. In viperine bites, evidence of increase of local swelling is an indication for antivenom.

Scorpion bites

The 'bite' occurs in the tail or telson. The tail can be brought forward, in front of the animal. The two most important types in Africa, Asia and the Middle East are the *Leiurus* and the *Buthus*.

Clinical

The venom causes an 'autonomic' storm, resulting in falling blood pressure and pulmonary oedema, which may cause death in some children. In India, disseminated intravascular coagulation has been reported.

Management

1. Local pain may be severe and this can be controlled by the injection of 2 ml 1 per cent lignocaine but i.v. pethidine (2 mg/kg) may have to be given.
2. If available, antivenom given i.v. will reverse symptoms.
3. Supportive treatment. The course of the illness is seldom more than 2−3 days.

Wild dogs, hyenas and dingos

These animals seldom approach humans but, as they may well have rabies, treatment with anti-rabies immunization should always be started when a child is bitten. Tetanus toxoid should also be given and the wound surgically cleaned.

Lions and tigers

These animals seldom attack humans unless they have been rejected by their 'tribe'.

Crocodiles

Small children playing by a river are at great risk from these animals, who always attack unprotected small children.

Child abuse

Child abuse is a major child health problem in the West, responsible for significant morbidity and mortality. In the United States alone, there are nearly three million cases of physical as well as sexual abuse annually; an estimated 1 per cent of abused children die. Although the extent and seriousness of the problem in the developing countries is not known, it does exist but is, perhaps, not always recognized and reported. Most cases are likely to come first to the primary care physician and it is essential that anyone involved with the care of children must be aware of the problems, how to recognize them and the basic approach to management.

Children have always been abused throughout history to some extent determined by cultural patterns and behaviour existing within different societies. It has taken various forms:

- physical punishment and beating for wrongdoing
- unwanted children have been abandoned, fostered out to unwilling relatives, or simply murdered
- neglect because of weakness, handicap, being unwanted or other reason.
- infanticide — the murder of an unwanted baby by a distraught, and often unmarried mother
- the second or weaker of twins was often deliberately abandoned or murdered at birth in some societies
- use of children as cheap labour from an early age
- childhood prostitution

Until recently, children were seen as the property of their parents, who were free to deal with them as they saw fit. Also their parents were responsible for their education and well-being as members of society. Only recently, with our increasing knowledge of the physical and emotional needs of growing children and their psychological development, has society become aware of the problem of child abuse. In the early 1960s, cases of deliberate physical injury to children were being increasingly identified and the term 'battered child syndrome' was used by Kempe to identify them. With increasing awareness, the extent and diversity of the problem was recognized and all intentional acts of commission or omission by an older person which could harm or threaten to harm the physical and emotional development of a child were included in the term 'child abuse'. It is now classified into:

- physical abuse
- neglect and nutritional deprivation
- emotional abuse
- sexual abuse
- drug abuse

Factors predisposing to child abuse

These are often a complex combination of parental factors and characteristics in the child, but abuse always occurs at a time of stress or crisis in the family relationship. However, the child may be abused by a close relative or someone who cares for the child while parents are away or at work.

Parental characteristics
These include family disruption, frequent absences by father, either because of work or simple neglect; personality traits especially poor impulse control; rigid or authoritarian parents; alcoholism, parents with psychiatric problems; an unstable personality or depression in the mother. Some parents have unreasonably high or unrealistic expectations of their children. Parents who themselves have been subjected to abuse as children are more likely to abuse their own children because of their inability to form a satisfying emotional relationship with them.

The child
The child is often unwanted; the child of a large 'child a year' family; it may be simply the wrong

sex, or a child with a handicap or chronic illness which many parents find frustrating and they are quite unable to cope with the demands and the care of such children (a common cause of child abuse in many developing countries). The baby may be difficult to manage, and the mother in-experienced in child rearing, and without support of relatives. Babies who have been separated from their mother at birth (premature sick infants) are more likely to be abused because of a lack of bonding – the mother feels that the baby does not belong to her.

Social factors
These include poverty and unemployment in the parents; unmarried and deserted mothers, father in prison. Children of divorced parents and children whose parents remarry and are rejected by the step-parent are at increased risk of abuse.

The crisis
This may appear an insignificant incident to out-siders, but always occurs at a breaking point in family relationships – a tense, anxious or frustrated parent who finally loses patience with the child. The parents are often isolated, with little or no lifeline of support; they cannot rely on each other, and have few relatives or friends to whom they can turn for help. They are often of low intellect and lack the ability to cope with the crisis when it arises.

Physical abuse

The commonest forms of physical injury are bruising and fractures, often multiple. The bruising has a character pattern, taking the form of 'finger tip' bruising – multiple small circular bruises from one to two centimetres diameter over the face, cheeks and head where the child has been pinched or slapped. Similar bruises may be seen over the shoulders, arms or trunk where the child has been gripped and held. Other bruises or marks over the body may result from bites or lashing with belts, ropes or shoes. Unexplained fractures, not resulting from road traffic accidents, or other accidents are likely to be the result of physical abuse. Sometimes however parents may explain an unusual injury by saying that the child was accidentally dropped or they fell while carrying the child.

Head injuries of any severity may result from direct physical trauma or from sudden violent shaking of the infant. The rapid acceleration and deceleration of the brain within the skull tears small blood vessels causing a subdural haematoma and retinal haemorrhages.

Burns may be caused by cigarettes or hot water, and are common on the extremities and buttocks.

Abdominal injuries are less common, and result from a blow to the abdomen, usually with a hand or fist, occasionally a kick, and cause contusion and laceration of the viscera, internal bleeding and perforation of the bowel.

Sexual abuse

This may be defined as a sexual act by an adult with a child which causes, or is likely to cause, physical or psychological trauma. Girls are abused much more frequently than boys, and generally by a close male relative. Others who may abuse children in their care include personnel in day care centres, schools and other institutions such as orphanages and involve children of lower socio-economic groups. These cases are seldom reported. Such children may themselves exhibit inappro-priate sexual behaviour for their age. Some may show an apparent irrational fear of men, while others may present with a variety of apparently inexplicable psychosomatic symptoms. Occasion-ally a child may be abused by a stranger.

Role of the primary care doctor

Abused children with serious injuries are often brought by parents for medical attention, but they seldom admit to having assaulted the child. The primary care doctor must be aware of this possibility whenever a child is brought to him with unusual injuries, and be able to identify abused children so that he can refer them for proper man-agement as well as for appropriate legal action.

Some factors which might suggest the possibility of child abuse include:

1. There may be a delay in taking the child for medical attention.
2. An inappropriate reaction by the parents to the child's injuries – this may be either over-anxiety or indifference.
3. A discrepancy between the explanation given by the parents and the extent or type of injury –

thus multiple small bruises on the face of a child unable to walk are not the result of a fall.

4. The reaction of the child towards the parents and doctor — the natural reaction of a child is to cling to the parents for comfort. A child who is repeatedly abused does not relate well to his parents and often looks afraid or is unresponsive, with 'watchful frozen awareness'.

5. Parents may be frequent attenders at a clinic, often for trivial complaints. This may be an unspoken request for sympathy and support.

Abuse must be differentiated from accidental injuries as well as medical causes. Mongolian blue spots may be mistaken for bruises. Bruises are common in bleeding disorders. Multiple fractures and eiphyseal injuries are often the result of abuse, and children who have had several fractures may be alleged to have 'brittle bones'. The X-ray appearances of osteogenesis imperfecta, however, are quite characteristic.

All children suspected to have been abused should have a clotting screen (platelet count, prothrombin time and thromboplastin generation time or equivalent) and skeletal survey (whole body X-ray) performed. The latter may reveal evidence of previous healed or healing fractures.

Non-accidental burns or scalds are usually caused by immersion and have definite linear demarcations with hands and feet burned in a 'glove and stocking' fashion. A child may be placed in a bowl of hot water or on a hot stove causing burns on the buttocks.

In cases of sexual abuse, as well as the physical and psychological trauma, there is the possibility of sexually transmitted diseases, and in post-pubertal girls pregnancy may have to be considered. Appropriate investigations must be done in each instance. Psychiatric or psychological counselling and help may be necessary.

All suspected cases of abuse must be reported to the competent health authority, social services, and if necessary law enforcing authority although in many countries the mechanism for dealing with this problem is not well established. The aim of management should be to help parents with their problem, not to punish them unless a criminal offence has been committed.

21

Notes on Prescribing for Children

I do not want two diseases — one nature-made, one doctor made.

Napoleon Bonaparte, 1820

The first principle is 'to do no harm'. All drugs have side effects, some of these are more serious than others. Use only the appropriate drug in the correct dosage for the minimum time.

1. Many disorders can be cured by the use of a single basic drug, or without drugs at all. Sometimes, however, it may be necessary to prescribe more than one drug (e.g. tuberculosis), but the number should be kept to a minimum.
2. The more drugs that are prescribed, the less likely is the mother to understand treatment regimes, and compliance will be poor. There is always the possibility of overdosage.
3. It has to be stressed to parents that the medicines prescribed are for a specific patient and must not be used for other children who may have similar symptoms. The medicines may not only be inappropriate but carry the risk of overdose and accidental poisoning.
4. To avoid the risk of accidental poisoning, all medicines should be dispensed in proper medicine bottles and not in empty soft drink bottles etc.
5. Some consider that all medication should be given in the hospital or clinic. This may involve daily visits and the use of intra-muscular injections of long-acting antibiotics, as the dangers mentioned above are so common. Much depends on the sophistication of the local population. The problems are not unknown in the UK.

However, some parents expect and demand to be prescribed a medicine after a visit to the hospital or clinic, and one is sometimes pressurized into doing this. If this happens, then use a harmless placebo such as multivitamin preparations. Avoid giving even relatively harmless cough medicines such as 'linctus simplex'.

Intramuscular injections

1. These should never be given into the buttocks of young children and infants, because of the danger of damaging the sciatic nerve, resulting in paralysis of the leg. Likewise avoid using the deltoid muscle in the arm.
2. Always use the outer aspect of the thigh.
3. Intramuscular injections should not be given for prolonged periods. They are painful and may cause local reactions such as subcutaneous fat necrosis or sterile muscle abscesses.
4. If prolonged treatment is necessary it should be remembered that most antibiotics are well absorbed orally and reach therapeutic levels in the blood stream, so sick patients can be treated with an indwelling nasogastric tube.

Intravenous drips

1. If careful and continuous observation is impossible and the maintenance of accurate fluid balance records is unreliable, then these should be avoided. In the experience of the authors, many mothers, although illiterate, are keen observers and can readily be taught to inform nursing staff when a drip has stopped or is running too fast, as well as when the bottle is nearly empty. The main danger, particularly in the case of young infants, is that of overhydration from a drip that is running too fast.
2. Intravenous drips should be used for the resuscitation of severely dehydrated babies and infants who are in shock. Once shock has been fully corrected, after about 1 or 2 hours, rehydration may be continued via the nasogastric route.

Feeding sick children in hospital

1. Breast feeding should be continued as far as possible, despite anorexia, poor sucking and nasal obstruction. If breast feeding is discontinued in hospital, it may be difficult or even impossible to re-establish when the baby returns home. This then introduces all the risks of artificial feeding in a poor and unhygienic environment. Weaned children should be given a good balanced diet in hospital. Nasogastric feeding may be necessary in a child that is too ill to suck. A polythene tube can be left *in situ* for several days. In breast fed babies milk should be expressed and given via the tube until breast feeding can be re-established.

2. Continuous milk drips are preferable to milk given directly as a 'bolus' from a syringe at regular intervals. If continuous milk drips are given the tube should be washed through with 2 to 3 ml of sterile isotonic saline every 6 or 8 hours. In the case of bolus feeding this should be done after every bolus.

3. Nasogastric feeding is not popular with or acceptable by many mothers, who may well remove the tube and try to forcefeed their babies with disastrous results. Mothers will also remove i.v. drips from time to time.

Table 21.1 Common drugs

Drug	Route	Total daily dose	Times/day	Notes
Antibiotics				
Penicillins				
Penicillin G	i.m./i.v.	50−100 mg/kg	4	600 mg = 1 000 000 units
(benzylpenicillin)	i.v.	300 mg/kg	6	Dose for severe infections
Procaine penicillin	i.m. only	25 mg/kg	1	Vials of 300 mg/ml
Benethamine penicillin (benzathine) penicillin	Deep i.m. only	¼ to ½ vial	Once every 3 days	Triplopen ™ − a long-acting mixture of benethamine penicillin G 475 mg, procaine penicillin 250 mg and penicillin G sodium 300 mg.
Phenoxymethylpenicillin (penicillin V)	Oral	50 mg/kg	4	
		25 mg/kg	2	As prophylaxis against rheumatic fever
Ampicillin	Oral i.m./i.v.	50 mg/kg	4	100 mg/kg in severe infections
Amoxycillin	Oral i.m./i.v.	50 mg/kg	3	100 mg/kg in severe infections
Cloxacillin sodium	Oral i.m./i.v.	50 mg/kg	4	100 mg/kg in severe infections
Flucloxacillin sodium	Oral i.m./i.v.	25 mg/kg	4	50 mg/kg in severe infections
Cephalosporins				
Cefotaxime	i.m./i.v.	100−150 mg/kg	2−4	In severe infections give 200 mg/kg
Ceftazidime	i.m./i.v.	50−100 mg/kg	3	In *Pseudomonas* infections increase to 150 mg/kg
Cefuroxime	i.m./i.v.	100 mg/kg	3	Give four doses daily in severe infections

Table 21.1(cont)

Drug	Route	Total daily dose	Times/day	Notes
Cephalexin	Oral	50 mg/kg	4	
Cephradine	Oral	50 mg/kg	4	
Other antibiotics				
Chloramphenicol	Oral i.m./i.v.	50 mg/kg	4	Use 100 mg/kg in bacterial meningitis. Danger of aplastic anaemia − restrict use to serious illness.
Co-trimoxazole (sulphamethoxazole 5 parts; trimethoprim 1 part)	Oral i.v. infusion	48 mg/kg 36 mg/kg	2 2	Avoid in G-6-PD deficiency and neonates Infusion 96 mg/ml in 5 ml ampoules Dilute with 25 to 35 times volume of normal (0.9%) saline or 5% dextrose before infusion
	Oral	48 mg/kg	1	Urinary infection prophylaxis
Erythromycin (stearate or ethylsuccinate)	Oral i.v./infusion	50 mg/kg	4	The estolate salt (Ilosone™) may cause cholestatic jaundice and should not be used
Ethambutol	Oral	15−25 mg/kg	1	Danger − visual disturbances. Use only in children over 6 years. Start with 25 mg/kg/day and reduce to 15 mg/kg/day after 2 months
Fusidic acid − see sodium fusidate				
Furazolidone	Oral	6 mg/kg	4	Avoid in G-6-PD deficiency.
Gentamicin sulphate	i.m./i.v.	6−7.5 mg/kg	3	Use half dosage or give only ONCE daily if renal function is impaired. Monitor blood levels if possible. Side effects − (1) Ototoxicity and VIII nerve damage − permanent and dose dependent. (2) Nephrotoxic − impairment of renal function is reversible.
	intrathecal or intraventricular	2 mg	1	
Griseofulvin	Oral	10 mg/kg	1−3	
Isoniazid (INAH)	Oral i.v.	10 mg/kg	1	Caution − should be given with pyridoxine
Metronidazole	Oral	22.5 mg/kg	3	
	Oral or i.v. infusion	22.5 mg/kg	3	For anaerobic infections. Change to oral as soon as possible.

Table 21.1(cont)

Drug	Route	Total daily dose	Times/day	Notes
	Rectal	Under 1 year 375 mg 1−5 years 750 mg Over 5 years 1.5 g	3	Suppositories 500 mg
Nalidixic acid	Oral	50 mg/kg	4	Causes haemolysis in G-6-PD deficiency Half dose in prophylaxis of urinary infections
Neomycin	Oral	50 mg/kg	4	
Nitrofurantoin	Oral	6−10 mg/kg	4	Do not give to neonates. Causes haemolysis in G-6-PD deficiency. Half dose in prophylaxis of urinary infections
Nystatin	Oral	100 000 units/kg	3−4	
Pyrazinamide	Oral	20−30 mg/kg	1	Danger − avoid in liver disease
Rifampicin	Oral	10−15 mg/kg	1	Danger − avoid in liver disease Note − colours urine orange-red
Sodium fusidate (fusidic acid)	Oral i.v. infusion	50 mg/kg 20 mg/kg	3 3	Reconstitute with buffer and dilute further Infuse slowly over several hours
Streptomycin	i.m. only intrathecal	40 mg/kg 1 mg/kg	2 Once daily	Side effects as for gentamicin Special preparation necessary Rarely used except in tuberculosis.
Trimethoprim	Oral i.v. infusion	10 mg/kg 8 mg/kg	2 2	Slow i.v. infusion

Note − tetracyclines should never be given to children. These drugs are deposited in growing bones and teeth, causing permanent staining and sometimes damage.

Other drugs

Drug	Route	Total daily dose	Times/day	Notes
Adrenaline	Subcutaneous injection	0.1−0.5 ml 0.01 ml/kg	Single dose	Subcutaneous injection only
Aminophylline	i.v.	5−7 mg/kg	First dose as slow infusion over 15−20 min.	
	i.v. infusion	0.7−0.9 mg/kg/hour	Continuous infusion	
Aspirin	Oral/rectal	50 mg/kg	3−4	Dosage for analgesia and antipyretic
	Oral	100 mg/kg	4	Dosage for rheumatic fever
Atropine sulphate	i.m.	0.01 mg/kg	Single dose	

Table 21.1(cont)

Drug	Route	Total daily dose	Times/day	Notes
Bisacodyl	Oral	5 mg	1	
Carbamazepine	Oral	10—20 mg/kg	2	Start with half dose and increase to full dose after 10—14 days
Chloral hydrate	Oral	50—100 mg/kg	2—3	
Chlorothiazide	Oral	25 mg/kg	1 or 2	
Chlorpheniramine maleate	Oral	0.3 mg/kg	3	
	s.c. i.m.	0.3 mg/kg		
Chlorpromazine	Oral	2—3 mg/kg	3	Dose may be doubled
	i.m.	1 mg/kg	Single dose	
	Rectal	10 mg/kg	1—3	
Clonazepam	Oral	100 µg/kg	2	Start with half dose and increase to full dose after 10—14 days
	Slow i.v.	50 µg/kg	Single dose	
	i.v. infusion	10 g/kg/hour	Continuous infusion	
Codeine phosphate	Oral	1—2 mg/kg	3	Risk of respiratory depression with prolonged use
Dexamethasone	i.m./i.v.	0.2—0.5 mg/kg	Single dose	Higher doses in cerebral oedema and malignancy
Diazepam	Oral	0.5 mg/kg	3	
	i.v.	0.2 mg/kg	Single dose Slow i.v.	For controlling convulsions
	Rectal	0.2—0.5 mg/kg	Single dose	Suppositories or single dose rectal tubes
Ferrous fumarate	Oral	20 mg/kg	2—3	
Ferrous gluconate	Oral	50 mg/kg	2—3	
Ferrous sulphate	Oral	20 mg/kg	2—3	
Frusemide	Oral i.m./i.v.	1 mg/kg	Single dose	Repeat if necessary
Hydralazine	Oral	0.75 mg/kg	4	
	i.m./i.v.	0.25—0.5 mg/kg	Single dose Infuse slowly	Increase to 20 mg/kg maximum as required. Repeat 2—3 hourly. Danger — do not give with dexamethasone. Reduce dose to 0.15 mg/kg if given with reserpine
Hydrochlorothiazide	Oral	2.5 mg/kg	1 or 2	

Table 21.1(cont)

Drug	Route	Total daily dose	Times/day	Notes
Ibuprofen	Oral	20 mg/kg	3	Total daily dose not to exceed 500 mg for children under 30 kg
Methyldopa	Oral	10 mg/kg	4	Range from 5–25 mg/kg
	i.v.	10 mg/kg	4–6	Range from 6–20 mg/kg infuse over 20 minutes
Metoclopramide	Oral i.m./i.v.	0.3 mg/kg	3	Danger of dystonic reactions
Morphine	s.c. or i.m.	0.1 mg/kg	Single dose	Increase to 0.2 mg/kg if necessary
Naloxone	s.c., i.m., i.v.	0.01 mg/kg	Single dose	
Paracetamol	Oral	60 mg/kg	4	
	Rectal	60 mg/kg	4	
Paraldehyde	Deep i.m.	0.1 ml/kg	Single dose	
	Rectal	0.3 ml/kg	Single dose	Mix with equal volume of arachis oil or olive oil
Pethidine hydrochloride	Oral, s.c., i.m., i.v.	1 mg/kg	Single dose	
Phenobarbitone	Oral	5–10 mg/kg	2	
	i.m.	10 mg/kg	2	
Phenytoin	Oral	5–8 mg/kg	2	
	i.v.	5–10 mg/kg	Single dose	Slow infusion
Prednisolone	Oral	1–2 mg/kg	3–4	Maximum dosage
	Rectal	20 mg	1	As retention enema
Prochlorperazine	Oral	0.25 mg/kg	2–3	Danger of dystonic reactions
	i.m.	0.3 mg/kg		
Propranolol	Oral	1–5 mg/kg	3	Start with low dose
	i.v.	0.02–0.05 mg/kg	Single dose Slow infusion	Preferably with ECG monitoring
Reserpine	Oral	0.01 mg/kg	1	
	i.m.	0.02–0.07 mg/kg	Up to 3 max.	Never give i.v. Avoid giving with hydralazine
Salbutamol	Oral	0.2–0.4 mg/kg	3–4	
	Aerosol inhalation	800 µg	4	100 µg in each metered inhalation Two metered inhalations per dose
	Nebulizer	2.5 mg	4–6	Respirator solution 5 mg/ml Single dose ampoules contain 1 mg/ml
	i.v. infusion	2.5–5 µg/kg/hour	Continuous	Danger – ventricular arrhythmias if given with i.v. aminophylline. Monitor with ECG
	s.c.	8 µg/kg	Single dose	

Table 21.1(cont)

Drug	Route	Total daily dose	Times/day	Notes
Sodium valproate	Oral	20–30 mg/kg	2	Start with half dose and increase to full dose after 14 days
Spironolactone	Oral	3 mg/kg	1	
Terbutaline	Oral	0.2 mg/kg	3	
	Aerosol inhalation	1 mg	3–4	One or two metered inhalations per dose 0.25 mg in each metered inhalation
	Nebulizer solution	0.2 mg/kg	3	Respirator solution 10 mg/ml Single dose ampoules contain 2.5 mg/ml
	s.c.	0.1–0.2 mg	Single dose	

Further reading

British National Formulary (use latest edition), British Medical Association and The Pharmaceutical Society of Great Britain, London.

Davidson, D.C. *et al.* (Eds) (1982). Alder Hey Book of Children's Doses 4th Edn. Pharmacy Office, Alder Hey Children's Hospital, Liverpool.

Forfar, J.C. and Forfar, J.O. (1984). Paediatric drug usage and dosage. In: *Textbook of Paediatrics* (Eds J.O. Forfar and G.C. Arneil) 3rd Edn, Churchill Livingstone, 2008.

Recommended Further Reading

Clinical

Ebrahim, G.J. (1981). *Paediatric Practice in Developing Countries.* Macmillan, Basingstoke.

Hendrickse, R.G. (Ed.) (1981). *Paediatrics in the Tropics — a Current Review.* Oxford Medical Publications, Oxford.

Insley, J. and Wood, B. (Eds) (1982). *A Paediatric VadeMedum.* 10th Edn, Lloyd-Luke, London.

Jelliffe, D.B. and Paget Stanfield, J. (Eds) (1978). *Diseases of Children in the Tropics and Sub-Tropics,* 3rd Edn, Edward Arnold, London.

Robinson, M.J. and Lee, E. (Eds) (1971). *Paediatric Problems in Tropical Countries.* Churchill Livingstone, Edinburgh.

Laboratory

Cheesborough, Monica (1987). *Medical Laboratory Manual for Tropical Countries* Vol. 1, 2nd Edn, Butterworth Scientific, Guildford.

Community Paediatrics

Morley, D. (1973). *Paediatric Priorities in Developing Countries.* Butterworth Scientific, Guildford.

Journals

Annals of Tropical Paediatrics. Publishers: Butterworth Scientific, Guildford. Four issues per year.

Children in the Tropics (L'enfant en milieu tropicale). Publishers: International Children's Centre, Chateau de Longchamp, Bois de Boulonge, 75016 Paris, France. (Each issue is devoted to a single topic at Primary Health Care level.)

Journal of Tropical Paediatrics. Publishers: Oxford University Press. Six issues per year.

Postgraduate Doctor. Publishers: Barker Publications Ltd., Richmond, Surrey. Twelve publications per year. Separate editions for Middle East, Asia and Africa. A general journal, but contains many useful articles on paediatric subjects.

Tropical Doctor. Publishers: Royal Society of Medicine. Four times per year.

Index

Reference numbers in brackets refer to figures and tables.

abdomen 145
  intussusception 145, 154
  swollen 147−8
abuse, of child 269−71
accidents 263−4
acidosis
  metabolic 35−6, 102, 104, 115
  diabetic 208, 209−11
acquired immunodeficiency disease
  61
acute miliary tuberculosis 64
adrenal steroid synthesis (219)
AIDS 61
albinism 246−7
alkalosis, metabolic 36
ammoniacal dermatitis 250
ameobiasis 236−7
anaemia
  aetiology (160)
  and breathlessness 115
  and growth 223
  haemolytic 161, (162)
  megaloblastic 159−60
  from tapeworm 232
  in renal failure   104
anthropometry 7
aorta, coarctation of 127
aortic stenosis 126
Arnold−Chiari malformation 199
arthritis 133, 155−7
ascaris 226, (226)
asthma 122
  drugs for (123)
  from worms 227
athlete's foot 252−3
atopic child 122
atrial septal defect 125

bedbugs 234
bilharzia 238
bladder, abnormalities 85−6
bleaches, and poisoning 264
bleeding disorders (169)
bleeding, in Wiscott−Aldrich
  syndrome 170
blepharitis, of eyelid 259, (259)
blindness 203
blood, in stool 148
blood sugar, control of 212
blood vessels, abnormally arranged
  127
breast feeding 10−13
breathlessness 115
bronchiolitis 106, 107, 116−7
bronchopneumonia 107, 117
burns 266−7, (266)

cancer 173−4
  drugs for (184−6)
cancrum orus, from measles 40
Candida albicans 251
cardiac disease
  and breathlessness 115
  congenital 223
  congestive 127−8
  cyanotic 125
  in infants 128−9
cardiac tamponade 135
cardiac-respiratory arrest (142−3),
  143−4
carditis (131)
  endocarditis, infective 133, 136
  myocarditis, diphtheritic 136
  pericarditis 133, 134−5
cataract 261
cellulitis 249
centile charts 16
  see also growth charts
cerebellar astrocytoma 183
cerebellar medulloblastoma 183
cerebral oedema 197
cerebral palsy 197−8
cerebrospinal fluid (199)
  in meningitis (75)
chalazia, of eyelid 259, (259)
chicken pox 44−5
child abuse 269−71
chorea 131, 134
  rheumatic 133
Christmas disease 171−2
chromosomal abnormalities, and
  growth 222
chronic/reactivation tuberculosis 65
cirrhosis, Indian childhood 149
coeliac disease
  complications 152−3
  and growth, 224
cold, common 106, 107−8
coma, classification (195)
congenital adrenal hyperplasia 219,
  (220), 222
congenital heart disease, and
  growth 223
congenital hypothyroidism 214−15
conjunctivitis 259−60
  epidemic 106
  from measles 39
convulsions
  febrile 62
  management of 193−4
  and meningitis 77
  see also seizure disorders; spasms
cornea, ulcered 261

cough 114−15
craniopharyngioma 184
cretinism 214
Crohn's disease, and growth 224
croup 49, 111
cyst, Meibomian 257
cystic fibrosis 149−51
cystinosis, in renal disorder 97
cytomegalic virus 60

dactylitis 249
Dandy−Walker malformation 200
dehydration 30−2, (30), (31)
dental development 7
deprivation, emotional 224
dermatitis 250−1
dermatosis, in kwashiorkor (18)
development, and growth 8−9
diabetes mellitus 207−8
  ketoacidosis during 208, 209−11
dialysis, peritoneal 102−3
diarrhoea, chronic 151−2
diet, for children 15−16
  see also feeding; nutrition
diphtheria 47−9, (47), 107
diphtheritic myocarditis 136
Diplococcus pneumonia, and
  meningitis 73
diuretics, for rheumatic fever (130)
ductus arteriosus, patent 125
dysmorphic syndromes, in growth
  222
dysplastic kidney 84

ECG changes (34)
ear and throat infections, and fever
  62
ecchymoses, from whooping cough
  (43)
eczema 254−5
electrolyte disturbances 33
11-hydroxylase deficiency 220−1
encephalitis 39, 40
endocarditis, infective 133, 136
endocrine system, and growth 4,
  223
endomyocardial fibrosis 138, (141)
enterococci 137
enzyme deficiencies
  glucose-6-phosphate-
    dehydrogenase 162, (163)
  11-hydroxylase 220−1
  21-hydroxylase 219−20
ependymoma 184
epiglottis, acute 106, 107, 112−13
epilepsy 189, (191)

erysipelas 249
erythema
  marginatum 132
  nodosum 66, (67), 71
  nuchae 247
erythroid hyperplasia 170
extrauterine growth 5
eye
  and chalazia 259
  lens disease 261
  structure (257)
  styes 257
  tumours of 262
  see also conjunctivitis
eyelid, diseases 259, (259)

Fallot's tetralogy 125, (126)
Fanconi's syndrome, in renal
  disorders 97
feeding
  artificial, of infants 13–14
  breast 10–13
  of sick children 273
  see also diet; nutrition
fevers in children 62
fleas 236
fluid requirements, daily (29)
folliculitis 249
furunculosis 249

gastro-enteritis 57
gastrointestinal disease, and growth
  223
genetic disorders
  albinism 246–7
  Christmas disease 172
  coeliac disease 152–3, 224
  thalassaemia 166–9
  Turner's syndrome 222–3, 224
  Von Willebrand's disease 172
  see also enzyme deficiencies
genetics, and growth 4
genital growth 5
giardiasis 237–8
glomerular disease 90
  nephritis, acute, 46–7, 234
glomerulonephritis 91–2, 97
glomerulosclerosis, focal segmental
  96
glucose-6-phosphate-dehydrogenase
  deficiency 162, (163)
goitre 216–17
granuloma, from toxocara 228–9
Graves' disease
  see thyrotoxicosis
growth
  delay 221–5
  dysmorphic syndromes in 222
  and endocrine system 4, 223
  stages 4–5
  tests for 225

growth charts 7
growth curves 5
growth hormone deficiency 224
growth hormone releasing hormone
  225
growth retardation, intrauterine
  222
gut, perforation of 147

haemangioma, cavernous 247,
  (247)
haematuria 90–1, 239
haemoglobinopathies 164, (165)
haemolytic streptococcus (45)
haemolytic uraemic syndrome 98
haemophilia 171–2
haemophilus influenzae, and
  meningitis 73
haemorrhagic fever
  South East Asian acute 171
  viral in renal syndrome 99
handicap, in children 202–6
health care, primary 1, 2–3, (2)
hearing loss 203
heart disease
  see cardiac disease
heart failure, congestive 127–8
height, gains in children 6
height and weight graph (7)
hepatitis, viral 54–6
hernia, strangulated 154
herpes simplex 254
Hodgkin's disease 176–8
hookworm (227–8)
Hurler's syndrome 200
hydatid disease 233–4
hydrocephalus 77, 198–201
hyperbilirubinaemia 163, 164
hyperglycaemia 34, 213
hyperkalaemia 34–5, 102
hyperlipidaemia 95
hypernatraemia 14–15, 33–4
hyperphosphataemia 104
hyperplasia
  congenital adrenal 219, (220),
  222
  erythroid 170
hyperpyrexia, from malaria 243,
  244
hypertension 141–2
  in renal failure 102, 104
hypocalcaemia 104
  in renal failure 102
hypoglycaemia 212–13
hypogonadism, and growth 224
hypokalaemia 34
hypopituitarism, and growth
  hormone deficiency 223
hypothyroidism 214–16, 224
hypovolaemia 94–5
hysteria, and breathlessness 115

immunity
  active 78
  passive 82–3
immunization
  complications 80–1
  contraindications 81
  schedule (79), (80)
  see also vaccines
immunoglobulins 82–3
impetigo 248–9
infantum roseola 41
injections, intramuscular 272
insulin 209, (210)
insulin test, for growth 225
intercranial pressure, raised 197
intrauterine growth 4–5
intravenous drips 272
intravenous fluids 32
intussusception 145, 154
iridocyclitis 261
iron, and poisoning 266
iron deficiency 160–1

jaundice 149

keloid formation 256, (256)
keratitis 260
keratomalacia 260
kerosene poisoning 264, (265)
kidney 84–5
  see also glomerular disease; renal
  disease
Kussmaul breathing 35–6
kwashiorkor
  acute 21
  dermatosis in (18)
  and fever 62
  malignant 19
  and oedema (18)
laryngo-tracheo-bronchitis 106,
  107, 111
Leishmaniasis 240–2
Lennox–Gastaut syndrome 189
lens, diseased 261
leprosy 70–2
leukaemia 174–6
lice 234–6
liver disease 148–9
lung abcess (121)
lupus erythematosis, systemic 133
Lyme disease 133
lymphoid growth 5
lymphoma 176
  Burkitt's 179, (179)
  non-Hodgkin's 178

malabsorption 154
malaria 62, 242–5
  chemoprophylaxis (245)
  parasites (243)
malnutrition 16–21, (17), 223

marasmic kwashiorkor (19)
marasmus 17–18, (17), 20–1
measles (37), 38–40, 62
megalencephaly 200
membranoproliferative
   glomerulonephritis 96
meningitis
   complications 77
   cerebrospinal fluid results (75)
   diplococcus pneumonia 73
   factors predisposing 73
   meningococcal, in Africa 74
   from mumps 40
   pyogenic 62
   treatment for 76–7
   tuberculous 69, (70)
meningococcal septicaemia 74
mental retardation 201, (202)
metabolic disorders 164, 219–21
milk analysis (13)
molluscum contagiosum 253–4
Mongolian blue spot 246
mononucleosis, infectious 58–9
mumps 40–1
myocarditis 48, 49, 133, (135)
   diphtheritic 136
myositis 158
myxoedema, juvenile
   see hypothyroidism

naevi 247
nappy rash 250–1
Neisseria meningitidis 73
nephritis 96–7
nephrotic syndrome 93, (93), 94–7
neural growth 5
neuritis 48, 49
neuroblastoma 180
nipple/teat comparison (11)
nutrition
   fetal 10
   and growth 4
   for infants 10–15
   and obesity 22
   see also diet; feeding
nutritional needs (14)
nutritional rehabilitation 26–7,
   (27)
nurtritional state, assessment 19
   see also growth charts

obesity, nutritional 22
obstructive lesions, in heart disease
   125
onchocerciasis 262
osseous maturation 6–7
osteitis 157
otitis media 107, 110–11
   acute 109

parasites 226

drugs for (240–1)
paronychia 249
pelvi-ureteric junction 85
pericardial effusion (140)
pericarditis 134–5
   viral 133
peritonitis 154
peritonsillar abcess 110
pertussis
   see whooping cough
pharyngitis 106, 107, 108–9
phenylketonuria 214
pigmentation, postinflammatory
   246
pityriasis versicolor 253
pleurisy 65
pneumonia
   acute 106
   atypical, non-bacterial 106
   diplococcus 73
   lobar, 107, 117–18, (119)
   mycoplasma 120–1
   right middle lobe 117, (118)
   staphylococcal 107, 119–20
   verminous 227
poisons 263–6
poliomyelitis 49–51
   development of (50)
polyarthritis 131, 133, 155
polyclinic 1, 3
port-wine stain 247–8
postnatal environment, and growth
   4
prenatal environment, and growth
   4
prescribing, for children 272
preventative medicine 1
prolactin, reflex 12
proteinuria 89–90
pulmonary stenosis 126
purpura 170–1
pyogenic meningitis 62
pyomyositis 157
pyruvate kinase deficiency 164

quinsy 109

rehydration, oral 31
renal agenesis 84
renal disease 84, 223
   failure (100)
      acute 99–102
      chronic 103–4
renal osteodystrophy 104
renal tract
   and glomerular disease 90
   and glomerulonephritis 91–2, 97
   and haematuria 90–1, 239
   and hyperlipidaemia 95
   and hypovolaemia 94–5
   and nephrotic syndrome 93, (93),

94–6
   and proteinuria 89–90
   and urinary calculi 88
renal tubular disorders 97–9
respiratory diseases, chronic, and
   growth 223
respiratory infections 105–6, (106),
   (107)
respiratory obstruction 113–4
respiratory paralysis 115
retardation, metal 201, (202)
retina, diseases of 261–2
retinoblastoma 181, 262, (262)
rhabdomyosarcoma 182
rheumatic chorea 133
rheumatic fever 46, 109–10
   acute 129–31, (132)
   diuretics for (130)
   prophylactic therapy (134)
rickets 24, (25)
ringworm 251–2
Ritter's disease 250
river blindness 262
rubella 41, 59

salicylates, and poisoning 264–6
scabies 234
scalds 266–7
scarlet fever 46, 250
schistosomiasis 238, (238), 239–40
scorpion bites 268
scrofuloderma 66
seborrhoeic dermatitis 251
seizure disorders
   absence 188
   and drugs (190)
   and EEG appearances (189)
   febrile 192–3
   focal 188–9
   Lennox–Gastaut 189
   myoclonic 188
   tonic-clonic 187
   see also convulsions; spasms
sex, and growth 4
sickle cell crisis 147
sickling disorders 164–5, (166)
snake bites 267–8, (268)
spasms, infantile 188
   see also convulsions, seizure
   disorders
spherocytosis, hereditary 162
staphylococcal scalded skin
   syndrome 250
staphylococcal scarlet fever 250
Staphylococcus 137
stenosis
   aortic 126
   congenital hypertrophic pyloric
   154
   pulmonary 126
   pyloric 153

steroid synthesis, adrenal (219)
stomatitis, ulcerative 106
stool, blood in 148
streptococcal disease 45—6
Streptococcus viridans 137
stridor 111
Strongyloides stercoralis 229, (229)
styes, of eye 257
subdural effusion, and meningitis 77
syphilis 60

tapeworm 231—3, (231), (233)
tetanus 56—7
thalassaemia 166—9
threadworms 230—1
throat, sore 108—9
thrombocytopenia 169—70
thrush 251
thyroid
    disorders 213
    function 214
    hormones (213)
thyroiditis, autoimmune 216
thyrotoxicosis 217, 218
tinea 251—3, (252)
tonsillitis 106, 107, 108—9
toxic epidermal necrolysis 250
toxic shock syndrome 250
Toxocara (226), 228—9

toxoplasmosis 60
tracheostomy (48), 112—13
trachoma 258, (258)
tuberculin test 67
tuberculosis
    abdominal 66
    chronic/reactivation 65
    drugs for (68)
    miliary 62, 64
    primary complex 63—4
    skeletal 65
    of skin 66
    treatment schedules (69)
tuberculous lymphadenitis 65
tuberculous meningitis 69, (70)
tubular disease 90
tumour
    of brain (183)
    of central nervous system 182—4
    Wilm's 179—80
Turner's syndrome, and growth 222—3, 224
21-hydroxylase deficiency 219—20
typhoid fever 51—4, 62
    development (52)

ulcer, of cornea 261
unconsciousness, in children (194)
ureter, abnormalities 85
urinary calculi 88

urinary tract, infections 62, 86—7

vaccines 82
    see also immunization
varicella 44—5
veno-occlusive disease 149
ventricular septal defect 125
verrucae vulgaris 253
vesico-ureteric reflux (86), 87—8
villi, damaged (151)
virilization 220—1
vitamins 22—6
vitiligo 246, (246)
vomiting, in children 153—4
Von Willebrand's disease 171—2

warts 253—4
weaning 14—15
weight, gains in children 5—6
wheezing 121—2
whipworm 230
whooping cough 41—4, (42)
wild animals, and injury 269
Wilm's tumour 179—80
Wiskott—Aldrich syndrome, and bleeding 170
worms 226—233

Yersinia enterocolitica 133